FROM M
TO ME

OSHO

FROM MEDICATION
TO MEDITATION

SAFFRON WALDEN
THE C. W. DANIEL COMPANY LIMITED

First published in Great Britain in 1994
by The C. W. Daniel Company Limited
1 Church Path, Saffron Walden
Essex, CB10 1JP, England

ISBN 085207 280 5

*All sections taken from spontaneous
discourses given by Osho*

Production in association with
Book Production Consultants plc, Cambridge
Typeset by Cambridge Photosetting Services
Printed and bound by Biddles, Guildford

CONTENTS

FOREWORD

Talk given to the Medical Association in Ahmedabad, Gujarat.

My beloved ones,

Man is a disease. Diseases come to man, but man himself is also a disease. This is his problem, and too, this is his uniqueness. This is his good fortune, and also his misfortune. No other animal on earth is such a problem, an anxiety, a tension, a disease, an illness, in the way man is. And this condition itself has given man all growth, all evolution, because 'disease' means that one cannot be happy with where one is; one cannot accept what one is. This disease itself has become man's dynamism, his restlessness, but at the same time it is his misfortune also, because he is agitated, unhappy, and he is suffering.

No other animal except man has the capacity to become mad. Unless man drives some animal insane, it does not go mad on its own – does not become neurotic. Animals are not mad in the jungle, they become crazy in a circus. In the jungle, the life of an animal is not warped; it becomes perverted in a zoo. No animal commits suicide; only man can commit suicide.

Two methods have been tried to understand and cure the disease called man. One is medicine, the other is meditation. Both these are treatments for the same disease. It will be good to understand here that medicine considers each disease in man separately – an approach of analysis of the part. Meditation considers man himself as a disease; meditation considers the very personality of man as the disease. Medicine considers that diseases come to man and then they go – that they are something alien to man. But slowly this difference has diminished and medical science too has started saying, "Do not treat the disease, treat the patient."

1

This is a very important statement, because this means that disease is nothing but a way of life which a patient lives. Every man does not fall sick in the same fashion. Diseases also have their own individuality, their personality. It is not that if I suffer from TB and if you also suffer from TB, we both will be patients of the same kind. Even our TBs will present themselves in two forms, because we are two different individuals. It may also happen that the treatment that cures my TB does not bring about any relief to your TB. So deep down the patient is at the root, not the disease.

Medicine catches the diseases in man very superficially. Meditation gets hold of man from deep within. In other words it can be said that medicine tries to bring about the health of a person from the outside; meditation tries to keep the inner being of a person healthy. Neither can the science of meditation be complete without medicine, nor can the science of medicine be complete without meditation, since man is both body and soul. In fact it is really a linguistic mistake to call man both of them.

For thousands of years man has thought that the body and the soul of a person are separate entities. This thinking has given rise to two very dangerous results. One of the results was that some people considered that man was only the soul and they neglected the body. Such people brought about developments in meditation but not in medicine – medicine could not become a science; the body was totally disregarded. In contrast, some people considered man as only the body and negated the soul. They did a lot of research and development in medicine but no steps towards meditation.

But man is both at the same time. I am also saying that this is a linguistic mistake: when we say both at the same time, it gives the impression that there are two things but connected together. No, in fact the body and the soul of man are two ends of the same pole. If it is seen in the right perspective, we will not be able to say that man is body plus soul – it is not so. Man is psycho-somatic or somato-psychic. Man is mind-body or body-mind.

According to me, that part of the soul which is within the grasp of our senses is the body, and that part of the body which is beyond the grasp of the senses is the soul. The invisible body is the soul, the visible soul is the body. They are not two different things, they are not two separate entities, they are two different states of vibrations of the same entity.

Actually, this notion of duality has harmed mankind badly. We always think in terms of two and land up with problems. Initially we used to think in terms of matter and energy; now we do not. Now we cannot say that matter and energy are separate. Now we say that matter *is* energy. The reality is that use of the old language is creating difficulties. Even to say that matter is energy is not right. There is something – let us call it X – which seen on the one end is matter while seen on the other end is energy; they are not two. They are two different forms of the same entity.

Similarly the body and the soul are two ends of the same entity. Illness can begin from either of the two ends. It can start from the body and reach to the soul; in fact, whatever transpires in the body, its vibrations are felt in the soul. That is why sometimes it happens that a man is physically cured of a disease but still he goes on feeling ill. The disease has left the body; the doctor says there is no disease, but the patient still feels ill and refuses to believe that he is not sick. All the various investigations and tests indicate that clinically everything is alright, but the patient keeps on saying that he does not feel well.

This type of patient has really bothered the doctors a lot, because all the modes of investigation indicate that there is no disease. But having no disease does not mean that you are healthy. Health has its own positivity. Absence of disease is only a negative state. We might be able to say that there is no thorn, but that does not mean the presence of a flower; that there is no thorn only indicates the absence of thorns. But the presence of a flower is another matter altogether.

The science of medicine has so far not been able to achieve anything in the dimension of what health is. Its whole work has been in the dimension of what disease is. If you question the science of medicine about diseases it tries to give definitions, but if you ask it what health is then it tries to deceive you. It says that when there is no disease, then whatever remains is health. This is deception, not a definition. How can you define health in relation to disease? It is like defining a flower in relation to thorns; it is like defining life in relation to death, or light in relation to darkness. It is like defining a man in relation to a woman, or vice-versa.

No, the science of medicine has not been able to say so far what health is. It can only tell us what disease is, naturally. There is a reason for it. The reason is that the science of medicine only grasps from the outside, only grasps the bodily manifestations – from the outside only the disease can be grasped. Health can be grasped only from that which is within the man, his innermost being and his soul. In this respect the Hindi word *swasthya* is really wonderful. The English word 'health' is not synonymous with swasthya. Health is derived from healing; illness is associated with it. Health means healed – the one who has recovered from illness.

Swasthya does not mean that, swasthya means the one who has settled within himself, the one who has reached himself. Swasthya means the one who is able to stand within himself, and that is why swasthya is not just health. Actually there is no word in any other language in the world comparable to the word swasthya. All the other languages of the world have words which are synonyms either with disease or with no-disease. The very concept of swasthya that we carry is that of no-illness. But

3

having no-illness is necessary but not enough for swasthya. Something else is required – something from the other end of the pole, from our inner being. Even if a disease starts from the outside, its vibrations are echoed all the way to the soul.

Suppose I throw a stone in a calm lake: the disturbance occurs only at the place where the stone hits the water, but the ripples produced reach the banks of the lake where the stone did not hit. Similarly, whatever happens to our body, its ripples reach the soul. And if clinical medicine treats only the body, then what will happen to those ripples which have reached far away to the banks? If we have thrown a stone in the lake and if we concentrate only at the place where the stone has hit the water and settled down, then what will happen to all those ripples which now have their own existence independent of the stone?

Once a man falls ill, the vibrations of the disease enter the soul, and that is why often the disease persists even after the body has been given the treatment and is cured. This persistence of the disease is there because of its vibrations which echoed all the way to the innermost being of the person and for which medical science has no solution so far. So medical science will always remain incomplete without meditation. We will be able to cure the disease but we will not be able to cure the patient. Of course, it is in the interest of the doctors that the patient is not cured; that only the disease is cured but the patient should always come back!

The disease can also originate from the other end. Actually, in the state in which man is, the disease is already present there. In the state in which man is, there is a lot of tension present within him. I have already said before that no other animal is dis-eased in this manner, is restless in this manner, is in such a tension – and there is a reason for this. No other animal's mind has this idea of becoming something else. A dog is a dog; it does not have to become one. But a man has to become a human being, he is not one already. That is why we cannot say to a dog that he is a little less dog. All dogs are equally dogs. But in the case of man, we can reasonably say to a man that he is a little less man. Man is never born in his completeness.

Man is born in an incomplete state; all other animals are born in their completeness. It is not so with man. There are certain things he will have to do in order to be complete. This state of incompleteness is his disease. That is why he is troubled throughout the twenty-four hours. It is not that only a poor man is in trouble because of his poverty – this is how we commonly think. But we do not realize that on becoming rich, only the level of trouble changes but the troubles remain.

The truth is that a poor man is never in such anxiety as a rich man gets into, because the poor man at least has a justification for his problems – that he is poor. A rich man does not have even this justification. He cannot even pinpoint the reason for his anxiety. And when an anxiety is without any apparent cause, it becomes terrible. A reason gives you some relief, some consolation, because then one has hopes that one may be able to remove the reasons. But when some trouble arises without any reason then difficulties increase.

The poor nations have suffered a lot, but the day they become rich they will realize that the rich countries have their own sufferings.

I would like humanity to choose the rich man's sufferings, not the poor man's. If it is a question of choosing sufferings, then it is better to choose those of a rich man. But the intensity of restlessness will be heightened.

Today, the amount of restlessness and anxiety faced by America is greater than any other country in the world. Although no other community has ever had the amount of facilities that are available in America today, actually it is in America that for the first time disillusionment has taken place. For the first time the illusions have been broken. Man used to think he was in anxiety due to some reason. In America, for the first time it has become clear that man is in anxiety not because of any reason; man himself *is* the anxiety. He invents new anxieties for himself. The personality that is there within him goes on demanding continuously for something that is not there. That which is there goes on becoming meaningless every day; that which has already been achieved becomes meaningless, futile. There is a continuous striving for those things which one does not have.

Nietzsche has said somewhere that man is a bridge stretched between two impossibilities — always eager to achieve the impossible, always eager to become complete. It is out of this eagerness to become complete that all the religions have been born.

It will be useful to note that there was a time on the earth when the priest was the physician also, when the religious leader was the doctor also. He was the priest and he was the doctor. And it will not be surprising if we end up with the same situation again tomorrow. There will only be a slight difference: the one who is a physician will be the priest! This has started happening in America, because for the first time it has become clear that the question is not of the body alone; and also it has come to light that if the body is completely healthy, then the problems increase manyfold, because for the first time the person starts sensing the disease which is present within, at the other pole from the body.

Our senses too need causes. If a thorn has pierced one's leg, only then does one feel the leg. As long as the thorn does not prick one's leg, one remains unaware of the leg. When the thorn is in the leg, then one's whole soul becomes like an arrow pointed towards the leg; it notices only the leg and nothing else — naturally. But if the thorn is removed from the leg, then too the being would need to notice something else. If your hunger is satisfied, good clothes are available to wear, your house is in proper order, you get the wife you wanted — although there is no bigger calamity in this world than this. There is no end to the sufferings of a person who gets the wife he wanted. If you do not get the wife you want, then at least you can derive some happiness out of hope. That too is lost when you get the wife you want.

I have heard about an asylum. A man had gone to see the asylum, and the superintendent of the asylum took him around on a tour. In front of a particular cell the man asked the superintendent what was wrong with the inmate. The superintendant replied that this person became mad because he could not get the woman with whom he was in love. In another cell the inmate was trying to break the bars, was beating his chest, was pulling at his hair. When asked what was wrong with this man, the superintendent replied that this man got the same woman the other person could not get, and he became mad. But because he could not get his beloved, the first person used to keep her photograph near his heart and was happy in his madness, while the second person was beating his head against the bars! Fortunate are those lovers who do not get their beloveds!

In fact, whatever we have not achieved, we hope for it and can go on living in that hope. Once we have achieved it our hopes are shattered and we become empty. The day the physician makes man free from his body-problems, that day he will have to take on the other part of the work. The day man becomes free of his bodily diseases, that day we are providing him with the situation in which he can become aware of his inner diseases. For the first time he will be troubled inside and will wonder that everything on the surface is alright, and yet nothing seems to be alright.

It is not surprising that in India, twenty-four *tirthankaras* were the sons of kings; Buddha was a king's son, Rama and Krishna were all from royal families. For these people the restlessness had disappeared from the level of the body; their restlessness had begun from within now.

Medicine tries to free man from diseases superficially, at the level of the body. But remember, even freed from all his diseases, man does not become free from the basic disease of being a man. That disease of being a man is a desire for the impossible. That disease of being a man is to be not satisfied with anything, that disease of being a man is making all that one achieves futile and attaching significance to whatever one has not got.

The cure for the disease of being a man is meditation. For all the other diseases, physicians have the cure, medicine has the cure; but for this particular disease of being a man only meditation has the cure. Medical science will be complete the day we understand the inner side of man and start working with that too, because according to my understanding, the dis-eased person who is sitting within us creates a thousand and one illnesses at the level of the body outside.

As I have already said, whenever the body becomes ill, the vibrations, the ripples are felt in the soul. Similarly, if the soul is diseased then the ripples reach the level of the body.

This is why there are so many kinds of pathies in the world. It should not be so if pathology is a science; then there cannot be thousands of pathies. But it becomes possible because man's diseases are of thousands of types. Some types of diseases cannot be cured with the help of allopathy. For those diseases which originate in the interiority of man and travel to his outside, allopathy is useless. For those diseases which start on the outside and move towards the interiority, allopathy is very successful. Those diseases which reach the outside from within are not bodily diseases at all. They just manifest at the body level. Their level of origin is always psychic, or still deeper – spiritual.

Now, if a person is suffering from a disease in his psyche, this means no clinical medicine can give him any relief. In fact it may be harmful, because it will try to do something and in the process, if it does not give relief, it is bound to do some harm. Only those medicines are incapable of causing harm which are incapable of giving any relief either. For example, homoeopathy does not harm anyone, because there is no question of any relief from it either. But homoeopathy *does* give relief. It is incapable of providing relief but that does not mean that people do not get relief.

But to get relief is entirely a different story; to give relief is again a different story. These two things are two separate phenomena. People do get relief because if the person is creating the disease at the level of his psyche then he needs some placebo for it. He needs some placebo for his disease, he needs some consolation, some assurance that he is not sick, but is just carrying the idea that he is sick. That can also be achieved through ashes from some mendicant; that can be achieved through the holy water of the Ganges, etcetera.

Nowadays a lot of experimentation is going on with what you may call illusory medicine, placebo. If ten patients are suffering from the same disease, and if three of them are treated by allopathy, three with homoeopathy and three of them by naturopathy, then an interesting result is seen: each of these pathies is affecting the same percentage of people for the good and for the bad. There is not much difference in the proportions. This *does* produce some reason for thought. What is going on?

According to me, allopathy is the only scientific medicine. But since something in man is unscientific, the scientific medicine alone will not do. Allopathy alone deals with the human body in a scientific manner. But allopathy cannot cure one hundred percent, because man in his inner being is imaginative, inventive, and projective also. Actually a person on whom allopathy does not work is sick due to some unscientific reason. What does it mean to be ill due to some unscientific reason?

7

These words may sound very strange. You know that there can be scientific medical treatment and there can also be unscientific medical treatment. I am saying to you that there can also be scientific sickness and unscientific sickness – unscientific ways of falling sick. All the diseases which start at the level of the psyche of a person and manifest at the level of the body, cannot be cured in a scientific way.

I know a young woman who went blind. But the blindness was psychological – actually her eyes were not affected. Eye specialists said that the eyes were alright, the girl was deceiving everyone. But the girl was not deceiving anyone, because even if you led her towards the fire she would go into the fire; she would stumble against a wall and injure her head. The girl was not fooling; she really could not see with her eyes. But this disease was beyond the physicians.

This girl was brought to me and I tried to understand her. I came to know that she was in love with somebody but her family members had stopped her from seeing that person. When I repeatedly questioned her, she replied that she had no desire to see anyone else in the world except her lover. This determination not to see anything except her lover...and if this sort of intensity is present in the determination, the eyes become psychologically blind. The eyes will become blind, the eyes will stop seeing anything. This cannot be understood by seeing the anatomy of the eyes, because the anatomy is normal, the mechanism of seeing is functional. Only the seer who used to be behind the eyes has slipped away, has removed itself from there. We experience this in our day-to-day life, only we are not aware of it. The mechanism of our body functions only while our presence is there behind it.

Now consider a young boy playing hockey who gets injured in his leg. He is bleeding but he does not realize it. Others can see that he is bleeding but he himself has no inkling of it. Then, when the play is over after half an hour, he grasps his leg and starts shouting and asking when he got hurt. It is hurting a lot. Now half an hour has passed since he was injured. The injury in his leg is a reality, the sensory mechanisms in his leg are working absolutely alright – since it is they that informed him about the pain after half an hour – so why was the information not conveyed earlier? His attention was not there with the leg, his attention was on the play, and so great was his attention that there was nothing of it left to notice his leg. The leg must have kept on informing him – the muscles, the nerves must have twitched – the leg must have knocked on all possible doors, it must have rung the exchange, but the man at the exchange was asleep. He was fast asleep or he was present somewhere else. He was absent, he was not present. When he returned after half an hour, then it was noticed that there was an injury to the leg.

I told the girl's family to do one thing. I told them that since she is not allowed to see the person she wants to see, she has committed a partial suicide – a suicide of her eyes. Nothing else is the matter with her except that she has gone into a phase of partial suicide. Let her lover meet her. They said, "What has that got to do with the eyes?" I asked them to just try it for once. And as soon as she was informed that she is allowed to meet her lover and that he would arrive at five o'clock, she came and stood at the door. Her eyes were alright!

No this is not deception. Now, experiments in hypnotism have shown us that there is no place for deception. This I am telling you from my own experiments. If a deeply hypnotized person is given an ordinary pebble in his hand and told that it is a piece of hot coal, he will behave exactly the way he would with a piece of ember in his hand. He will throw it away, he will start shouting, wailing that he has been burned. Up to this point it can be easily understood. But he will also get blisters on his hands – and then the difficulty arises. If by merely imagining that there is burning coal in your hand you can get blisters, then it is dangerous to begin the treatment of these blisters at the level of the body. The treatment for these blisters should start at the level of the mind.

Since we consider only one end of man, we have been able to slowly eliminate diseases which affect the body, but at the same time diseases originating from the mind have increased. Today, even those who think only in terms of science have started agreeing that at least fifty percent of diseases are of the mind. This is not so in India, because for diseases of the mind, first a strong mind is required. In India we still see that about ninety-five percent of diseases are of the body, but in America incidents of diseases of the mind are increasing.

Diseases of the mind usually begin from within and spread to the outside; they are outgoing diseases, while those of the body are ingoing. If you try to treat the bodily manifestations of the mental disease, then it will immediately find some other means of manifestation. We might be able to stop the small trickles of the mental disease from one place or a second or third place, but it will certainly manifest at a fourth or fifth place. It will try to manifest from the weak spot in the personality of the individual. That is why so many times a physician is not only unable to treat a disease but also is responsible for multiplying the various forms of the disease. What can come out through one source alone starts pouring from various sources, because we have built dams at different sites.

According to me, meditation is the cure at the other end of the human being. Naturally, medicines depend on matter, their chemical constituents; meditation depends on the consciousness. There are no tablets available for meditation, though people are trying. LSD, mescalin, marijuana – thousands of things are being tried. Thousands of efforts are going on to produce pills for meditation. But you can never have any pills for meditation. Actually, trying to make such pills is the same old stubbornness of only treating from the level of the body, of making all the treatments only from the outside. Even if our psyche is affected inside, we will still treat from the outside, never from within. Drugs like mescalin and LSD can only produce an illusion of inner health, they cannot create it. We cannot reach man's innermost being through any chemical means. The deeper we go inside, the less will be the effect of chemicals. The deeper we go within man, the less meaningful the physical and material approach starts becoming. A non-material approach, or we could say a psychic approach, has meaning there.

But it has not been achieved so far because of some prejudices. Interestingly, doctors are one of the two or three most orthodox professions in the world. Professors and medical doctors list highest among the most orthodox people. They do not let go of old ideas easily. There is a reason for it – perhaps it is quite a natural reason. If doctors and professors drop old ideas, become flexible, then they will have a difficult time teaching the children. If things are fixed, then they are able to teach efficiently. Ideas should be definite, solid, not shaky and fluid; then they can have confidence while teaching them.

Even criminals do not require the amount of confidence that a professor requires. He should have self-confidence that what he is saying is absolutely right, and who-ever requires this kind of confidence about being right in their profession becomes orthodox. Teachers become orthodox. This does great harm, because in all senses education should be the *least* orthodox; otherwise there will be obstacles in the path of progress. This is the reason why usually no teacher is an inventor. There are so many professors in all the universities but inventions, discoveries are made by people from outside. More than seventy percent of Nobel prizewinners are people from outside the universities.

The other profession that is full of orthodoxy is that of the doctors. That too has its professional reason. Doctors have to make decisions very fast. If they start contemplating when the patient is on the deathbed, then only the ideas will remain, the patient will be dead. If the doctor is very unorthodox, liberal, and practices new theories, does new experiments every time, then too there is danger. He has to make instant decisions, and all those who have to make instant decisions rely mainly on past knowledge; they do not want to get caught up in new ideas.

These people who are making decisions on the spot every day have to rely on past knowledge, and that is why the medical profession runs behind medical research by about thirty years. This results in many patients dying unnecessarily, because what should not be practiced today is actually being followed. But this is a professional hazard. And so some of the concepts of the doctors are deep down very funda-mentalist. One of them is their faith in medicine more than in the man himself – more faith in the chemicals than in the consciousness, more importance is given to chemistry than consciousness. The most dangerous outcome of this attitude is that while chemistry is given more importance, no experiments will be done on consciousness.

Here I would like to talk about a few such examples so that you might get some idea. To have painless labour during the birth of a child has been a very old problem; how to bear a child without pain has long been a question. Of course the priests are against this. Actually the priests are against the very idea that the world should become free from pain and suffering, because they will be out of a job if there is no pain in this world. Their profession will have no meaning. If there is pain, suffering and misery, then there is a call, a prayer. Maybe even God might get totally neglected if there is no suffering in the world. People may hardly pray, because we remember God only in suffering. Priests have always been against painless labour. They say that the pain during labour is a natural process.

But it should not be there. To call it an arrangement by God is a false idea. No God wants to give pain during childbirth. The doctor believes that for the painless birth of a child some medicine should be given, some chemicals should be arranged for, anaesthesia should be given. All these remedies by the doctors start at the level of the body, meaning that we get the body in such a state that the mother does not realize that she is in pain. Naturally women themselves have been experimenting with this on their own for centuries....

That is why seventy-five percent of babies are born during the night. It is difficult in the daytime because a woman is very active and aware at that time. When the woman is asleep she is more relaxed and it is easier for the baby to be born. During the night they go to sleep, they are more relaxed, and so seventy-five percent of babies do not get a chance to be born when the sun is shining; they have to take birth in the darkness. A mother starts creating obstacles for the child right from the moment it is about to be born. Of course later on she manages so many obstacles for the child, but she begins causing hindrances for the child even before it is born.

One of the remedies is to do something through medication so that the body becomes relaxed as it is during sleep. These remedies are being followed but they have their own drawbacks. The biggest drawback is that we do not trust at all in the consciousness of the person. And as this trust in the human consciousness goes on decreasing, the consciousness starts disappearing.

A doctor called Lozem has trusted in human consciousness and he has managed thousands of painless deliveries of babies for women. This method is of conscious cooperation – that the mother tries to cooperate meditatively, consciously, during

11

the delivery, that she welcomes it, does not fight against it or try to resist it. The pain that is produced is not because of the childbirth but because of the fight the mother makes against it. She tries to constrict the whole mechanism of childbirth. She is in fear that it will be painful, she is afraid of the labour. This fear-centred resistance is preventing the child from being born. While the child is trying to be born, there is a tussle between the two; there is a clash between the mother and the baby. This conflict is responsible for the pain. This pain is not natural: it is only from the clash, from the resistance.

There are two possible ways to solve this problem of resistance. We can sedate the mother, if we are working at the level of the body. But the thing to remember here is that a mother who delivers her child in a state of unconsciousness can never become a mother in the fullest sense. And there is a reason for it. When a child takes birth, not only is a child born but a mother too is born. The birth of a child actually is two births: on the one hand a child is born and on the other an ordinary woman becomes a mother. And if the baby is born in the state of unconsciousness, we have managed to distort the basic relationship between the mother and the child. The mother will not be born, only a nurse will be left behind in the process.

I am not in favour of delivering a child by sedating the mother with the help of chemicals or using superficial means. The mother should be fully conscious during the delivery, because in that very consciousness the mother is born too. If you realize the truth of this matter, then it means that the mother's consciousness should be trained for the delivery. The mother should be able to take the childbirth meditatively.

Meditation has two meanings for the mother. One is that she should not resist, should not fight. She should cooperate with whatever is going on. Just like a river which flows wherever there is a depression in the earth, just as the winds are blowing, just like the falling of the leaves – no one gets an inkling of it and the dry leaf just falls off the tree – similarly she should be in total cooperation with all that is unfolding before her. And if the mother gives her total cooperation during the delivery, does not fight against it, does not become afraid, becomes fully immersed meditatively in the event, then there will be painless birth, the pain will just vanish.

I am telling you this on a scientific basis. Many experiments have been done using this method. She will become free from pain. And remember, this will have far reaching results.

Firstly, we start harbouring an ill feeling towards the thing or person that produces pain in us from the very first moment of contact. We fall into a sort of enmity with the person with whom we encounter a struggle in our very first experience. This becomes an obstacle in forming a friendly relationship. It is difficult to create a bridge of cooperation with a person with whom we fell into conflict in the very beginning. It will be superficial. But that moment when we will be able to deliver a child with cooperation and in full awareness....

This is very interesting: until now we have only heard the expression 'labour pains', but we have never heard the expression 'labour bliss' – because it has not taken place so far. But if there is full cooperation, then 'labour bliss' will also happen. So I am not in favour of painless birth, I am in favour of blissful birth. With help from medical science, at the most we can achieve painless birth but never blissful birth. But if we approach it from the side of consciousness, then we can have blissful birth. And right from the first moment we will be able to build a conscious inner connection between the mother and the child.

This was only an example to put across to you that something can be done from within also. Whenever we fall sick, we are trying to fight the sickness only from the outside. The question is, is the patient really ready from the inside to fight the sickness? And we never bother to find this out. It is quite possible that it is a self-invited disease. The number of self-invited sicknesses is large. Actually very few diseases come on their own, most of them are invited. Of course, we had invited them long before they came; hence we are unable to see any connection between the two.

For thousands of years so many societies in this world could not form a connection between physical intercourse and childbirth because the time difference was big – nine months. It was difficult for them to relate such a distant cause and effect. And then not all intercourse leads to childbirth, so obviously there was no reason for thinking in terms of connecting the two. It was much later that man understood that what had occurred nine months back is resulting in a childbirth today. He could form a cause and effect relationship. The same happens to us regarding illness. We invite it sometime, but it will come later on. Much time passes between the two events, and that is the reason we are unable to see any connection between the two.

I have heard of a man who was on the verge of becoming bankrupt. He was afraid to go to the market, to his shop. He was afraid to even walk on the streets. One day as he was coming out of his bathroom he fell down and was paralyzed. Now all sorts of treatments are being done for him. But we do not want to accept that the man *wanted* to become paralyzed. He did not think about this consciously, but that is not the point. Nor does it matter whether he had made up his mind or not to get paralyzed – most probably he never thought of it. But somewhere inside his mind, in his unconscious, he must have wanted that he should not have to go to the market or to the shop or on the streets. This is the first thing.

Secondly, he also wanted people to be less hostile towards him and wanted them to start showing some sympathy – these were his deep desires. Obviously his body will support him. The body always follows the mind like a shadow; it will always support the mind. The mind makes the arrangements. Actually we never realize what arrangements the mind has in its store. If you have fasted for the whole day, then you will have a meal in the night – the mind will see to that. It will tell you in your dreams that you have fasted for the whole day, you must be uncomfortable; let's go to a feast at the king's palace. And you will eat there in the night in your dream.

The mind arranges for everything that the body could not do. So most of the dreams we see are just like these – just substitutes. What we could not do in the day we do in the night. Mind arranges all these things. If suddenly in the night you feel like going to the bathroom, then it means that the mind is sounding an alarm. It will send you to the bathroom in your dream and you will feel less strain on your bladder. You will think that that is alright and that you have been to the bathroom. The mind arranges so that your sleep is not disturbed. Throughout the day and night, the mind is constantly making arrangements so that all your desires are fulfilled.

This man had an attack of hemiplegia and he fell down. Now we are trying to treat that. But actually the medicines might harm him, because he does not have hemiplegia; he has brought the disease upon himself. Even if we treat his paralysis then he will manifest a second or a third, or maybe a fourth disease. Actually, until he gathers courage to go to the market he will suffer from one disease or another. And as soon as he falls ill he realizes that the whole situation has changed. Now he has some justification for going bankrupt. What can I do? – I am paralyzed! Now he can tell his creditors, "How can I repay you? You can see the condition I am in." Actually, when the creditor will come to him, he himself will feel ashamed to ask for the money. His wife will take better care of him, his children will serve him better, his friends will come to meet him, people will surround his bed.

In reality we never show our love to anyone until he falls sick. So whoever wants to be loved has to fall sick. Women are always falling sick, and the main reason is that for them this is the way of getting love. They know there is no other way of keeping their husbands at home. The wife cannot keep him there but the illness can. Once we realize this, and if this gets fixed in our minds, then every time we want some sympathy we will fall sick. Actually it is dangerous to show sympathy to a sick man; you should only treat him. It is dangerous because through sympathy you may be adding flavour to his disease and this will be harmful.

No medicine will cure this person who has had paralysis; at the most he will keep changing diseases, because in reality he does not have the disease, it is just deep auto-suggestion. The hemiplegia is mental in origin.

A similar story is that of another man who was also suffering from hemiplegia. For two years he was suffering and he could not even get up. One day his house caught fire and everybody ran out of the house. Suddenly they panicked and wondered what would happen to the sick man. But then they saw him coming – he was running – and this person could not even sit before. And when his family pointed out to him that he could walk, he said that that was not possible and he collapsed then and there.

What has happened to this man?…and he is not fooling anybody. The disease is mind-oriented, not body-oriented. That is the only difference. And that is the reason why when a physician tells a patient that his disease is in the mind, the patient does not like it because it seems to convey that he is unnecessarily trying to show that he is sick. This is not right. No one wants to show that he is ill for no reason. There are mental reasons for falling sick, and these reasons are as important or maybe more important than the reasons for falling sick because of some actual physical problem. And it will be mistreatment on the part of the physician to tell someone, even by mistake, that he is mentally ill. The patient does not feel better with this statement; in fact he feels bitter towards the doctor.

We haven't yet been able to develop a kindly attitude towards mind-oriented diseases. If my leg is hurt then everyone will be sympathetic, but if my mind is hurt then people will say that this is a mental disease – as if I have done something wrong. If my leg is hurt then I get sympathy, but if I have a mind-oriented disease then I am blamed as if it is my fault! No, it is not my fault.

Mind-oriented diseases have their own place, but the physicians don't accept it. This reluctance is because they have treatment only for body-oriented diseases; there is no other reason. It is beyond him, so he just says that this is not a disease. Actually he should say that this is beyond his scope. He should advise you to find a different type of doctor. This person actually needs a treatment which will start from within and then come outwards. And it is possible that a very small thing can change his inner life.

According to me, meditation is a treatment that spreads from the inside out.

One day somebody went to Buddha and asked, "Who are you? Are you a philosopher, or a thinker or a saint or a yogi?" Buddha replied, "I am only a healer, a physician."

This answer of his is truly marvellous: Only a healer – I know something about the inner diseases and that is what I discuss with you.

The day we understand that we will have to do something about these mind-oriented diseases – because anyway we will never be able to eradicate all the body-oriented diseases completely – that day we will see that religion and science have come closer to each other. That day we will see that medicine and meditation have come nearer to each other. My own understanding is that no other branch of science will help as much as medicine in bridging this gap.

Chemistry does not have any reason to come close to religion as yet. Similarly physics and maths have no reason to come close to religion as yet. Maths can survive without religion and I think this will remain true forever, because I do not see a situation where maths will need the help of religion. Nor can I conceive of a moment when maths will feel that it cannot develop without religion. Never will that day come. Maths can keep its game going for eternity, because maths is only a game, it is not life.

But a physician is not playing a game, he is dealing with life. Most probably it is the medical doctor who will become the first bridge between religion and science. Actually it has already started happening, especially in the more developed and understanding nations. The reason is that the doctors have to deal with human lives. It is what Carl Gustav Jung said just before dying. He said that on the basis of being a physician I can say that of all the patients who came to me after the age of forty, basically their illness was because of lack of religion. It is a very surprising point. If somehow we can give them some kind of religion then they will become healthy.

This is worth understanding. As the life of a person declines...until the age of thirty-five it is on the rise, then it starts moving down. Thirty-five is the peak. So it is possible that up to the age of thirty-five a person may not find any value in meditation, because until then man is body-oriented; the body is still on the rise. Perhaps all the diseases in this stage are of the body. But after the age of thirty-five the diseases will take a new turn, because now life has started moving towards death. And when life grows it spreads towards the outside, but when man dies he shrinks withinwards. Old age is to have shrunk withinwards.

The truth is that most probably all the diseases of old people are deep down rooted in death.

Usually people say that such and such person died because of such and such sickness. But I think it would be more appropriate to say that such and such person is sick *because* of death. What happens is that the possibility of death makes a person vulnerable to all kinds of diseases. As soon as a person feels that he is moving towards death, all the doors open up to various diseases and he starts catching hold of them. Even if a healthy person comes to know for sure that he is going to die tomorrow, he will fall sick. Everything was alright, all the reports were normal; X-ray was normal, the blood pressure was within normal limits, the pulse was alright; the stethoscope was conveying that everything was perfect. But if a person becomes convinced completely that tomorrow he is going to die, then you will see that he starts catching a variety of diseases. He will catch so many diseases in twenty-four hours that it is difficult to catch them in twenty-four lifetimes.

What has happened to this person? He has opened himself up to all kinds of diseases. He has stopped resisting. Since he was sure of his death, he has moved away from his consciousness which was within him acting as a wall and forming a barrier against all the diseases. Now he has become ready for his death and the diseases start coming. And that is why a retired person dies soon.

So everybody wishing to retire should understand this before they retire. They die sooner by as much as five or six years. The one who would have died at the age of seventy, will die when he is only sixty-five; the one who would have died at the age of eighty, will die when he is seventy-five. Those ten, fifteen years of retirement will be spent in the preparation for death; he will not accomplish anything else, because now he knows that he is of no use in life. There is no work for him, no one greets him on the road.

It was different when he was in the office. Now no one even looks at him, because now they have to greet someone else. Everything works on economics. New people are there in the office, so people will have to greet them. They cannot afford to go on greeting this man as well. They will forget him. Now he suddenly realizes that he has become useless. He feels uprooted. He is of no use to anybody. Even the children are busy with their wives, going out to movies. The people he knew have slowly started ending up at the burning ghats. He has become useless for the same people who needed him earlier. Suddenly he becomes vulnerable, he opens up completely for death.

When does the consciousness of man become healthy from within? Firstly, when he starts feeling his inner consciousness. Usually we do not feel the inner; all our feelings are for the body – for the hand, for the leg, for the head, for the heart. There are no feelings of "I am." Our whole awareness is concentrated on the house and not on the dweller in the house.

This is a very dangerous situation, because if the house starts falling down tomorrow then I will think that I am falling, and this itself will become my sickness. But if I understand that I am different from the house, I am only residing in it – even if the house collapses I will still remain – then this will make a big difference, a basic difference. Then the fear of death will fade away.

Without meditation the fear of death never vanishes. So the first meaning of meditation is awareness of oneself. As long as we are in consciousness, our consciousness is always an awareness about something, it is never about itself. That is why when we are sitting alone we start feeling sleepy, because there is nothing to do. If we are reading a paper or listening to the radio, then we feel that we are awake. If we leave a person alone in a dark room then he will feel sleepy, because since you cannot see anything you do not require your consciousness. If you cannot see anything, then what can you do except sleep? There does not seem to be any other solution. If you are alone, there is darkness, no one to talk to, nothing to think about, then sleep will envelop you. There is no other way.

Remember that sleep and meditation are alike in one sense, and different in another. Sleep means that you are alone but you are in a slumber. Meditation means that you are alone but awake. This is the only difference. If you can remain awake about yourself when you are alone....

One day a person sitting with Buddha was fidgeting with his toe. Buddha asked him, "Why are you moving your toe?"

The person replied, "Forget it, it was just moving. I was not even aware of it."

Buddha said, "Your toe is moving and you do not even know? Whose toe is it? Is it yours?"

The man said, "It is mine – but why have you deviated from what you were saying? Please continue."

Buddha said, "I will not continue with my talk anymore because the person I was talking to is unconscious. And remain aware of your toe movement in future. That will create double awareness in you. In the awareness of the toe will be born the awareness of the watcher as well."

Awareness is always double-pointed. If we experiment with it, then one side of it will go outwards and the other one will pierce within you. So the basic meditation is that we start becoming aware of our bodies and ourselves. And if this awareness can increase then the fear of death will fade away.

And the medical science which cannot free man from the fear of death can never cure this disease which is man. Of course medical science tries hard; it tries to increase the lifespan. But increasing your lifespan increases only the waiting period for death and nothing else. And it is better to wait for a shorter period of time than a longer one. You make death even more pitiful by increasing the lifespan.

Do you know, there is a movement going on in those countries where medical science has increased the lifespan of people. This movement is for euthanasia. The old people are demanding that they should be given a right to die in the constitution. They say that life has become arduous for them and you are just keeping them hanging on in the hospitals. It has become possible: you can put a man on an oxygen cylinder and keep him hanging on endlessly. You can keep him alive, but that life will be worse than death. God knows how many people in Europe and America are lying in hospitals in upside down or other strange positions, hooked up to oxygen cylinders. They have not the right to die, and they are demanding to be given the right to die.

My understanding is that by the end of this century most of the developed countries in the world will have the right to die as one of the constitutional rights of man, because the doctor has no right to keep a person alive against his wishes.

By increasing the age of a person you cannot remove the fear of death from him. By making a person healthy you can make his life more happy but not fearless. Fearlessness comes in only one situation, which is when one comes to understand from within that there is something in him that never dies. This understanding is absolutely essential.

Meditation is the realization of this immortality, that that which is within me never dies. Only that dies which is on the outside. And that is why you should treat the body medically so that it lives happily for as long as it lives, and at the same time try to be aware of what is inside you so that even if death is at your doorstep, you are not afraid. This inner understanding is fearlessness.

Meditation from within and medication on the outside; then you can make medical science a complete science.

According to me, meditation and medicine are two poles of the same science where the connecting link is still missing. But slowly, slowly they are coming closer to each other. Today, in most of the major hospitals of America, a hypnotist has become essential. But hypnotism is not meditation. However, this is a good step. At least it shows that there is an understanding that something needs to be done about the consciousness of man, and that only treating the body is not enough.

And I think that if a hypnotist has entered the hospitals today, then tomorrow a temple will also enter. It will come later, it will take some time. After the hypnotist every hospital will have a department of yoga, of meditation. It should happen. Then we will be able to treat man as a whole. The body will be taken care of by the doctors, the mind by the psychologists, and the soul by yoga, meditation.

The day the hospitals accept man as a whole, as a totality, and then treat him as such, will be a day of rejoicing for mankind. I request you to think in that direction so that this day will come soon.

I am grateful that you listened to my talk with love and silence. In the end I offer my salutations to the God enthroned within all of you. Accept my salutations.

Osho

CHAPTER 1
DEFINITION OF HEALTH

You have recently said that most of humanity is vegetating, not living. Please explain to us the art of living so that death may become also a celebration.

Man is born to achieve life, but it all depends on him. He can miss it. He can go on breathing, he can go on eating, he can go on growing old, he can go on moving towards the grave – but this is not life. This is gradual death from the cradle to the grave, a seventy-year-long gradual death. And because millions of people around you are dying in this gradual, slow death, you also start imitating them. Children learn everything from those who are around them, and we are surrounded by the dead. So first we have to understand what I mean by 'life'. It must not be simply growing old. It must be growing up. And these are two different things. Growing old, any animal is capable of. Growing up is the prerogative of human beings. Only a few claim the right.

Growing up means moving every moment deeper into the principle of life; it means going further away from death – not towards death. The deeper you go into life, the more you understand the immortality within you. You are going away from death; a moment comes when you can see that death is nothing but changing clothes, or changing houses, changing forms – nothing dies, nothing *can* die. Death is the greatest illusion there is.

For growing up, just watch a tree. As the tree grows up, its roots are growing down, deeper. There is a balance: the higher the tree goes, the deeper the roots will go. You cannot have a tree one hundred and fifty feet high with small roots; they could not support such a huge tree. In life, growing up means growing deep within your-self – that's where your roots are.

To me, the first principle of life is meditation. Everything else comes second. And childhood is the best time. As you grow older, it means you are coming closer to death, and it becomes more and more difficult to go into meditation. Meditation means going into your immortality, going into your eternity, going into your godliness. And the child is the most qualified person because he is still unburdened by knowledge, unburdened by religion, unburdened by education, unburdened by all kinds of rubbish. He is innocent. But unfortunately his innocence is being condemned as ignorance. Ignorance and innocence have a similarity, but they are not the same. Ignorance is also a state of not knowing, just as innocence is. But there is a great difference too, which has been overlooked by the whole of humanity up to now. Innocence is not knowledgeable – but it is not desirous of being knowledgeable either. It is utterly content, fulfilled....

The first step in the art of living will be to create a demarcation line between ignorance and innocence. Innocence has to be supported, protected – because the child has brought with him the greatest treasure, the treasure that sages find after arduous effort. Sages have said that they become children again, that they are reborn....

Whenever you understand that you have missed life, the first principle to be brought back is innocence. Drop your knowledge, forget your scriptures, forget your religions, your theologies, your philosophies. Be born again, become innocent – and it is in your hands. Clean your mind of all that is not known by you, of all that is borrowed, all that has come from tradition, convention, all that has been given to you by others – parents, teachers, universities. Just get rid of it. Once again be simple, once again be a child. And this miracle is possible by meditation.

Meditation is simply a strange surgical method which cuts you away from all that is not yours and saves only that which is your authentic being. It burns everything else and leaves you standing naked, alone under the sun, in the wind. It is as if you are the first man who has descended onto earth – who knows nothing, who has to discover everything, who has to be a seeker, who has to go on a pilgrimage.

The second principle is the pilgrimage. Life must be a seeking – not a desire, but a search; not an ambition to become this, to become that, a president of a country or a prime minister of a country, but a search to find out "Who am I?" It is very strange that people who don't know who they are, are trying to become somebody. They don't even know who they are right now! They are unacquainted with their being – but they have a goal of becoming. Becoming is the disease of the soul. Being is you, and to discover your being is the beginning of life. Then each moment is a new discovery, each moment brings a new joy; a new mystery opens its doors, a new love starts growing in you, a new compassion that you have never felt before, a new sensitivity about beauty, about goodness.

You become so sensitive that even the smallest blade of grass takes on an immense importance for you. Your sensitivity makes it clear to you that this small blade of grass is as important to existence as the biggest star; without this blade of grass, existence would be less than it is. And this small blade of grass is unique, it is irreplaceable, it has its own individuality.

And this sensitivity will create new friendships for you – friendships with trees, with birds, with animals, with mountains, with rivers, with oceans, with stars. Life becomes richer as love grows, as friendliness grows....

As you become more sensitive, life becomes bigger. It is not a small pond, it becomes oceanic. It is not confined to you and your wife and your children – it is not confined at all. This whole existence becomes your family, and unless the whole existence is your family you have not known what life is – because no man is an island, we are all connected. We are a vast continent, joined in millions of ways. And if our hearts are not full of love for the whole, in the same proportion our life is cut short.

Meditation will bring you sensitivity, a great sense of belonging to the world. It is our world – the stars are ours, and we are not foreigners here. We belong intrinsically to existence. We are part of it, we are *heart* of it.

Secondly, meditation will bring you a great silence – because all rubbish knowledge is gone, thoughts that are part of the knowledge are gone too... an immense silence, and you are surprised: This silence is the only music there is. All music is an effort to bring this silence somehow into manifestation.

The seers of the ancient East have been very emphatic about the point that all the great arts – music, poetry, dance, painting, sculpture – are all born out of meditation. They are an effort to in some way bring the unknowable into the world of the known for those who are not ready for the pilgrimage – just gifts for those who are not ready to go on the pilgrimage. Perhaps a song may trigger a desire to go in search of the source, perhaps a statue.

The next time you enter a temple of Gautam Buddha or Mahavira, just sit silently, watch the statue...because the statue has been made in such a way, in such proportions that if you watch it you will fall silent. It is a statue of meditation; it is not concerned with Gautam Buddha or Mahavira....

In that oceanic state the body takes a certain posture. You have observed it yourself, but you have not been alert. When you are angry, have you observed? – your body takes a certain posture. In anger you cannot keep your hands open; in anger –

22

the fist. In anger you cannot smile – or can you? With a certain emotion, the body has to follow a certain posture. Just small things are deeply related inside....

A certain secret science has been used for centuries so the coming generations could come in contact with the experiences of the older generations – not through books, not through words, but through something which goes deeper – through silence, through meditation, through peace. As your silence grows, your friendliness, your love grows; your life becomes a moment-to-moment dance, a joy, a celebration....

Have you ever thought about why, all over the world, in every culture, in every society, there are a few days in the year for celebration? These few days for celebration are just a compensation – because these societies have taken away all celebration of your life, and if nothing is given to you in compensation your life can become a danger to the culture. Every culture has to give some compensation to you so that you don't feel completely lost in misery, in sadness.... But these compensations are false. But in your inner world there can be a continuity of lights, songs, joys.

Always remember that society compensates you when it feels that the repressed may explode into a dangerous situation if it is not compensated. The society finds some way of allowing you to let out the repressed. But this is not true celebration, and it cannot be true. True celebration should come from your life, *in* your life.

And true celebration cannot be according to the calendar, that on the first of November you will celebrate. Strange, the whole year you are miserable and on the first of November suddenly you come out of misery, dancing. Either the misery was false or the first of November is false; both cannot be true. And once the first of November is gone, you are back in your dark hole, everybody in his misery, everybody in his anxiety.

Life should be a continuous celebration, a festival of lights the whole year round. Only then you can grow up, you can blossom. Transform small things into celebration.... Everything that you do should be expressive of you; it should have your signature on it. Then life becomes a continuous celebration.

Even if you fall sick and you are lying in bed, you will make those moments of lying in bed moments of beauty and joy, moments of relaxation and rest, moments of meditation, moments of listening to music or to poetry. There is no need to be sad that you are sick. You should be happy that everybody is in the office and you are in your bed like a king, relaxing – somebody is preparing tea for you, the samovar is singing a song, a friend has offered to come and play flute for you. These things are more important than any medicine. When you are sick, call a doctor. But more important, call those who love you because there is no medicine more important than love. Call those who can create beauty, music, poetry around you because there is nothing that heals like a mood of celebration.

Medicine is the lowest kind of treatment. But it seems we have forgotten everything, so we have to depend on medicine and be grumpy and sad – as if you are missing some great joy that you were having in the office! In the office you were miserable – just one day off, and you cling to misery too; you won't let it go.

Make everything creative, make the best out of the worst – that's what I call 'the art'. And if a man has lived his whole life making every moment and every phase of it a beauty, a love, a joy, naturally his death is going to be the ultimate peak of his whole life's endeavour.

The last touches...his death is not going to be ugly as it ordinarily happens every day to everyone. If death is ugly, that means your whole life has been a wastage.

Death should be a peaceful acceptance, a loving entry into the unknown, a joyful good-bye to old friends, to the old world. There should not be any tragedy in it....

Start with meditation, and things will go on growing in you – silence, serenity, blissfulness, sensitivity. And whatever comes out of meditation, try to bring it out in life. Share it, because everything shared grows fast. And when you have reached the point of death, you will know there is no death. You can say good-bye, there is no need for any tears of sadness – maybe tears of joy, but not of sadness.[1]

?   *What is the relationship between medicine and meditation?*

The word 'meditation' and the word 'medicine' come from the same root. Medicine means that which heals the physical, and meditation means that which heals the spiritual. Both are healing powers.

Another thing to be remembered: the word 'healing' and the word 'whole' also come from the same root. To be healed simply means to be whole, not missing anything. Another connotation of the word – the word 'holy' also comes from the same root. Healing, whole, holy, are not different in their root.

Meditation heals, makes you whole, and to be whole is to be holy.

Holiness has nothing to do with belonging to any religion, belonging to any church. It simply means that inside you, you are entire, complete; nothing is missing, you are fulfilled. You are what existence wanted you to be. You have realized your potential....

Religion is a journey inwards, and meditation is the way. What meditation actually does is, it takes you, your consciousness, as deep as possible. Even your own body becomes something outside. Even your own mind becomes something outside.

24

Even your own heart – which is very close to the centre of your being – becomes outside. When your body, mind and heart, all three, are seen as outside, you have come to the very centre of your existence.

This coming to the centre is a tremendous explosion which transforms everything. You will never be the same man again, because now you know the body is only the outer shell; the mind is a little bit inner but not really your inner core; the heart is a little bit more inner, but still not the innermost centre. You are disidentified with all the three.

You start feeling, for the first time, crystallized...not that old wishy-washy person you had always been. For the first time you start feeling a tremendous energy, inexhaustible energy that you were not aware of. For the first time you know that death will happen only to the body, to the mind, to the heart, but not to you.

You are eternal. You have always been here, and you will be always here – in different forms, and ultimately in a state of formlessness. But you cannot be destroyed – you are indestructible. That takes all fear from you. And the disappearance of fear is the appearance of freedom. The disappearance of fear is the appearance of love. Now you can share. You can give as much as you want, because you are now at the inexhaustible source of living waters....

Meditation makes you whole, makes you holy, and makes you an inexhaustible source for all those who are hungry, thirsty, seeking, searching, groping in the dark. You become a light.... Meditation is the way to the mastery of your own being. No God is needed, no catechism is needed, no holy book is needed. Nobody is needed to become a Christian or a Jew or a Hindu – all that is sheer nonsense. All that is needed is to find your centre, and meditation is the simplest way to find it.

It will make you whole, healthy spiritually, and it will make you so rich that you can destroy all the spiritual poverty of the world. And that is the real poverty.

The poverty of physical bodies in food, in clothes, in shelter, can be easily helped by science and technology. But science and technology cannot help to give you blissfulness – that is beyond their scope. And you may have everything that the world can offer, but if you don't have peace, serenity, silence, ecstasy, you will still remain poor.

In fact, you will feel your poverty more than ever, because the contrast will be there. You are living in a golden palace, and you know you are a beggar. The golden palace will become a contrast: now you can see inside there is nothing, you are just empty.

That's why as humanity becomes more intelligent, more mature, more and more people start feeling meaninglessness, more and more people start feeling life is accidental, that it is just futile to go on living.

The latest developments in philosophy in the West all indicate one thing, that perhaps suicide is the only solution. And of course, if you don't know your inner world, and you have everything available that the outside world can give to you, suicide will appear to be the only solution.

Meditation can make you inwardly rich. Then suicide is out of the question; even if you want to destroy yourself, there is no way. Your being is indestructible. And to know this immortality is a great freedom – from death, from disease, from old age. All those things will come and go, but you remain untouched, unscratched. Your inner health is beyond any sickness.

And it is there, just to be discovered.[2]

Medical science, physiology, psychology, are very immature in the sense that they are only doing their work on the surface of human beings – they are not finding a way to man's centre. And because they do not accept the existence of some consciousness beyond mind, of some consciousness beyond death, they are completely closed, prejudiced against the whole tremendous effort mystics have made in finding the centre of consciousness.

Many times the diagnosis of a physiologist or a physician may be absolutely wrong for the simple reason that the vision is not comprehensive enough. He understands man only as matter, and mind as just by-product of matter, a shadow phenomenon with nothing beyond it, nothing eternal, nothing that is going to remain forever. They have created a picture of human beings which creates despair in intelligent people. And because of their outright rejection, their approach is not scientific; it is as superstitious as any other fanatic religious or political person's.

Science has no right to deny consciousness unless it has explored the inner sky of human consciousness and found that it is dream stuff, not a reality but only a shadow.

They have *not* explored – they have simply assumed. Materialism is the assumption, the superstition of the world of science, just as God, heaven and hell are superstitions of the religious world.

Science is not yet pure science and it cannot be, because the scientist is not yet innocent, unprejudiced, ready to go with the truth in spite of himself and his conditioning.[3]

? *You have talked about the need for Western medicine to take man as a whole organism, and that man needs not only the treatment of the part that is sick. Can you please comment further on this?*

For example, you have a headache; they will give you 'Aspro'. Aspro is not a cure, it simply makes you unaware of the symptom. The aspirin does not destroy the headache; it simply does not allow you to know about it. It confuses you. The headache remains there but you are no longer aware of it. It creates a kind of oblivion.

But why in the first place was the headache there? Ordinary medicine does not bother about it. If you go to a doctor he is not going to be bothered why in the first place you have a headache. You have a headache! – the problem is simple for him: "The symptom is there, take this medicine – some drug, some chemical – and that symptom will disappear." The headache may disappear and you may have a disturbed stomach the next day; another symptom has come up.

Man is one; man is a totality – an organic unity. You can push a problem from one side, it will assert itself from another side. It may take time to come to the other side, to travel to that point, but it is bound to come. And then pushed from that side it moves to another side...and man has many sides. It goes on being pushed from one corner to another.

Out of all this you become more and more ill rather than healthy. And sometimes it happens that a very small disease becomes a big disease. For example, if the headache is not allowed, and the stomachache is not allowed, and the backache is not allowed, and *no* ache is ever allowed, immediately the ache comes and you take something and you stop it.... If for years together you have gone on with this repression – this is repression – then one day all that disease gathers together, asserts itself in a more organized way. It can become cancer. All that has gathered together and now it asserts itself almost like an explosion.

Why have we not yet been able to find a drug for cancer? Maybe cancer is an expression of all the repressed diseases of man. We know how to repress single diseases up to now; now this is not a single disease, this is a very collective attack. It is a total attack – *all* the diseases have gone together, joined hands together. They have made an army...and they attack you. That's why drugs are failing; there seems to be no possibility right now that any drug will be found.

Cancer is a new disease. It does not exist in primitive societies. Why? – it has to be asked why it does not exist in primitive societies – because the primitive man does not repress, there is no need. It is a *rebellion* of your very system. If you don't repress, there is no need for any rebellion. Small things happen and go.

The religious attitude is to look, not for the symptom but for the source. That's what I call 'the psychology of the buddhas.' If you have a headache, that is not your illness, that is not your disease. In fact, that is a signal from your body that something is going wrong in the source – run to the source! Find out what is going wrong. The head is simply giving you a signal, a danger signal, an alarm: "Listen to the body. Something is going wrong, you are doing something which is not right, which is destroying the harmony of the body. Don't do it anymore; otherwise the headache will go on reminding you."

The headache is not the disease, and the headache is not your enemy – it is your friend. It is in your service. It is very, very essential for your existence that the body should make you alert when something goes wrong. Rather than changing that wrong, you simply put the alarm off – you take an Aspro. This is absurd. This is what is happening in medicine and this is what is happening in psychotherapies – symptomatic treatment.

That's why the essential is missing. The essential is: look into the source. Next time you have a headache try a small meditation technique, just experimentally, then you can go on to bigger diseases and bigger symptoms.

When you have a headache just try a small experiment. Sit silently and watch it, look into it – not as if you are looking at an enemy, no. If you are looking at it as your enemy, you will not be able to look rightly. You will avoid – nobody looks at the enemy directly; one avoids, one tends to avoid. Look at it as your friend. It is your friend, it is in your service. It is saying, "Something is wrong – look into it." Just sit silently and look into the headache with no idea of stopping it, with no desire that it should disappear, no conflict, no fight, no antagonism. Just look into it, into what it is.

Watch, so if there is some inner message the headache can give it to you. It has a coded message. And if you look silently you will be surprised. If you look silently three things will happen. First: the more you look into it, the more severe it will become. And then you will be a little puzzled: "How is it going to help if it is becoming more severe?" It is becoming more severe because you have been avoiding it. It was there but you were avoiding it; you were already repressing – even without the aspirin you were repressing it. When you look into it, repression disappears. The headache will come to its natural severity. Then you are hearing it with unplugged ears, no wool around your ears; it will be very severe.

First thing: it will become severe. If it is becoming severe, you can be satisfied that you are looking rightly. If it does not become severe, then you are not looking yet; you are still avoiding. Look into it – it becomes severe. That is the first indication that yes, it is in your vision.

The second thing will be that it will become more pin-pointed; it will not be spread over a bigger space. First you were thinking, "It is my whole head aching." Now you will see it is not the whole head, it is just a small spot. That is also an indication that now you are gazing more deeply into it. The spread feeling of the ache is a trick — that is a way to avoid it. If it is in one point then it will be more severe. So you create an illusion that it is the whole head which is aching, spread all over the head, then it is not so intense at any point. These are tricks that we go on playing.

Look into it, and the second step will be that it comes to be smaller and smaller and smaller. And a moment comes when it is just the very point of a needle — *very* sharp, immensely sharp, very painful. You have never seen such pain in the head — but very much confined to a small spot. Go on looking into it.

And then the third and most important thing happens. If you go on looking at this point when it is very severe and confined and concentrated at one point, you will see many times that it disappears. When your gaze is perfect it will disappear. And when it disappears you will have the glimpse of where it is coming from — what the cause is. It will happen many times. Again it will be there. Your gaze is no longer that alert, that concentrated, that attentive — it will come back. Whenever your gaze is *really* there, it will disappear; and when it disappears, hidden behind it is the cause. And you will be surprised: your mind is ready to reveal what the cause is.

A thousand and one causes there can be. There are different causes. The same alarm is given because the alarm system is simple. There are not many alarm systems in your body. For different causes the same alarm is given. You may have been angry lately and you have not expressed it. Suddenly, like a revelation, it will be standing there. You will see all your anger that you have been carrying, carrying...like pus inside you. Now this is too much, and that anger wants to be released. It needs a catharsis. Cathart! — and immediately you will see the headache has disappeared. And there was no need for the aspirin, no need for any treatment.*

And when the anger has disappeared, a totally different quality of well-being will arise in you that can never arise out of the aspirin. Aspirin represses — anger remains hidden inside you, violence goes on raging inside you. You only keep the alarm shut, that's all. Nothing changes, only the alarm is no longer there.

This goes on and on, and it becomes more and more accumulated. It may give you ulcers, it may give you tuberculosis — one day it can give you cancer. When a great quantity gathers, there are qualitative changes. There is a certain limit for the body to tolerate anything, beyond that limit it starts feeling ill. So is the case with mind. And never think of body and mind as two separate things; they are not. Man is body-mind, psychosomatic.[6]

---

* **OSHO'S DYNAMIC MEDITATION**

The Dynamic Meditation lasts one hour and is in five stages. It can be done alone, but the energy will be more powerful if it is done in a group. It is an individual experience so you should remain oblivious of others around you and keep your eyes closed throughout, preferably using a blindfold. It is best to have an empty stomach and wear loose, comfortable clothing.

First stage: 10 minutes

Breathing rapidly in and out through the nose, let breathing be intense and chaotic. The breath should move deeply into the lungs. Be as fast as you can in your breathing, making sure breathing stays deep. Do this as totally as you possibly can; without tightening up your body, make sure neck and shoulders stay relaxed. Continue on, until you literally become the breathing, allowing breath to be chaotic (that means not in a steady, predictable way). Once your energy is moving, it will begin to move your body. Allow these body movements to be there, use them to help you build up even more energy. Moving your arms and body in a natural way will help your energy to rise. Feel your energy building up; don't let go during the first stage and never slow down.

Second stage: 10 minutes

Follow your body. Give your body freedom to express whatever is there .... EXPLODE! .... Let your body take over. Let go of everything that needs to be thrown out. Go totally mad.... Sing, scream, laugh, shout, cry, jump, shake, dance, kick, and throw yourself around. Hold nothing back, keep your whole body moving. A little acting often helps to get you started. Never allow your mind to interfere with what is happening. Remember to be total with your body.

Third stage: 10 minutes

Leaving your shoulders and neck relaxed, raise both arms as high as you can without locking the elbows. With raised arms, jump up and down shouting the mantra HOO!...HOO!...HOO! as deeply as possible, coming from the bottom of your belly. Each time you land on the flats of your feet (making sure heels touch the ground), let the sound hammer deep into the sex centre. Give all you have, exhaust yourself completely.

Fourth stage: 15 minutes

STOP! Freeze where you are in whatever position you find yourself. Don't arrange the body in any way. A cough, a movement, anything will dissipate the energy flow and the effort will be lost. Be a witness to everything that is happening to you.

Fifth stage: 15 minutes

Celebrate!...with music and dance express whatsoever is there. Carry your aliveness with you throughout the day.[4]

Remain a witness. Don't get lost. It is easy to get lost. While you are breathing you can forget. You can become one with the breathing so much that you can forget the witness. But then you miss the point. Breathe as fast, as deep as possible, bring your total energy to it, but still remain a witness. Observe what is happening, as if you are just a spectator, as if the whole thing is happening to somebody else, as if the whole thing is happening in the body and the consciousness is just centred and looking. This witnessing has to be carried in all the three steps. And when everything stops, and in the fourth step you have become completely inactive, frozen, then this alertness will come to its peak.[5]

This is a meditation in which you have to be continuously alert, conscious, aware, whatsoever you do. If you feel pain, be attentive to it, don't do anything. Attention is the great sword – it cuts everything. You simply pay attention to the pain.

For example, you are sitting silently in the last part of the meditation, unmoving, and you feel many problems in the body. You feel that the leg is going dead, there is some itching in the hand, you feel that ants are creeping on the body. Many times you have looked and there are no ants. The creeping is inside, not outside. What should you do? You feel the leg is going dead? – be watchful, just give your total attention to it. You feel itching? – don't scratch. That will not help. You just give your attention. Don't even open your eyes. Just give your attention inwardly, and just wait and watch. Within seconds, the itching will have disappeared. Whatsoever happens – even if you feel pain, severe pain in the stomach or in the head. It happens because in meditation the whole body changes. It changes its chemistry. New things start happening and the body is in a chaos. Sometimes the stomach will be affected, because in the stomach you have suppressed many emotions, and they are all stirred. Sometimes you will feel like vomiting, nauseous. Sometimes you will feel a severe pain in the head because the meditation is changing the inner structure of your brain. Passing through meditation, you are really in a chaos. Soon, things will settle. But for the time being, everything will be unsettled.

So what are you to do? You simply see the pain in the head, watch it. You be a watcher. You just forget that you are a doer, and by and by, everything will subside, and will subside so beautifully and so gracefully that you cannot believe unless you know it. Not only does the pain disappear from the head – because the energy which was creating pain, if watched, disappears – the same energy becomes pleasure. The energy is the same.

Pain or pleasure are two dimensions of the same energy. If you can remain silently sitting and paying attention to distractions, all distractions disappear. And when all distractions disappear, you will suddenly become aware that the whole body has disappeared.[7]

Osho has warned against turning this witnessing approach to pain into another fanaticism. If unpleasant physical symptoms – aches and pains or nausea – persist beyond three or four days of daily meditation, there is no need to be a masochist – seek medical advice. This applies to all Osho's meditation techniques.

 In your understanding, what does it mean to be truly healthy?

Real health has to happen somewhere inside you, in your subjectivity, in your consciousness, because consciousness knows no birth, no death. It is eternal. And to be healthy in consciousness means: first, to be awake; second, to be harmonious; third, to be ecstatic; and fourth, to be compassionate. If these four things are fulfilled, one is inwardly healthy. And sannyas can fulfill all these four things. It can make you more aware, because all the meditation techniques are methods to make you more aware, devices to pull you out of your metaphysical sleep. And dancing, singing, rejoicing, can make you more harmonious. There is a moment when the dancer disappears and only the dance remains. In that rare space one feels harmony. When the singer is completely forgotten and only the song remains, when there is no centre functioning as 'I' – the 'I' is absolutely absent – and you are in a flow, that flowing consciousness is harmonious.

And to be awake and harmonious creates the possibility for ecstasy to happen. Ecstasy means the ultimate joy, inexpressible; no words are adequate to say anything about it. And when one has attained to ecstasy, when one has known the ultimate peak of joy, compassion comes as a consequence. When you have that joy, you like to share it; you cannot avoid sharing, sharing is inevitable. It is a logical consequence of having. It starts overflowing; you need not do anything. It starts happening of its own accord.

These four are the four pillars of inner health. Attain to it. It is our birthright, we just have to claim it. [8]

What is meant by health? This we must try to understand. Ordinarily, if we ask a physician what the definition of health is, he will only say that health is the absence of sickness. But this definition is negative. It is unfortunate that we must define health in terms of illness. Health is a positive thing, a positive state. Illness is negative. Health is our nature; illness is an incursion upon nature. So it is very strange that we must define health in terms of illness.

That we must define the host in terms of the guest – this is very strange. Health coexists with us; illness comes occasionally. Health accompanies us at birth; illness is a superficial phenomenon. But if we ask a physician what is the meaning of health, he can only say that health is present when illness is absent. Paracelsus used to say that this interpretation is wrong – that the concept of health needs to be positively defined. But how can we arrive at a positive definition, at an interpretation of the concept of health that will be creative?

Paracelsus used to say, "Until we know the state of your inner harmony, we can at the most release you from your illness – because your inner harmony is the source of your health. But when we release you from one illness, you will immediately catch another, because nothing has been done with regard to your inner harmony. The fact of the matter is that it is your inner harmony which must be supported." [9]

There is only one kind of health – you don't need any adjective with it. If somebody asks, "How is your health?" you say, "I am perfectly healthy." He does not ask you, "What kind of health?" If he asks you, "What kind of health?" you will be surprised. You will say, "Simply health! Health is just health, a sense of well-being, that nothing is wrong, that everything is running smoothly, that I am happy, that I can't think that things can be better than this."

Are there many kinds of health? No, there is only one kind: healthiness. But diseases are millions.

The same is the case with truth: truth is one. But lies are millions because lies depend on you; you can go on inventing as many as you want. Diseases depend on you. You can go on living wrongly, eating wrong things, doing wrong things, and you can go on creating new diseases.

Health is the same – always new, but it has always been the same. You can call it the ancientmost and yet the latest, the newest.

Five thousand years ago somebody was healthy, and now you are healthy; do you think there will be some difference? He was not your colour, he did not know your language, and five thousand years have passed; but if somebody was healthy, whoever he was, whatever his language, whatever his colour, man or woman, young or old – if he was healthy then you know at least one thing that he was: healthy. That feeling of health you can experience. You need not know anything about that man – beautiful, ugly, short, tall, does not matter; one thing is similar, that he was healthy and you are healthy. One experience is exactly the same.

But diseases…every day new diseases go on being produced. There are millions of diseases, and there will be many more as man becomes more inventive.

You never go to the doctor because you are feeling healthy, or do you? saying, "For two weeks I have been feeling healthy – something must be wrong."

In fact in ancient China there was one thing worth remembering; perhaps some time in the future it may be used again. Confucius impressed China the most. One of his ideas was…and it became implemented, for centuries it remained functioning. The idea was: the doctor should be paid for keeping the patient healthy, not for curing him. If a doctor is paid for curing you then his vested interest is that you remain sick. The more you fall sick, the better; the more people are sick, the better. You are creating a dichotomy in the physician's mind.

First you teach the physician that his work is to keep people healthy: "Your function is to lengthen their life, vitality, youth." But the doctor's vested interest is that if everybody remains healthy, young, nobody falls sick, then he will die of hunger. If everybody is healthy then doctors will be sick, completely sick, sick unto death. What are they going to do?

33

No, a doctor's vested interest is against the philosophy that he has been taught. His interest is that people should remain sick, the more sicknesses the better. Hence you will see one strange thing: if a poor man falls sick, he gets well sooner than the rich man. Strange...why does the poor man get well soon? – because the doctor wants to get rid of him, he is unnecessarily wasting time....

Confucius' idea is of great importance; he says that every person should pay the doctor a monthly salary for keeping him healthy. If he remains healthy the whole month then he has to pay a certain amount to the doctor. If he falls sick then accordingly the salary will be cut.

Very strange in the beginning, because we are doing just the opposite all over the world – but very logical, very sane. And Confucius is, in many ways, a sane man. Everybody should have his physician, and he should pay the physician for keeping him healthy, not for curing him. If he falls sick then the expenses go on the doctor; the medicines and all the expenses – and his salary will be cut too because he has not been taking care of the man.

For centuries it continued. And it worked well, tremendously well, for both; for the doctors, for the patients, for both it worked well. Doctors were not so heavily burdened. And patients were perfectly happy because now the vested interest of the doctor was not against them, it was in their favour.

So the doctor was not interested that they should in any way fall sick and should depend on medicine. He was prescribing more exercises – walking, swimming, sports – so they would remain healthy. And for centuries, while Confucius' influence lasted, China must have been the healthiest country in the world.[10]

? *Western societies have developed the costliest health system that ever existed. People spend billions of dollars a year for it and it is really successful in some fields of surgery or in transplantation and preventing infections. But it seems that people are more sick than they ever were before. What is health?*

Western medical science has viewed man as a separate unit – apart from nature. That is one of the biggest faults that has been committed. Man is part of nature; his health is nothing but being at ease with nature.

Western medicine takes a mechanical view of man, so wherever mechanics can be successful, it is successful. But man is not a machine; man is an organic unity, and man needs not only the treatment of the part that is sick. The sick part is only a symptom that the whole organism is going through difficulties. The sick part is only showing it because it is the weakest.

You treat the sick part, you are successful...but then somewhere else the disease appears. You have prevented the disease from expressing itself through the sick part; you have made it stronger. But you do not understand that man is a whole: either he is sick or he is healthy, there is no station between the two. He should be taken as a whole organism. I will give you a few examples which can make it clear to you.

Acupuncture was developed in China nearabout seven thousand years ago by accident. A hunter was trying to kill a deer, but as his arrow was moving towards the deer, a man not knowing what was happening came in between and the arrow hit the man's leg. The man had been suffering from migraine his whole life; the moment the arrow hit his leg, the migraine disappeared. This was very strange. Nobody had thought about it in that way.

Out of that accident the whole of acupuncture developed, and developed to a full science. So if you go to an acupuncturist and you say, "Something is wrong with my eyes, or something is wrong with my head, or something is wrong with my liver," he may not bother about your liver, your head or your eyes. He will think of the whole organism; he will try to heal *you* – not just the part that is sick.

Acupuncture has developed seven hundred points which were discovered in man's body. Man's body is a bio-electric phenomenon, alive. It has a certain electricity – hence we call it bio-electricity. This bio-electricity has seven hundred points in the body, and each point relates to some part of the body which may be far away from it. That's what happened in that accident: the arrow hit a bio-electric point which related to the head, and the migraine disappeared.

Acupuncture is more holistic. The difference has to be understood. When you take man as a machine you take a partial view of him. If his hand is sick, you just treat the hand; you don't bother about his whole body of which the hand is only a part. The mechanical outlook is partial. It succeeds, but its success is not real success because the same disease which has been repressed in the hand by medicine, surgery and other things, starts expressing itself somewhere else in a worse form. So medicine has developed tremendously; surgery has become a great science – but man is suffering from more diseases, sicknesses, than ever.

This dilemma can be understood. Man should be taken as a whole, treated as an organic unity. But the problem with modern medicine, Western medicine, is that it does not think you have any soul, that you have anything more than a body-mind structure. You also are a machine: your eyes can be replaced, your hands can be replaced, your legs can be replaced – and sooner or later brains will be replaced.

But do you think if we can take Albert Einstein's brain while he is dying, remove it before death is certain and transplant it, for example in the skull of Polack the Pope, do you think he will become an Albert Einstein? The brain is only a part. He would become a strange phenomenon, a crossbreed between a Polack and Albert Einstein. At least right now he is perfectly a Polack; then he would be in a limbo, not knowing who he is – a pope or a physicist.

This we are already doing: we transfuse blood and we change people's other parts; we have mechanical hearts. A man with a mechanical heart cannot be the same as a man with a real, authentic heart. The man with the mechanical heart will not have anything like love. Even if he loves, he will love through the mind. His love will be, "I think I love you"; it will not be direct from the heart, because he has no heart.

In India, medical science developed almost five thousand years ago. And you will be surprised to know that whatever surgery we have today is exactly described by Sushrut, one of the greatest surgeons in the East, in ancient scriptures five to seven thousand years old. But it was abandoned – and that is the point I want you to notice. Why was a developed science abandoned? – because it was found that surgery takes man as a mechanism, and man is not a mechanism; so rather than destroying man they abandoned surgery.

All the finest instruments that surgery uses are described by Sushrut in his scripture. All the operations, even the brain operations, are described in full detail as if it is a modern textbook on surgery. But it is seven thousand...or at least five thousand years old. They developed it to the same point where we are, and they must have faced the same problem that we are facing. They must have found that something is basically wrong.

We go on working so much...and the sickness and the disease go on increasing. Even if we make a person without sickness, that does not mean that he is healthy. Absence of sickness is not health; that is a very negative definition. Health should have something more positive, because health is the positive thing and sickness is the negative thing. Now the negative is defining the positive.

Health is the feeling of well-being, your whole body functioning at its peak without any disturbance. You feel a certain well-being, a certain at-onement with existence. That was not happening through surgery.

India abandoned the whole science and developed a totally different approach, ayurveda, which means science of life. It is significant. In the West we call it medicine, and medicine simply indicates sickness. Health has nothing to do with medicine. Medicine means that the whole science is devoted to curing you from sicknesses.

Ayurveda has a different approach. It is the science of life; it helps you, not to cure sicknesses but to prevent sicknesses from happening – to keep you so healthy that the sickness becomes impossible. The ways of the East and the West are different on this point, whether man is a machine or a spiritual entity with a wholeness....

Secondly, what Western medicine has done is make people less immune....

Real medicine should give you immunity rather than take it away. It should make you stronger, able to fight any infection rather than make you weak so that you are vulnerable to all kinds of infections....

One very famous psychologist, Delgado, has been working on animals. He was surprised to know that if rats are given one meal a day, they live twice as long; the lifespan of the rats who are given two meals a day is cut in half. He himself was surprised: less food and longer life; more food and less life. Now he has come up with the theory that one meal is perfectly enough; otherwise you are loading the system of digestion, and that causes the cut in your lifespan. But what about people who are taking five meals a day...? Medicine will not allow them to die but will not allow them to live either. They will simply vegetate.

Man has to reconsider all traditions, all different sources; whatever facts have become available have to be reconsidered. A totally new medical approach has to be evolved which takes note of acupuncture, which takes note of ayurveda, which takes note of Greek medicine, which takes note of Delgado and his researches – which takes note of the fact that man is not a machine. Man is a multidimensional spiritual being, and you should behave with him in the same way.

Health should not be defined negatively: you don't have any sickness so you are healthy. Health should find some positive definition. I understand why they have not been able to find a positive definition – because sickness is objective, and the feeling of well-being is subjective.

Western medicine does not accept that there is any subject in you. It only accepts your body; it does not accept *you*.

Man has to be accepted in his totality.

All other methods that have been used around the world should be brought into a synthesis; they are not against each other. Right now they are functioning as if they are against each other. They should be brought to a synthesis and that will give you a better view of man and a better life for human beings....

It is now well known, by brain surgeons particularly, that everything has its centre in the brain. If your hand becomes paralyzed, it is stupid to treat the hand; you cannot treat it. Then the only suggestion, the mechanical suggestion, will be to cut it off and put on a mechanical hand which will at least be movable, you can do something with it. This hand is absolutely useless, it has died. It has *not* died. Some centre in your head controls this hand, and that centre has to be cured. The hand has not to be touched at all; that centre is not working, there is some problem with the centre.

Sooner or later the whole of medicine is going to become dominated by the brain centres. Those centres have control of everything in the body. When something goes wrong in the centre it is only symbolically represented by the outer part of the body. You start treating the outer part; you don't go deep enough.

Modern Western medicine is superficial. You should go to very root: why has this hand suddenly become paralyzed? The centre in the brain is in some trouble, and that centre can be cured very easily. It is a bio-electric centre....

Perhaps when you are not feeling well-being it is just that your battery is running out – you need some recharging. If your hand has gone paralyzed, perhaps the centre has lost its electricity; it can be recharged. No medicine is needed, no surgery is needed. We are in a position now to look at man from different angles: how different societies, in different cultures, in different times have treated man. And sometimes if strange things seem to be working, they should be accepted rather than rejected.

For example, seventy percent of diseases are only in your mind: you don't have them, you just think you have them. Now, to give you allopathic medicines for these diseases is dangerous, because all allopathic medicine is somehow or other connected with many poisons. If you have a disease, medicine is good; but if you don't have the disease but only the idea, then homoeopathy is the best because it harms nobody. It has nothing in it, but it is a great help to humanity. Thousands of people are getting cured by homoeopathy.

The question is not whether homoeopathy is real medicine or not. The question is: if people are having unreal diseases, you need some unreal medical system for them. Homoeopathy has nothing in it, but there are people who don't have any sickness but are getting tortured with the idea that they have. Homoeopathy will help them immediately. It cures people but it never harms anybody. It is bogus medicine – but what to do with a bogus humanity?

The Indian physician and the practical nurse don't have any instruments, sophisticated mechanisms, X-rays or other things; they don't have even the stethoscope. They just check your heartbeat – and this has been functioning perfectly well for thousands of years. They check it because the heartbeat is your very centre of life; if something is not perfect it gives them indications of what has to be done. Rather than treating the disease, they will try to make your heartbeat more harmonious. Their medicine will help your heartbeat be more harmonious, and immediately the disease disappears. You think the disease has been treated – but the disease was only a symptom.

That's why in ayurveda they could discard surgery completely: it was reducing man to a machine. When things can be done very easily with minerals, herbs, natural things, without poisoning the system of man, then why unnecessarily go on giving man poisons, which are going to have their side effects?

Perhaps that is one of the reasons why medicine has grown and evolved, and side by side disease goes on growing. You treat one disease, but you treat it with poison; the disease will be gone but the poison will be left in the system. And that poison is going to create its own effects. So all herbal medicines, all minerals and things like homoeopathy should be combined.

There should be only one science with different branches, and the medical person has to decide to which branch this man has to be sent. It is no use telling somebody, "You don't have the disease"; it is no use at all. He will simply change the doctor, that is the only effect. He will love the doctor who says, "You have the disease...."

A few people have lost the will to live; then no medicine can help because the basic will to live is no longer there. They have already died; they are only waiting for the funeral time. These people do not need medicine, they need a different kind of therapy which gives them the will to live again. That is their basic thing – only then will any other medicine help.

All these things have to be combined together into a synthesis, a whole, and man can be completely free from diseases. Man will be able to live at least three hundred years; that is a scientific estimate. His body has the possibility to go on renewing itself for three hundred years. So whatever we have been doing is basically wrong because man dies at seventy.

And there are proofs.... In a part of Kashmir which is now part of Pakistan – Pakistan has occupied it – people live very easily to one hundred and fifty years. In Russia there are many people who are one hundred and fifty years old, and there are people who have even reached one hundred and eighty. Now, these people's foods, their habits should be studied, and those foods and those habits should be made known. A person one hundred and eighty years old in Soviet Russia, in a particular part of the Caucasus, still works in the field just like any young man; he is not even old. His food, his way of living has to be looked into very deeply. And there are many people in that area – only in that area, Caucasia. That area has produced really strong people. Joseph Stalin himself was from that area; George Gurdjieff was from that area – tremendously strong people.

Medicine needs a totally new orientation. It is possible now because everything is known that has happened around the world; we just should not be prejudiced from the very beginning.[11]

?
In medicine today, we talk about the subjectivity of therapy; the same medicine has different results with different doctors.

Can you comment about the subjectivity of a science that claims to be an objective one?

Anything that has to do with human beings can never be totally objective; it will have to allow a certain space for subjectivity.

It is not only true that the same medicine from different doctors has different effects; it is also true that the same medicine has different effects on different patients from the same doctor. Man is not an object.

First you have to understand the word 'subject'. A piece of stone is just an object. There is no interiority, there is no innerness to it. You can cut it in two; then there are two objects. You can cut it in four, and there are four objects. But you will not find any interiority.

Subjectivity means that from the outside a man is just as objective as any other object – a statue, a dead body, a living body, what is the difference? The statue is simply an object, it has no subjectivity. The dead body has once been a house for a subjective phenomenon, but now it is empty. Now it is an empty house; the person who used to live in it has left.

The living man has all the objectivity of the statue, the dead body, and something more – an interior dimension – which can change many things because it is the most powerful thing in existence. For example, it has been noted that three persons can be suffering the same disease, but the same medicine will not work. On one person it is working; on another it is just fifty-fifty, working and not working; but on the third it is not working at all. The disease is the same, but the interiorities are different. And if you take the interiority into consideration, then perhaps the doctor will make a different impact on different people for different reasons.

One of my friends was a great surgeon in Nagpur – a great surgeon but not a good man. He never failed in his surgery, and he charged five times more than any other surgeon would charge. I was staying with him and I told him, "This is too much. When other surgeons are charging a certain amount for the same disease, you charge five times as much."

He said to me, "My success in many other things also has this basis: when a person gives me five times more, he is determined to survive. It is not only because of money that I am greedy. If he is willing to give me five times more – when he could get the operation at cheaper rates – he is determined to survive whatsoever the cost. And his determination is almost fifty percent of my success."

There are people who don't want to survive; they are not willing to cooperate with the doctor. They are taking the medicine, but there is no will to survive; on the contrary, they are hoping that the medicine does not work so they will not be blamed for suicide, yet they can get rid of life. Now, from the inside that person has withdrawn already. Medicine cannot help his interiority, and without his interior support, the doctor is almost helpless – the medicine is not enough.

I came to know from this surgeon.... He said, "You don't know. Sometimes I do things which are absolutely immoral, but to help the patient I have to do them."

I said, "What do you mean?"

He said, "I am condemned by my profession...." And all the doctors of Nagpur condemned him – "We have never seen such a cheat."

He would put the patient on the table in the operating theatre – doctors would be ready, nurses would be ready, students would be watching from the gallery above. And he would whisper in the patient's ear, "We had agreed on a fee of ten thousand – that will not do. Your problem is more serious. Only if you are ready to give me twenty thousand, am I going to take the instruments in my hands; otherwise, you get up and get out. You can find cheaper people."

Now, in such a situation.... And the person has money, otherwise, how can he say yes? And he accepts it: "I will give twenty thousand, but save me."

And he told me, "Any surgeon could have saved him, but not with such certainty. Now that he is paying twenty thousand, he is absolutely with me; his whole interior being is supportive. People condemn me because they don't understand me. Certainly it is immoral to agree on ten thousand and then put the person in the operating theatre and whisper in his ear, 'Twenty thousand, thirty thousand; otherwise, get up and get out – because I had not realized that the disease had gone so deep. I am taking a risk, and I am putting my whole reputation on the line. For ten thousand I will not do that. And I have never failed in my life, success is my rule. I operate only when I am absolutely certain to succeed. So you decide. And I don't have much time, because there are other patients waiting. You just decide within two minutes: either agree, or get up and get lost.' Naturally, the person will say, 'I will give you anything you want, but please do the operation.' It is illegal, immoral, but I cannot say that it is unpsychological."

Anything to do with man cannot be purely objective.

I used to have another friend, a doctor who is now in jail because he was not qualified at all. He had never been to any medical college; all the degrees that he had written on his sign were bogus. But still I am of the opinion that an injustice has been done to the man – because it does not matter whether he had degrees or not. He helped thousands of people, and particularly those who were becoming hopeless, going from one doctor to another – all with degrees – and getting tired. And this man was able to save them. He had a certain charisma – no degree. And he made his hospital almost a magic land. The moment a patient entered his office, immediately he would be surprised. He had been everywhere...because people used to go to him only as a last resort. Everybody knew that the man was bogus, it was not something hidden. It was an open secret. But if you are going to die, what is the harm in trying?

And as you entered his garden – he had beautiful garden – and then his office....
He had beautiful women as his receptionists, and it was all part of his medical treatment – because even if a person is dying, looking at a beautiful woman his will to live
takes a jump; he wants to live. After the reception, the person would pass through
his lab. It was absolutely unnecessary to take him through the lab, but he wanted
the person to see that he was not an ordinary doctor. And the lab was a miracle
– absolutely useless, there was nothing significant, but so many tubes, flasks,
coloured water moving from one tube into another tube, as if great experiments were
going on.

Then you would reach the doctor. And he never used the ordinary methods of
checking your pulse, no. You would have to lie down on an electric bed with a remote
control. The bed would move far up into the air, and you are lying there looking up
and hanging over you there are big tubes. And wires would be attached to your pulse
and the pulse would make the water in the tubes jump. The heart would be checked
in the same way – not by ordinary stethoscope. He had made all his arrangements
visual for the patient – so that he could see he had come to some genius, an expert.

The man had no degrees, nothing at all. His pharmacist had all the degrees, and
he used to prescribe the medicines because the man had no idea about medicine. In
fact, he never did any criminal thing. He never prescribed medicines, he never signed
for them. This was done by a man who had degrees, who was absolutely qualified to
do it. But because he arranged all this, and because he had written strange degrees
on his sign...and since those degrees don't exist I don't think they can be illegal. He
was not claiming that they were from any university that exists. It was *all* fiction –
but the fiction was helpful.

I have seen patients half cured just in the examination. Coming out, they said,
"We feel almost cured, and we have not taken the medicine yet. The prescription is
here – now we will go and purchase the medicine."

But because he had done all this.... This is when I saw that the law is blind. He
had not done anything illegal, he had not harmed anybody – but he is in jail because
he was "cheating people." He has not cheated anybody. To help somebody to live
longer, if that is cheating, then what is medical help?

Because of human beings, medicine can never become an absolutely solid, one
hundred percent objective science. That's why there are so many medical schools –
ayurveda, homoeopathy, naturopathy, acupuncture, and many more – and they *all* help.
Now homoeopathy is simply sugar pills, but it helps. The question is whether the
person believes. There are people who are fanatic naturopaths – nothing else can help
them, only naturopathy can help them. And it has no connection with the disease.

One of my professors was madly into naturopathy. Any problem...and a mud pack on your stomach. I used to go to him to enjoy, because it was very relaxing, and he had a very good arrangement – a beautiful bath and showers.... And without any difficulty I used to go and say, "I have a very bad migraine."

He said, "Don't be worried. Just a mud pack on your stomach." Now a mud pack on the stomach is not going to help a migraine. But it used to help me, because I had no migraine! A mud bath, the full bathtub, and you are drowned in the mud, just your head is out – it is very comfortable and very cool. Soon he realized: "You come again and again with new diseases."

I said, "That's true...because I have got a book on naturopathy; from the book I get the disease, and then I come to you. First I read it, to see what you will do. If I want it to be done to me, I bring that disease; otherwise, unnecessarily lying down in the mud for half an hour...."

He said, "So you have been cheating me?"

I said, "I am not cheating you. I am your most prominent patient. In the university everybody else laughs at you, I am the only one who supports you. And the others who come here, come here because of me – because I say that my migraine disappeared."

He said, "My God, now *I* am suffering from migraine. Go!"

People used to become angry with me. They would tell me, "My migraine, instead of going, has become more intense – because a cold stomach does not help migraine!"

I would say, "Then your system must work differently. With my system, it helps me!"

There are homoeopaths, fanatics who believe that homoeopathy is the only right medicine and all other medicines are dangerous – particularly allopathy is poison. If you go to a homoeopath, the first thing he will do is inquire about your whole history from your birth up to now. And you are suffering from a headache.

One of the homoeopathic doctors used to live near me. Whenever my father came to see me, I would take him to the homoeopath. The homoeopath told me, "I pray you don't bring your father because he starts back three generations, that his grand-father had a disease...."

I said, "He is also a homoeopath. He goes deeper into the roots."

He said, "But he wastes so much time, and I have to listen – and he just has a headache! About his grandfather and all his diseases, then his father and all his diseases...then himself. By the time *he* comes, almost the whole day is finished. My other patients are gone, and I am listening to him telling me what kind of diseases he has suffered from his childhood, and finally it comes out that he has a headache."

"I say, 'My God, why didn't you tell me before?' and he says, 'Just as you are a homoeopath, I am also a homoeopath. And I want to give you a complete picture.'"

The first thing they will ask is about all your diseases because they believe that all diseases are connected, your whole life is one single whole. It does not matter whether you had something in your leg or your head – they are part of one body, and for the doctor to understand, he has to know everything. The homoeopath will ask you what kind of allopathic medicines you have been taking – because that is the root cause of all your diseases; all allopathic medicines are poison. That is the attitude of naturopathy too, that allopathy is poison. So first you have to do fasting, enemas...just to clean you of all allopathy. Once you are clean of allopathy....

Man is a subjective being. If the patient loves the doctor, then water can function as medicine. And if the patient hates the doctor, then no medicine can help. If the patient feels the doctor is indifferent – which is ordinarily the case with doctors, because they are also human beings, the whole day long seeing patients, the whole day long somebody is dying.... They slowly, slowly, become hard, they create a barrier to their emotions, sentiments, humanity. But this prevents their medicine from being effective. It is given almost in a robot-like way, as if a machine is giving you medicine.

With love the patient is not only getting medicine, around the medicine something invisible is also coming to him. Medicine will have to understand man's subjectivity, his love, and will have to create some kind of synthesis in which love and medicine together are used to help people.

But one thing is absolutely certain: that medicine can never become entirely objective. That has been the effort of medical science up to now, to make it absolutely objective.[12]

A new kind of therapy is arising they call placebo therapy. A placebo is false, pseudo medicine, with no medicinal qualities in it, but is has to be given in such a way that the patient thinks it is medicine. Not only that the patient thinks it is medicine, even the doctor has to think it is medicine, otherwise his gestures may show, may reveal the truth. The doctor is kept in ignorance; he is given just water to inject, or given just sugar pills with all the marks and names and labels of the true medicine. He knows that this is medicine. The patient knows this is medicine. And the miracle is that it works – and there is no medicine in it. The patient is healed. The very belief of the doctor that it is medicine creates an atmosphere, a psychology, a hypnosis, and the whole paraphernalia of the hospital.... The patient *wants* to get rid of his illness, and when a famous doctor gives the medicine it is bound to help; whether it is medicine or not doesn't matter much.

It has been found that medicine or no medicine functions almost in the same proportion. If seventy percent of patients are cured by medicine, real medicine, then seventy percent of patients are cured by unreal medicine, placebo medicine. It is creating a great stir in the medical world. What is happening?

What is really happening is this, that in the first place the illness has been created, it is a mind phenomenon. And in the second place, if the mind is convinced that it is going to be cured, then it is going to be cured. That's why if the doctor's fee is not really big, medicine is not going to affect you much. The bigger the fee, the better the medicine. If the therapist has a big fee and you are paying fortunes, then it is going to affect you more, because then you want to be affected. When it is free, who bothers whether it works or not? "If it works, good; if it doesn't work, okay – because we have not paid for it." When you pay for it you are intent that it should work – and it works!

Buddha says mind is a conjurer; it creates illnesses, it can create cures. Mind creates all kinds of illusions – beauty and ugliness, success and failure, richness and poverty...mind goes on creating. And once the idea settles in you, your whole life energy functions to create it, to make it a reality. Every thought becomes a thing, and every thing in the beginning was only a thought and nothing else. You live in a kind of hypnosis. Buddha says this hypnosis has to be broken, and no other religion has tried so hard to break this hypnosis. Man has to be de-hypnotized. Man has to be made aware that *all* is mind: pain and pleasure both, birth and death both. All is mind. And once this has been seen absolutely, the conjurer disappears...and then what is left is truth. And that truth liberates. [13]

In all the medical 'pathies' developed around the world – homoeopathy or ayurveda or acupuncture – except allopathy, nobody has exactly understood the inner function of nature in man's body and mind. I say, except allopathy, because others may be sometimes helpful, but they are not scientific. And others are helpful not in a small way either; if you look at their help, it is tremendous.

In almost seventy percent of the cases ayurveda will be successful, acupuncture may be successful, homoeopathy may be successful, naturopathy may be successful. But remember the seventy percent – it is no more than that because seventy percent of diseases are false. They are just in your mind, they don't really exist. That's why you don't need real medicine; any hocus-pocus will do. And seventy percent is not a small percentage so I would not like these 'pathies' to disappear from the world. I want them to be recognized, because seventy percent is a big percentage.

And strangely enough, those seventy percent of the cases are the most difficult as far as allopathy is concerned. Allopathy finds itself in a difficulty: how to deal with a person who has no disease but believes he has? Allopathy has no way to help such a person. So only thirty percent remain to be helped by allopathy. It is a strange world.

Thirty percent to the most scientific approach and seventy percent to all kinds of hocus-pocus – superstitious approaches which really don't make any change, but they help. The most scientific approach of allopathy is based on a deep understanding of nature, and that is that the body has a resistance of its own.

Because of this fact, naturopathy condemns allopathy. Allopathy goes on injecting viruses into patients because the allopathic understanding is, the moment the body gets a virus, it immediately creates antibodies. It immediately starts fighting, it has a resistance of its own. The whole body immediately goes on red-alert to destroy the disease. Naturopathy condemns it because they think you are poisoning people with diseases. You are supposed to take out diseases and you are, on the contrary, putting poisonous viruses into people's bodies.

Naturopathy cleans people's bodies by fasting, by strange methods that you cannot believe. But they can help only those people who are not suffering from any real disease.[14]

CHAPTER 2

THIS-OPATHY AND THAT-OPATHY

? *I understand that the science of Yoga regards man as having not one but several types of body. If this is so, does it follow that for different individuals, one kind of medicine might work more effectively than another, depending from where the illness is originating?*

The science of man does not exist yet. Patanjali's Yoga is the closest effort ever made. He divides the body into five layers, or into five bodies. You don't have one body, you have five bodies; and behind the five bodies, your being. The same as has happened in psychology has happened in medicine. Allopathy believes only in the physical body, the gross body. It is parallel to behaviourism. Allopathy is the grossest medicine. That's why it has become scientific, because scientific instrumentation is only capable yet of very gross things. Go deeper.

Acupuncture, the Chinese medicine, enters one layer more. It works on the vital body, the *pranamayakos*. If something goes wrong in the physical body, acupuncture does not touch the physical body at all. It tries to work on the vital body. It tries to work on the bioenergy, the bioplasma. It settles something there, and immediately the gross body starts functioning well. If something goes wrong in the vital body, allopathy functions on the body, the gross body. Of course, for allopathy, it is an uphill task. For acupuncture, it is a downhill task. It is easier because the vital body is a little higher than the physical body. If the vital body is set right, the physical body simply follows it because the blueprint exists in the vital body. The physical body is just an implementation of the vital.

47

Now acupuncture is gaining respect, by and by, because a certain very sensitive photography, Kirlian photography, in Soviet Russia, has come across the seven hundred vital points in the human body as they have always been predicted by acupuncturists for at least five thousand years. They had no instruments to know where the vital points in the body were, but by and by, just through trial and error, through centuries, they discovered seven hundred points. Now Kirlian has also discovered the same seven hundred points with scientific instrumentation. And Kirlian photography has proved one thing: to try to change the vital through the physical is absurd. It is trying to change the master by changing the servant. It is almost impossible because the master won't listen to the servant. If you want to change the servant, change the master. Immediately, the servant follows. Rather than going and changing each soldier, it is better to change the general. The body has millions of soldiers, cells, simply working under some order, under some commandment. Change the commander, and the whole body pattern changes.

Homoeopathy goes still a little deeper. It works on the *manomayakos,* the mental body. The founder of homoeopathy, Hahnemann, discovered one of the greatest things ever discovered, and that was; the smaller the quantity of the medicine, the deeper it goes. He called the method of making homoeopathic medicine 'potentizing'. They go on reducing the quantity of the medicine. He would work in this way: he would take a certain amount of medicine and would mix it with ten times the amount of milk sugar or with water. One quantity of medicine, nine quantities of water; he would mix them. Then he would again take one quantity of this new solution, and would again mix it with nine times more water, or milk sugar. In this way he would go on; again from the new solution he would take one quantity and would mix it with nine times more water. This he would do, and the potency would increase.

By and by, the medicine reaches to the atomic level. It becomes so subtle that you cannot believe that it can work; it has almost disappeared. That is what is written on homoeopathic medicines, the potency: ten potency, twenty potency, one hundred potency, one thousand potency. The bigger the potency, the smaller is the amount. With ten thousand potency, a millionth of the original medicine has remained, almost none. It has almost disappeared, but then it enters the most deep core of *manomaya*. It enters into your mind body. It goes deeper than acupuncture. It is almost as if you have reached the atomic, or even the sub-atomic level. Then it does not touch your body. Then it does not touch your vital body; it simply enters. It is so subtle and so small that it comes across no barriers. It can simply slip into the *manomayakos,* into the mental body, and from there it starts working. You have found an even bigger authority than the *pranamaya*.

Ayurved, the Indian medicine, is a synthesis of all three. It is one of the most synthetic of medicines.

Hypnotherapy goes still deeper. It touches the *vigyanmayakos:* the fourth body, the body of consciousness. It does not use medicine. It does not use anything. It simply uses suggestion, that's all. It simply puts a suggestion in your mind – call it animal magnetism, mesmerism, hypnosis or whatsoever you like, but it works through the power of thought, not the power of matter. Even homoeopathy is still the power of matter in a very subtle quantity. Hypnotherapy gets rid of matter altogether, because howsoever subtle, it is matter.... Ten thousand potency, but still, it is a potency of matter. It simply jumps to the thought energy, *vigyanmayakos:* the consciousness body. If your consciousness just accepts a certain idea, it starts functioning.

Hypnotherapy has a great future. It is going to become the future medicine, because if by just changing your thought pattern your mind can be changed, through the mind your vital body, and through the vital body your gross body, then why bother with poisons, why bother with gross medicines? Why not work it through thought power? Have you watched any hypnotist working on a medium? If you have not watched, it is worth watching. It will give you a certain insight.

You may have heard, or you may have seen – in India it happens; you must have seen fire-walkers. It is nothing but hypnotherapy. The idea that they are possessed by a certain god or a goddess and no fire can burn them, just this idea is enough. This idea controls and transforms the ordinary functioning of their bodies. They are prepared: for twenty-four hours they fast. When you are fasting and your whole body is clean, and there is no excreta in it, the bridge between you and the gross drops. For twenty-four hours they live in a temple or in a mosque, singing, dancing, getting in tune with God. Then comes the moment when they walk on the fire. They come dancing, possessed. They come with full trust that the fire is not going to burn, that's all; there is nothing else. How to create the trust is the question. Then they dance on the fire, and the fire does not burn.

It has happened many times that somebody who was just a spectator became so possessed. Twenty persons walking on fire are not burned, and somebody would immediately become so confident: "If these people are walking, then why not I?"; and he has jumped in, and the fire has not burned him. In that sudden moment, a trust arose. Sometimes it has happened that people who were prepared, were burned. Sometimes an unprepared spectator walked on fire and was not burned. What happened? – the people who were prepared must have carried a doubt. They must have been thinking whether it was going to happen or not. A subtle doubt must have remained in the *vigyanmayakos,* in their consciousness. It was not total trust. So they came, but with doubt. Because of that doubt, the body could not receive the message from the higher soul. The doubt came in between, and the body continued to function in the ordinary way; it got burned. That's why all religions insist on trust.

Trust is hypnotherapy. Without trust, you cannot enter into the subtle parts of your being, because a small doubt, and you are thrown back to the gross. Science works with doubt. Doubt is a method in science because science works with the gross. Whether you doubt or not, an allopath is not worried. He does not ask you to trust in his medicine; he simply gives you medicine. But a homoeopath will ask whether you believe, because without your belief it will be more difficult for a homoeopath to work upon you. And a hypnotherapist will ask for total surrender; otherwise, nothing can be done.

Religion is surrender. Religion is hypnotherapy. But, there is still one more body. That is the *anandmayakos:* the bliss body. Hypnotherapy goes up to the fourth. Meditation goes up to the fifth. Meditation – the very word is beautiful because the root is the same as 'medicine'. Both come from the same root, medicine and meditation are off-shoots of one word: that which heals, that which makes you healthy and whole is medicine – and on the deepest level that is meditation.

Meditation does not even give you suggestions because suggestions are to be given from the outside. Somebody else has to give you suggestions. Suggestion means that you are dependent upon somebody. They cannot make you perfectly conscious because the other will be needed, and a shadow will be cast on your being. Meditation makes you perfectly conscious, without any shadow – absolute light with no darkness. Now even suggestion is thought to be a gross thing. Somebody suggests – that means something comes from the outside, and in the ultimate analysis that which comes from the outside is material. Not only matter, but that which comes from the outside is material. Even a thought is a subtle form of matter. Even hypnotherapy is materialistic.

Meditation drops all props, all supports. That's why to understand meditation is the most difficult thing in the world, because nothing is left – just a pure understanding, a witnessing.[15]

? *Could you talk further on acupuncture?*

Acupuncture is utterly Eastern. So when you approach any Eastern science with the Western mind you miss many things. Your whole approach is different: it is methodological, it is logical, analytical. And these Eastern sciences are not really sciences but arts. The whole thing depends on whether you can shift your energies from the intellect to the intuition, whether you can shift from male to female, from yang to yin; from the active, aggressive approach. Can you become passive, receptive? Only then do these things work; otherwise you can learn all about acupuncture, and it will not be acupuncture at all. You will know all *about* it, but not *it*. And sometimes it happens that a person may not know much about it and *knows* it, but then it is a knack – just an insight into it.

So this is happening to many Eastern things: the West becomes interested – they *are* profound. The West becomes interested in an Eastern thing, but then it brings in its own mind to understand it. The moment the Western mind comes into it, the very base of it is destroyed. Then only fragments are left and those fragments never work. And it is not that acupuncture was not going to work, acupuncture *can* work, but it can work only with an Eastern approach.

So if you really want to learn acupuncture, it is good to know about it but remember that is not the most essential thing. Learn whatsoever information is possible, then forget all the information and start groping in the dark. Start listening to your own unconscious, start feeling en rapport with the patient. It is different....

When a patient comes to a Western medical man, the Western medical man starts reasoning, diagnosing, analyzing, finding out where the illness is, what the illness is, and what can cure it. He uses one part of his mind, the rational part. He attacks the disease, he starts conquering it: a fight starts between the disease and the doctor. The patient is just out of the game – the doctor does not bother about the patient. He starts fighting with the disease – the patient is completely neglected.

When you come to an acupuncturist the disease is not important, the patient is important, because it is the patient who has created the disease: the cause is in the patient, the disease is only a symptom. You can change the symptom and another symptom will come up. You can force this disease by drugs, you can stop its expression, but then the disease will assert itself somewhere else and with more danger, more force, with a vengeance. The next disease will be more difficult to tackle than the first. You drug it too, then the third disease will be even more difficult.

That's how allopathy has created cancer. You go on forcing back the disease on one side, it asserts itself from another, then you force it on that side – the disease starts becoming very, very angry. And you don't change the patient, the patient remains the same; so because the cause exists, the cause goes on creating the effect.

Acupuncture deals with the cause. Never deal with the effect, always go to the cause. And how can you go to the cause? Reason cannot go to the cause – the cause is too big for the reason – it can only tackle the effect. Only meditation can go to the cause. So acupuncture will feel the patient. He will forget his knowledge, he will just try to get in tune with the patient. He will feel en rapport; he will start feeling a bridge with the patient. He will start feeling the disease of the patient in his own body, in his own energy system. That is the only way for him to know intuitively where the cause is, because the cause is hidden. He will become the mirror and he will find the reflection in himself.

This is the whole process of it, and this is not being taught because it cannot be taught. It is really worth going into, so my suggestion is first learn in the West for two years, then for at least six months go to some Far Eastern country and be with some acupuncturist. Just be in his presence – just let him work and you watch. Just absorb his energy, and then you will be able to do something; otherwise it will be difficult.[16]

And if you start feeling your own energy by and by, or the working of the energy in your own body, acupuncture will not remain just a technique, it will become an instrument. And it is an insight – you can learn the technique and nothing will come out of it – it is more a hunch than an art. That is one of the most difficult things about ancient techniques: they are not scientific, and if you approach them with a scientific outlook you may get some inkling but the major part will be missing. And whatsoever you will be able to get hold of will not be much, and it will be frustrating.

The whole ancient approach was totally different: it was not logical at all, it was more feminine, more intuitive, more illogical. One was not thinking in syllogism as the scientific mind thinks; rather, one was in a deep participation with existence – more in a sort of dreaming state, in a reverie, and allowing nature to release its secrets and mysteries. It was not aggression on nature...a persuasion at the most. And the approach is from the interior.

One has to approach one's own body from the interiormost core. Those seven hundred points were not known objectively, they were known in deep meditation. When one goes deep inside and looks from inside – a tremendous experience – one can see all the acupuncture points surrounding oneself, as if the night is full of stars. And when you have seen those energy points, then only are you ready. Now you have an inner grasp, and just by touching the body of the other person you will be able to feel where the body energy is missing and where it is not; where it is moving, where it is not moving; where it is cold and where it is warm; where it is alive and where it has gone dead. There are points at which it responds, and there are points at which it has no response at all.

You will be able to know acupuncture only to the extent that you become capable of knowing yourself, and when both coincide there is a great light. In that light you can see everything – not only about yourself, but about the bodies of others. A new vision arises as if a third eye has opened.[17]

Acupuncture is not a science but an art, and every art demands of you a deep surrender. It is not like any other technique that a technician can manipulate. It needs your whole heart in it. You have to forget yourself just as a painter forgets while painting, or a poet forgets while composing, a musician forgets while playing. It is that kind of a thing. A technician can practice acupuncture but he will never be exactly what is needed. He will never be that. He may help a few people, but it is a great art, a great skill. It has to be imbibed. The secret is surrender. If you can surrender yourself totally into it, if it becomes a devotion, a dedication – and it can become – go into it, go wholeheartedly, with joy.[18]

Start being on your own. And you will have to find your own knack. Acupuncture is a knack and an art, and there is no need to follow anybody like a rule. There are none. Rules do not exist, just insights. So start working on your own…. In the beginning you will feel a little unconfident, and you will be worried many times about whether you are doing the right thing or not. But this is how one has to begin. It is a kind of groping. Sooner or later you will find the door. Once you have started finding the door then less and less groping is needed. Then you know the door. Start working![19]

When you touch anybody's body or you work with needles, you are working on God. One has to be very respectful, very hesitant. One has to work not out of knowledge but out of love. Knowledge is never adequate, it is not enough. So feel for the person. And always feel inadequate, because knowledge is limited and the other person is an entire world, almost infinite…. People touch you but they never touch *you*. They touch only the periphery, and you are there somewhere deep in the centre where nobody enters except love. Man is a mystery and is going to remain a mystery forever. It is not something accidental that man is a mystery. Mystery is his very being.[20]

Would you speak on the transformation of hypnosis into meditation? I have noticed that the line between therapy and meditation is dissolving.

There was a day when hypnosis was a recognized door towards meditation, but Christianity in the Middle Ages condemned hypnosis alongside witchcraft. That condemnation still lingers on, even in the minds of those who are not Christians but who are influenced without their knowing by Christian ideas. Why was Christianity against hypnosis? You will be surprised to know it was against hypnosis because it leads directly to meditation; neither the priest is needed nor the church is needed – not even God is needed. This was the trouble.

If meditation succeeds in the world there are not going to be any religions anymore, for the simple reason that you will be in direct contact with existence and yourself. Why should you go through brokers and all kinds of agents who know nothing, except that they are knowledgeable, except that they have been disciplined for years in how to influence people and win friends? It is not something religious that they are doing. What they are doing is the politics of numbers: gather as many numbers as possible into your fold; that becomes your strength and your power.

Hypnosis was a danger to the priesthood, and Christianity is absolutely based from the very beginning on priesthood. Jesus does not declare himself to be enlightened, nor has any other Christian after him declared him to be enlightened. He declares something nonsensical – that he is the only begotten son of God. God is a hypothesis, and hypotheses are not Indians who go on producing children. Hypotheses are barren; they produce nothing....

Christianity never wanted you to be directly connected with existence. You have to go via the priest, the pope, the son, and *then* God. In between, the mediators are many. And nobody knows who is lying.... Of course you can never discover, because you don't have any direct line with God. The priest has a direct line with the pope, the pope has a direct line with Jesus, Jesus has a direct line with God – and the numbers are not given in the telephone directories.

Hypnosis was the door, has always been the door to meditation. Once a man enters into the world of meditation he has such clarity, such a strength, so much life arising in him that he no longer needs any father in heaven. He no longer needs any priest to pray for him. He himself has become prayer – not prayer to any God, but simply a prayerfulness, a gratitude to the whole.

It was absolutely necessary for Christianity to condemn hypnosis and to condemn it as something created by the devil. For the same reasons witchcraft was brutally destroyed; millions of women were burnt alive because they were also doing the same thing. They were trying to contact the ultimate on their own without going through the proper channel of the Church....

Hypnosis in itself can be used dangerously unless it is used in the service of meditation. I will have to explain to you what exactly is meant by hypnosis and how it can be misused if it is not used singularly in the service of meditation.

Hypnosis literally means deliberately created sleep. It is now known that thirty-three percent, that is one-third of humanity is capable of going into the deepest layers of hypnosis. It is a strange number, thirty-three percent; strange because only thirty-three percent of people have the aesthetic sense, only thirty-three percent of people have sensitivity, only thirty-three percent of people have friendliness, only thirty-three percent of people are creators. And my own experience is that these thirty-three percent of the people are the same, because creativity and sensitivity *are* meditation, *are* love, *are* friendliness. All need essentially one thing: a deep trust in oneself, in the existence, and a receptivity and opening of the heart.

Hypnosis can be created in two ways. Because of the first, people became impressed by the Christian propaganda that it is dangerous. That is hetero-hypnosis: somebody else hypnotizes you, a hypnotist hypnotizes you. There are so many wrong ideas attached, and the most fundamental is that the hypnotist has the power to hypnotize you. That is absolutely wrong. The hypnotist has the technique, not the power.

Nobody can hypnotize you against yourself, unless you are willing. Unless you are ready to go into the unknown, untravelled darkness, no hypnotist can manage to hypnotize you. But in fact hypnotists don't deny that they have the power; on the contrary, they claim that they have the power to hypnotize people. Nobody has the power to hypnotize anyone. Only you have the power to hypnotize yourself or to be hypnotized by somebody else – the power is yours. But when you are hypnotized by somebody else it can be misused.

The process, the technique, is very simple. The hypnotist hangs a crystal from a chain just over your eyes, and tells you, "Don't close your eyes until you cannot keep them open. Fight to the last, keep your eyes open!" And the crystal shines in your eyes. Naturally, eyes have to blink continuously to keep themselves from getting dry. They are the most delicate part of your body. You blink your eyes because your eyelids function like windscreen wipers on a car: they bring liquid to your eyes and they clean your eyes of any dust, or anything that may have entered. They keep your eyes fresh and always showering.

The hypnotist says, "Stop blinking; just stare at something shiny!" – shiny because anything shiny will soon make your eyes tired. If you are told to look at a powerful enough electric bulb just hanging above your head, naturally your eyes will get utterly tired. And you are told that you are not to close them unless you feel they are closing by themselves.

This is one part. The other part is that the hypnotist is continuously saying that your eyes are becoming very heavy, your eyelids seem to be utterly tired…. Just by your side he is repeating these words continuously, that your eyes are becoming tired, the lids want to close – and to you just the opposite direction has been given so that you go on fighting to the last. But how long can you fight? It takes no more than three minutes at the most, because double processes are going on. You are focused on the light which is tiring your eyes, and the hypnotist goes on repeating like a parrot, in a very sleepy voice, that sleep is coming over you. You cannot resist; it is impossible now to keep your eyes open.

Now these suggestions…and the person is fighting, he knows that his eyes are becoming tired, and the eyelids are becoming heavy, burdened. A point comes within three minutes, not more than that, when he cannot resist the temptation to let them close. The moment the eyes are closed, the man starts repeating, "You are going into deep sleep, and you will be able only to hear my voice and nothing else. I will remain your only contact."

The person goes deeper and deeper into sleep, with continuous suggestions. There is a point when he stops hearing anything else except the sleepy voice of the hypnotist saying, "You are going deeper, deeper, deeper" – and then he tests whether you have gone deeper or not. He will prick your hand with a safety pin, but you are so asleep that you cannot know about it, you will not feel it.

In fact, in the Soviet Union they have started hetero-hypnosis even for operations; no anaesthesia is needed. A person can go so deep given the right conditions: a very sleepy atmosphere, dim, neither dark nor light, and a shining, forcefully shining light focused on his eyes; a very subtle music in the room, beautiful fragrance…all these help him to go into such a deep sleep that operations can be done, have been done, and the person knows nothing.

So the hypnotist tries a few things: he takes your hand up and lets go of it, and the hand falls because you cannot hold it, you are fast asleep; in sleep you cannot hold it up high. He lifts your eyelids up, he looks into your eyes and only the white of your eyes is seen; your pupils have moved upwards.

The deeper the hypnosis, the higher your pupils will move upwards. That happens in deep sleep every day, and that also happens when somebody dies. That's why all over the world people immediately close the eyelids of a dead person, for the simple reason that it is so frightening to see somebody with completely white eyes. In India it has been known for centuries that when a man is going to die, his eyes start slowly moving upwards, and the sign and symbol is that he cannot see the tip of his own nose. Remember, the day you cannot see your nose – because when the pupils of the eyes are moving upwards; they cannot see the tip of the nose – six months at the most….

So the hypnotist opens the eyelid and sees whether underneath it is white, and all that used to be there, your pupil, has moved upwards. Then he is certain that you are no longer capable of hearing anybody, you are no longer capable of disobeying him;

whatever he will say, you will do. This is the danger. He can say to you, "Just take out all your money and hand it over to me," and you will immediately take out all your money and hand it over to him. He can take your ornaments or he can tell you to sign any document that may create trouble for you, for example that you have sold your house, or donated your house.

There is one thing more to be understood, which is very dangerous: he can give a post-hypnotic suggestion. A post-hypnotic suggestion means that he can say to you, "After ten days you will come to me, you will have to come to me, bringing all your money, all your ornaments, anything valuable that you have. Leave it on my table and simply go back." It is possible to give a post-hypnotic suggestion that after twenty-four hours you will shoot somebody. All these orders will be followed because the person does not know...as far as his consciousness is concerned, he has no idea what has happened under deep hypnosis. Deep hypnosis reaches your unconscious.

These were the dangers that Christianity exaggerated, saying that this is against religion, against morality. A woman can be raped and she will not know, or a woman can be told, "You have fallen in love with me," and a great romance will begin from the moment she wakes up. She will feel a little hesitant because her conscious mind will not understand what has happened, but there is no communication between the conscious mind and the unconscious. The unconscious is so powerful – nine times more powerful – that when the unconscious wants to do something, the conscious may start protesting but that protest is futile.

All these things were spread, wildly exaggerated among man. But the purpose of the church was not to save you from these dangers; the purpose was that hypnosis should become condemned so that nobody can enter from that door into the ultimate realm of meditation.

Christianity kept people completely ignorant about another kind of hypnosis; that is self-hypnosis, not hetero-hypnosis. Only hetero-hypnosis can be misused; auto-hypnosis or self-hypnosis cannot be misused. There is nobody; you are alone. You can do the same thing by yourself. You can put an alarm clock on, and then repeat three times that within fifteen minutes, when the alarm goes off, you will come back from your deep hypnotic sleep. And then the procedure is the same.

You look at the light, and you do what the hetero-hypnotist was doing. Looking at the light, you go on repeating inside, "My eyes are becoming heavy, heavy... heavier, heavier. I am falling into sleep. I cannot keep my eyes open anymore; I am trying my best, but it is impossible" – and it also takes exactly three minutes. That is the maximum; it may happen in two minutes, it may happen in one minute, but the longer you struggle, the deeper will be the hypnosis.

I have heard about a man, an old man, who was torturing his family. Every day he would figure out how many diseases he had. The doctors were tired; they said he had no diseases. He listened to the medical programme on the television and learned the names of the diseases. Then he started torturing the family: "I am suffering from this, I am suffering from that. Nobody is taking care of me." This was simply a way for an old man to attract attention. Nobody gives attention to the old people, so they find their own ways. They become more irritable, more angry, more fussy; they have their own techniques to attract attention. Their whole lives they were nourished by attention, but now nobody looks at them, nobody even bothers whether they exist or are finished.

One Indian singer, who loves me, Jagjit Singh, tells a beautiful joke. One of his friends who lives in London had come, so he asked him, "How are you?"

He replied, "Alright."

Jagjit Singh said, "And how is your wife?"

He replied, "She is also alright."

"And how are your children?"

"They are also alright."

Jagjit Singh finally asked, "And what about Daddy?"

And the man said, "Daddy? – he has been alright for almost four years." Four years ago he had died, so the friend is saying that he has been alright, completely alright, *forever* alright since four years ago!

Old people have only these methods to attract attention – that they are suffering from migraine, that they have a stomachache. The greater their medical vocabulary is, the more they will manage.

Finally, doctors started refusing, saying, "He is a mad person. He has no sickness, no disease; we have checked him so many times."

But the son said, "What can we do? – we should bring the doctor."

So the doctors finally suggested that perhaps a hypnotist may be helpful: "Bring the hypnotist, so he can hypnotize him and tell him that he is absolutely alright. That is the only medicine he needs. If his unconscious grips the idea of being alright, then there is no problem."

The sons were very happy, and they brought the hypnotist. He looked like a doctor with his bag and paraphernalia, with his small Sigmund Freud beard, with one glass on one eye – one has to be properly dressed according to one's profession, and this is impressive! – and he asked the old man, "What are your troubles?"

The old man listed so many troubles. The hypnotist said, "Okay, you just lie down. I will be holding this pendulum which shines because it has a battery attached. You have to keep your eyes on it until you cannot keep them open."

Old people become very cunning and very clever after a long life's experience.

The old man thought, "This seems to be a con man by the way he is dressed…and what kind of treatment is going on?" He thought, "Let us see." He did not wait for three minutes, he immediately closed his eyes, and when the hypnotist took his hand, he dropped it. He knew all the tricks…an old man, he has seen everything in the world!

The hypnotist said, "He is completely at ease and asleep. Now I will give him the suggestion that he is perfectly alright, he doesn't have any disease and he will not harass his children with diseases that don't exist!" And the old man remained silent.

His sons were very happy: "Why have we never thought of the hypnotist? We have been wasting so much money paying the doctors, and all that they say is, 'You harass us. Although you give us money, it is sheer harassment. The man is not sick at all.' This man is the right man!"

The old man was lying completely still. All suggestions over, the hypnotist collected his fee. One of the sons went out the door to see him off to his car, but even before he returned, the old man opened one eye and asked, "Has that crackpot gone or not?"

If you immediately close your eyes, nothing will happen because you will remain conscious. Whatever the hypnotist is saying, he will look like a crank: What nonsense is he talking? "Your eyes are becoming heavy" – they will not become heavy. "You are falling deep in a sleep" – you are not falling, you are perfectly alert. And he is cheating; he is saying that you don't have any diseases!

But if you are doing a session of self-hypnosis, there is no danger. You just go through the whole process, looking at a bright thing that tires your eyes – that is its only function – and you go on repeating what the hypnotist was repeating, but inside your being. Finally, you will find you cannot keep your eyes open; they are closing. You have lost control over them. That feeling of losing control over your eyelids immediately gives you the feeling that you are certainly falling into deep sleep. As long as you are aware, you go on repeating, "I am going deeper, deeper," and a moment comes when you have gone deepest into your unconscious. And after ten minutes the alarm will go off, and you will come back from your unconscious to the conscious. You will be surprised how fresh, how young you are feeling within yourself – how clean, as if you have passed through a beautiful garden full of flowers, with a cool breeze.

You can also give yourself post-hypnotic suggestions. They have to be given at the last moment when your eyes are closing and you feel that now you will be going deeper. Before going deeper you start saying, "From tomorrow my health will be better." Just choose one thing, not too many; don't be greedy! And just a fifteen-day session or three-week session just on yourself, whatever you are saying…perhaps that your meditation will go deeper from tomorrow. You will find that your meditation is going deeper and you can create a very beautiful link.

When the meditation goes deeper, then you can suggest to yourself, "Tomorrow my hypnosis will go even deeper." You can use both to bring you to the very depths of your unconsciousness.

Once you have touched the depths of your unconsciousness, then you can start a second suggestion: "Although I will be in the dark unconscious, a slight awareness will remain so that I can see what is happening." And then go on repeating, "My awareness which was slight is becoming bigger and bigger and bigger...." And one day you will find the whole unconscious is lighted with your alertness – and that's what meditation is.

Hypnosis can be used, should be used, without any fear. Either together, by people who trust each other and love each other, so there is no fear that they will exploit...you are with your very intimate friends; you know that they cannot harm you, you can open yourself, you can be vulnerable. Or just yourself...by yourself it will take a little longer, because you have to do two persons' work yourself. That is a little disturbance.

But now, because tape recorders are available you can dispose of the other person completely, and give the suggestion part to the tape recorder. And the tape recorder certainly cannot misuse it; it cannot tell you to kill your wife, unless you have put that on the tape. Then I cannot help; whatever you put in the tape recorder it will repeat! You can put the whole process in the tape recorder, all the suggestions of falling into sleep, heaviness of the lids, going deeper. And then when you are deepest – a gap of four, five minutes, so you settle in your deepness – then from the tape recorder comes the voice saying that your meditation will become deeper from today, that you will not have to struggle with your thoughts. The moment you close your eyes, the thoughts will start dispersing themselves.

The tape recorder can be immensely helpful because there is no question of anybody to trust. You can trust your tape recorder without any fear. And you can lock the door so that nobody plays with your tape recorder – otherwise somebody may trick you!

Self-hypnosis has to be in the service of meditation; that is its greatest use. But it can serve health, it can serve long life, it can serve love, it can serve friendliness, it can serve courage. All that you want, self-hypnosis can help you with. It can dispel your fears of the unknown, it can dispel your fear of death; it can make you ready for being alone, silent, peaceful. It can make you able to continue an undercurrent of meditation the whole twenty-four hours.

You can even suggest, "While I am asleep my small flame of awareness will continue all through the night without disturbing my sleep."

In your question you are saying, "I have noticed that the line between therapy and meditation is dissolving." That has been my deep desire for a long time: therapy should dissolve into hypnosis, and hypnosis should dissolve into meditation. Then we have created one of the greatest forces for enlightenment, which has never been used in the past.

Therapy has never been used. Therapy will cleanse you of all garbage, it will take away all your conditionings; therapy will help you to cathart anything that has been there and you have been repressing inside. Therapy will throw it out. Therapy is a beautiful cleansing process, and a mind cleansed will fall into hypnosis more easily, without any struggle. Perhaps even those who are not easily available to self-hypnosis or to hypnosis – the people who don't belong to the thirty-three percent – with therapy, even they may start belonging to the group which is available for hypnosis. Therapy can change one hundred percent of people into authentic candidates for hypnosis. So therapy has to be used in such a way that it slowly dissolves into hypnosis, and then hypnosis has to be used so that it can become steps going towards meditation.

These three things together I propose to be my trinity. God and the Holy Ghost and Jesus Christ...forget all that nonsense. That is not a trinity. But something scientific, something that you can do yourself, something that is possible to be practiced – except for that, religion is so full of garbage, and people have become more interested in the garbage and forgotten the essential. In fact, the essential has become so small in comparison to the Himalayan garbage that has accumulated on top of it down the centuries that it is even difficult to find where it is.

What I am proposing is a simple thing: you don't need any priest, you don't need any church, you don't need any holy scripture. All that you need is a little under-standing and a little courage. Cathart totally in therapy. You don't know how much crap there is inside you. When you start catharting, then you will know – "My God, is this me or somebody else? What am I doing? What am I saying?" Sometimes what you say does not even make any sense. But it has been there, otherwise it cannot come to you. It has been a hindrance to your meditation, and it will be a hindrance to your going deep into hypnosis. It will become a barrier somewhere in between.

So therapy has to be the first thing. The second thing is hypnosis, and the third thing will grow out of it – your meditation.

The ultimate in meditation is enlightenment.

When meditation comes to its completion, then your whole being becomes full of light, full of blissfulness, full of ecstasy.[21]

CHAPTER 3

RELATIONSHIP BETWEEN MIND, BODY AND HEALTH

? *Would you talk about the connection between the mind and health?*

Seventy percent of diseases are mind-oriented. Through hypnosis those diseases can be prevented before they occur. Through hypnosis it can be found out what kind of sickness is going to happen in the near future. There are no symptoms on the body; the routine physical examination of the person will not show any indication that he is going to be sick or ill, he is perfectly healthy. But through hypnosis we can find that within three weeks he is going to fall sick, because before anything comes to the body, it comes from the deep cosmic unconscious. It travels from there to the collective unconscious, to the unconscious, and only then, when it comes to the conscious mind, can it be checked and found in the body. Sicknesses can be prevented even before the person has any idea that he is going to be sick.

In Russia, one genius photographer, Kirlian, has even photographed people.... His whole life he has been working in photography, with very sensitive plates, sensitive lenses, to find something which is not available to ordinary eyes and ordinary instruments. And he was puzzled that he could see in his photographs at least six months ahead. If he takes a picture of a rosebud with his special sensitive plates, the picture is not of a rosebud, the picture is of a rose. Tomorrow it is going to be a rose. No other camera can do that miracle. First he himself was puzzled how the sensitive plate can take a picture of something which has not happened yet – and when tomorrow the bud opens up, it is exactly similar to the photograph, there is no difference at all. Then he discovered more and more that there is a certain aura surrounding the bud – just an energy aura, and that energy aura has the whole program of how the bud is going to open. The sensitive plate gets the picture of the energy aura that we cannot see with our bare eyes. Then he started working on diseases, and in Soviet medicine he has created a revolution.

You need not first become sick, and then be cured. You can be cured even before you have any knowledge of any sickness, because Kirlian photography will show in what part the sickness is going to show, because the energy aura will be sick, already sick. It is six months ahead. It is connected with your cosmic unconscious. Through hypnosis and deeper experiments with it, you can find sicknesses that are going to happen and they can be treated. The children can be more happy.

It has been a topic of concern to the psychoanalysts why, all over the world except in a few places, seventy years has become the routine idea of the length of life, because there are a few tribes in Kashmir, in India – now that part has been occupied by Pakistan, a very small part – where people have always lived one hundred and thirty years, one hundred and forty years, one hundred and fifty. And even at the age of one hundred and fifty they were as energetic as any young man. They never became old, they remained young until they died…. Psychologists have been concerned to find the reason why in a few places people live long and in most of the world people live only the routine seventy years.

It seems to be that it is just a psychological programming. For centuries we have been programmed: seven decades and you are finished. That has gone so deep that you die, not because your body is not capable of living, but because your psychology insists, "Follow the routine. Follow the crowd." And in everything else you are following the crowd, so naturally you follow the crowd psychology in this too.

Scientists say that man's body is capable of living at least three hundred years. Just as it goes on rejuvenating itself for seventy years, in fact it can go on for three hundred years, but the program has to be changed. Scientists think in a different way how to change the program, and it will take very long for them. They think the program is in the cells of the body. So unless we split the human cell, just as we have been able to split the atom, and reprogram it, which seems to be far away, because even the scratch work has not started….

But my understanding is that there is no need to go through physiology, you can go through psychology. If your hypnosis goes deep enough…the more you go into it, if it becomes an everyday thing, slowly, slowly, you will touch the cosmic unconscious, and there is the real programming; you can change it.

Our children can live longer, our children can live healthier, our children can live without old age. All this is possible, and we have to make it, to show to the world, but it is dangerous in the sense that if politicians get hold of hypnotic methods they are going to use it for their own purposes.[22]

People can be helped with diseases, because almost seventy percent of diseases are mental. They may be expressed through the body, but their origin is in the mind. And if you can put in the mind the idea that the disease has disappeared, that you need not worry about it, it does not exist anymore, the disease will disappear....

Mind has tremendous power over your body. The mind directs everything in your body. Seventy percent of your diseases can be changed by changing the mind, because they start from there; only thirty percent of diseases start from the body. You fall down, and you have a fracture – now, that fracture cannot be helped by hypnosis saying that you don't have any fracture. You will still have the fracture. The fracture has started from the body and the body cannot be hypnotized – the body has its own way of functioning. But if the process starts from the mind and extends to some point in the body, then it can be easily changed.

Religions have exploited it. There are many religions in India – Mohammedans do it, Tibetans do it, Burmese do it...dancing in the fire without being burned. But these are not ordinary people, they are monks. For years they have been hypnotized, and this thing has settled in their unconscious – that fire cannot burn them. But remember, only seventy percent....

There used to be a sect in America...I think it still survives in a few places, but in the beginning of this century it was very prominent. It was a Christian group, they used to call themselves Christian Scientists. They believed that everything can be cured, you just have to believe in Jesus Christ, and that your diseases are nothing but your beliefs – you believe that you have tuberculosis, so you *have* tuberculosis.

One young man met on the road with one old woman and she asked, "I don't see your father in the meetings...." They used to have meetings every Sunday.

He said, "He's sick, very badly sick."

The old woman said, "Nonsense – because we are Christian Scientists. He is a Christian Scientist; he only *believes* that he is sick."

The young man said, "If you say so, perhaps he only believes that he is sick."

After two, three days, he came across the same woman again and she asked, "What happened?"

The young man said, "Now he believes he is dead, so we had to take him to the graveyard. We tried to shake him and shouted, 'Don't believe such a thing – you are a Christian Scientist. Believe that you are alive!' But nothing happened and the whole neighbourhood laughed. Now the poor man is in a grave, still believing that he is dead."

The body does not have beliefs or disbeliefs, but the mind has. And the mind has immense control over the body.[23]

Now medical science has become aware of certain phenomena. One of them is really very peculiar, and the phenomenon is this – that every country has different types of diseases prevalent, and every community, every religious sect, has different diseases occurring more. For example, Eastern people are more prone towards epidemics: plague, cholera – more prone towards communal diseases; infections, and diseases which spread by infection, because in the East the individual doesn't exist much. Only the community exists.

In an Indian village, the village exists; nobody exists as an individual – a community exists. When the community is too much, then infectious diseases will be prevalent, because nobody has a protective aura around himself. If one becomes ill, then the whole community by and by will become victim to the illness. And in the same community, there can be a few Westerners – they will not be affected by the infection. In fact just otherwise should be the case, because a Western man in India should be more prone to diseases because he is not immune. He is not immune to this climate, to such diseases: he should become a victim sooner. But no. For the last hundred years it has been studied and found that whenever there is an infectious disease Europeans are protected by some unknown force; Indians become victim.

The Indian mind is more a communal mind, the European mind is more egoistic and personal. So in the West certain other diseases are prevalent. For example, heart attack; it is an individual disease, non-infectious. In the East heart attack is not so common – unless you are Western, unless you are educated in a Western way and you have become almost Western.

In the East, heart attack is not a big problem; diabetes is not a big problem; blood pressure is not a big problem – these are non-infectious diseases. Christians are more prone to them. The Western mind lives as an individual unit. Of course, when you live as an individual unit, the community cannot impress you too much. You will be protected from infections.

In the West, infections have disappeared by and by. But people are becoming more and more personally ill. Heart attacks, suicide, blood pressure, madness –

these are individual diseases; they don't carry any infection – tenseness, anguish, anxiety....

In the East people are more at ease. You don't find them too tense. They don't suffer from insomnia, they don't suffer from heart illnesses. For that they are protected by the community, because the community has no heart. If you live a communal life you cannot suffer from a heart disease.

This is a rare phenomenon. It means your mind makes you available to certain diseases, and makes you protected against certain diseases.

Your mind is your world. Your mind is your health, your mind is your illness. And if you live with the mind, you continue to live in a capsule, and you cannot know what reality is. That reality is known only when you drop all types of minds – communal, individual, social, cultural, personal...when you drop all types of minds. Then your mind becomes universal. Then your mind becomes one with the mind of the universe.

When you don't have your own mind, your consciousness becomes universal.[24]

All problems are psychosomatic because the body and the mind are not two things. The mind is the inner part of the body, and the body is the outer part of the mind, so anything can start in the body and can enter into the mind, or vice versa: it can start in the mind and enter into the body. There is no division, there is no water-tight compartment.

So all problems have two edges to them: they can be tackled through the mind and through the body. And up to now this has been the practice in the world: a few believe that all problems are of the body – the physiologists, the Pavlovians, the Behaviourists.... They treat the body, and of course in fifty percent of cases they succeed. And they hope that as science grows they will be succeeding more, but they will never succeed more than fifty percent; it has nothing to do with the growth of science.

Then the other party is there which thinks that all problems are of the mind – which is as wrong as the first. Christian Science people and hypnotists and mesmerists, psychotherapists, they all think problems are of the mind. They also succeed in fifty percent of cases; they also think that sooner or later they will succeed more and more. That is nonsense. They cannot succeed more than fifty percent; that is the limit.

My own understanding is that each problem has to be tackled from both sides together, simultaneously. It has to be attacked from the doors, a double-fronted attack; then man can be cured one hundred percent. Whenever science becomes perfect it will work both ways....

The first is the body, because the body is the portal to the mind – the porch. And because the body is gross it is still easily manipulatable. First the body has to be freed of all its accumulated structures. If you have lived for so long with the feeling that you are weak, then it must have entered into the body, into the very structure of the body. First it has to be relieved from there; and simultaneously your mind has to be inspired so that it can start moving upwards and can start dropping all the loads that keep it down.[25]

CHAPTER 4

THE HEALER

? *What exactly is the function of a healer?*

The healer is not really a healer because he is not a doer. Healing happens through him; he has just to annihilate himself. To be a healer really means not to be. The less you are, the better healing will happen. The more you are, the more the passage is blocked. God, or the totality, or whatsoever you prefer to call it, is the healer: the whole is the healer....

An ill person is one who has simply developed blocks between himself and the whole, so something is disconnected. The function of the healer is to reconnect him. But when I say the function of the healer is to reconnect him, I don't mean that the healer has to do something. The healer is just a function. The doer is God, the whole.[26]

Medicine is not an ordinary profession. It is not just technology, because human beings are involved. You are not repairing mechanisms, it is not only a question of know-how, it is a deep question of love....

You are playing with human beings and their lives, and it is a complex phenomenon. Sometimes one can commit errors, and those errors can prove fatal to somebody's life. So go with deep prayer. Go with humanity, humbleness, simplicity.

People who simply go into medicine as if they are going into engineering are not the right people to be doctors and physicians – they are the wrong people. Those who are not ambivalent are the wrong people. They will operate on human beings as a motor-mechanic does with a car. They will not feel the spiritual presence of the patient. They will not treat the person, they will treat the symptoms. Of course, they can be very certain; a technician is always certain.

But when you are involved with human beings you cannot be so certain; hesitation is natural. One thinks twice, thrice, before doing anything, because a precious life is involved – life which we cannot produce, life which once gone is gone forever. And it is an individual, who is irreplaceable, unique, the like of whom has never been there, and the like of whom there is never going to be again. You are playing with fire – hesitation is natural. Go into it! Go with tremendous humbleness. Have a deep reverence for the patient. And while treating him, just become a vehicle of the divine energy. Don't become a doctor, simply become a vehicle of the divine healing energy – just instrumental. Let there be the patient – have great reverence for the patient, don't treat him like a thing – and let there be God, and with deep prayer allow God to flow through you and reach the patient. The patient is ill; he cannot connect with God. He has fallen far away. He has forgotten the very language of how to heal himself. He is in a desperate state. You cannot blame him; he is in a helpless state.

Somebody who is healthy can be of tremendous help if he becomes a vehicle. And if the healthy person is also a man who knows, it can be of more importance, because the divine energy can give you only very subtle hints – they have to be decoded by you. If you know medicine, you can decode them very easily. And then you are not doing anything to the patient, it is God who is doing it. You make yourself available to God and you make all your knowledge available. It is God's healing energy in conjunction with your knowledge that helps. And it never harms. *You* can be harmful. So drop yourself, let God be there. Go into medicine, and go on meditating.[27]

Everybody can become a healer. Healing is something like breathing; it is natural. Somebody is ill; it means he has lost his capacity to heal himself. He is no longer aware of his own healing source. The healer is to help him to be rejoined. That source is the same from which the healer draws, but the ill man has forgotten how to understand the language of it. The healer is in relationship with the whole, so he can become a via-media. The healer touches the body of the ill person and becomes a link between him and the source. The patient is no longer connected directly with the source so he becomes indirectly connected. Once the energy starts flowing, he is healed.

And if the healer is really a man of understanding…because it is possible that you can become a healer and you may not be a man of understanding. There are many healers who go on doing it but they don't know how it happens; they don't know the mechanism of it. If you understand also, you can help the patient to be healed and you can help him to be aware of the source from where the healing is happening. So not only is he healed of his present illnesses, he is prevented from future illnesses. Then the healing is perfect. It is not only curative, it is also preventative.

Healing almost becomes an experience of prayer, an experience of God, of love, of the whole.[28]

?   *I am a member of the healing profession, and I would like to know your views on how best to care for the ill. Religions have been saying, "Love the sick, love the diseased. Go to the hospitals, make hospitals, serve the poor." Please comment.*

It seems all religions are concerned with the sick, with the diseased, with the poor. Nobody is concerned with you and your riches and your greatness and your grandeur.

I say unto you: Unless you love yourself, unless you have found your own riches, your own heights, you will not be able to share your love with anybody. Certainly the sick and the diseased need care, but they don't need love. This has to be understood, because Christianity has made it almost a universally accepted truth – that it is the greatest religious thing, the most spiritual thing, to love the sick and the diseased. But it is absolutely against psychology and against nature. The moment you love the sick you are not helping him to recover from his sickness, because the moment he is healthy nobody loves him. Sickness is a good excuse for others to be provoked to love him.

You may have seen it, but you may not have thought about it. The wife is working the whole day, perfectly healthy, but as the husband comes home, looking from the window, she immediately goes to bed. She has a headache – because unless she has a headache the husband does not show any love. But if she has a headache, reluctantly the husband sits by her side, massages her head, shows some phony kind of love, talks sweet and beautiful words. For months he has not called her 'darling', but when the headache is there he has to call her 'darling'. And that's what she wants to hear, "I love you. And I love you not just today, I will love you forever."

It is strange that you show your love to your children when they are sick. But you don't understand a simple psychology of association – sickness and love become associated. Whenever the child needs your love he has to be sick. Who cares about the healthy child, who cares about the healthy wife, who cares about the healthy husband? Love seems to be something like a medicine; it is needed only by the sick.

I want it to be clear to you – take care of the sick, but never show love. Taking care of the sick is a totally different thing. Be indifferent, because a headache is not something great. Take care, but avoid your sweet nothings; take care in a very pragmatic way. Put the medicine on her head, but don't show love, because that is dangerous. When a child is sick, take care, but be absolutely indifferent. Make the child understand that by being sick he cannot blackmail you. The whole humanity is blackmailing each other. Sickness, oldness, disease have become almost demanding, "You have to love me because I'm sick, I'm old...."

When somebody is sick you show love.... And that's the routine that humanity has followed. To the sick person you don't show anger, even if you are angry. To the sick person, even if you don't feel any love, you show love; if you cannot show love, at least sympathy. But these are dangerous, and very much against psychological findings....

You should love yourself without thinking whether you deserve it or not. You are alive – that is enough proof that you deserve love, just as you deserve breathing. You don't think whether you deserve breathing or not. Love is a subtle nourishment to the soul, just as food is to the body. And if you are full of love for yourself you will be able to love others. But love the healthy, love the strong.

Take care of the sick, take care of the old; but care is a totally different matter. The difference between love and care is the difference between a mother and a nurse. The nurse takes care, the mother loves. When the child is sick it is even better for the mother to just be a nurse. When the child is healthy, pour as much love as you can. Let love be associated with healthiness, strength, intelligence – that will help the child a long way in his life.[29]

I am a psychiatrist. Can meditation help me in my work with patients?

A psychiatrist needs to be meditative more than anybody else – because your whole work is dangerous in a way. Unless you are very calm and quiet, unless you can remain unaffected by things that happen around you, it is very dangerous. More psychiatrists go mad than any other professional people, and more psychiatrists commit suicide than any other professional people. This is something to be pondered over. The proportion is really too much. Twice as many commit suicide. That simply shows that the profession is full of dangers. It is – because whenever you are treating a person who is psychologically disturbed, in a mess, he is constantly broadcasting his vibes. He is constantly throwing out his own energy, his negative waves upon you, and you have to listen to him. You have to be very attentive. You have to care, you have to love and be compassionate towards him; only then can you help him. He is constantly throwing negative-charged energy – and you are absorbing it. In fact the more attentively you listen, the more you absorb it.

Living continuously with neurotic and psychotic people, you start thinking, in an unconscious way, that this is what humanity is. We become by and by like the people we live with, because nobody is an island. So if you are working with sad people, you will become sad. If you are working with happy people, you will become happy, because everything is infectious. Neurosis is infectious; suicide also is infectious.

If you live around people who are enlightened, very aware, then something in you starts responding to this higher possibility. When you live with people who are very low, abnormally low, in a perverted state, then something morbid in you starts corresponding and relating to them. So to be continuously surrounded by ill people, is in a way dangerous, unless you protect yourself. And there is nothing like meditation to give you protection. Then you can give more than you are giving and yet you will remain unaffected. You can help more than you are helping, because the higher your energy, the more is the possibility to help. Otherwise the psychiatrist, the healer and the healee are almost on the same ground; maybe a little difference of degrees, but the difference is so small that it is not worth considering.

The psychiatrist can go into madness very easily – just a slight push, some accidental thing, and he can move into the condemned territory. People who are neurotic were not always neurotic. Just two days ago they were normal people, and again they can become normal. So normality and abnormality are not qualitative distinctions, just quantitative: ninety-nine degrees, one hundred degrees, one hundred and one degrees – that type of difference.

In fact, in a better world, every psychiatrist should be trained deeply in meditation, otherwise he should not be allowed to practice. That is the only way that you can protect yourself and not be vulnerable – and you can really help. Otherwise even great psychiatrists, great psychoanalysts, even they become in a way very hopeless about humanity...even Freud. After a whole life's experience he finally said that he could not hope for man; he felt hopeless. And it is natural – forty years of being with people who are in a mess; the only experience of humanity being of people who are mad. By and by it started to look to him as if abnormality is normal...as if man is bound to remain neurotic, as if there is something natural in man which drives him towards neurosis.

So at the most the healthy person is one who is a little more adjusted to the world, that's all. Adjustment becomes the standard of health. But it cannot be. If the whole society is mad you can be adjusted to it and you will still be mad. In fact in a mad society, a person who is not mad will be maladjusted. And that's what is really the case.

When a Jesus walks in this world he is maladjusted. We have to crucify him. He is such a stranger – we cannot tolerate him. We are not concerned with him, we are simply concerned with ourselves. Because of his presence, only two things are possible – either he is mad or we are mad. Both cannot be healthy. We are many and he is alone. Of course we will kill him; he cannot kill us. When a Buddha walks, he looks strange – a healthy man, a really natural, normal man, moving in an abnormal society.

So Freud came to conclude that there is no future for humanity. At the most we can hope that man can be adjusted with the social pattern, that's all. But there is no possibility for man to be blissful. There cannot be, by the very nature of things. Why such a pessimistic conclusion? – because of his whole experience.

Freud's whole life is a long nightmare of mad people, of working with them. And by and by he himself became abnormal. He was not really healthy. He was not a blissful person. He had never known what wholeness is. He was afraid of small things – so much so that it looks absurd. He was afraid of death. If somebody talked about ghosts, he would start perspiring. Twice he fainted because somebody started talking about death! This seems to be a very unbalanced mind, but in a way it can be accounted for. Even this is a miracle – that he remained sane for his whole life.

One of the most penetrating psychiatrists, Wilhelm Reich, went mad. And the only reason that he went and others have not, was because he was really penetrating. He had a really deep talent to go into the roots of things – but it is dangerous. Freud or Reich or others' whole lives show one thing – that had they been trained in deep meditation, the whole world would have been different. Then these neurotic people would not become the standard.

Maybe it is very difficult to become a Buddha, but he is the norm. And a normal person is one who comes closer to the norm. It has nothing to do with adjustment. One comes closer to the idea of wholeness, happiness, health.[30]

?
Is taking the role of a therapist dangerous to my own spiritual growth?
Is it possible to help people and still let my own ego dissolve at the same time? I feel that a subtle fight goes on inside me between one part that is clear and another part that wants nothing to do with clarity.
Under your guidance I have learned not to dominate others when I use my capacity to see, but am I still dominating myself?

The role of a therapist is a very delicate and complex affair.

First, the therapist himself suffers from the same problems that he is trying to help others with. The therapist is only a technician. He can manage to pretend and to deceive himself that he is a master – that is the greatest danger in being a therapist. But just a little understanding, and things won't be the same.

First, don't think in terms of helping others. That gives you the idea of being a saviour, of being a master – and from the back door the ego enters again. You become important, you are the centre of the group, everybody is looking up to you.

Drop the idea of help. Instead of 'help' use the word 'sharing'. You share your insight, whatsoever you have. The participant is not someone who is inferior to you. The therapist and the therapee are both in the same boat; the therapist is just a little more knowledgeable. Be conscious of the fact that your knowledge is borrowed. Never for a moment forget that whatever you know is still not your experience, and this will help the people who are participating in your group.

Man is a very subtle mechanism. It works on both sides: the therapist starts becoming the master, and rather than helping he is destroying something in the participant, because the participant will also learn only the technique. There will not be a loving, sharing friendliness, an atmosphere of trust, but, "You know more, I know less…. By participating in a few therapy groups I will also know as much as you know."

The participants slowly, slowly start becoming therapists themselves, because there is no degree required – at least in many countries. In a few countries they have started to outlaw all kinds of unaccepted therapies; only a man who has a university qualification in therapeutics, in psychoanalysis, in psychotherapy will be able to help people in therapy groups.

This is going to happen in almost every country of the world, because therapy has become a business, and people who are unqualified are dominating it. They know the technique, because technique they can learn; by participating in a few groups they know all the techniques, then they can make a concoction of their own. But there is no way of controlling….

But remember: the moment you play the role of a helper, the helped is never going to forgive you. You have hurt his pride, you have hurt his ego. That was not your intention…your intention was just to inflate your own ego, but this can happen only if you hurt other people's ego. You cannot inflate your ego without hurting others. Your bigger ego will need more space, and the others have to shrink their space and their personality to exist with you.

From the very beginning be an authentic loving person…and I make it an absolutely necessary point that there is nothing more therapeutic than love. Technique can help, but the real miracle happens through love. Love the people who participate in therapy and be one amongst them, with no pretensions of being higher or holier.

Make it clear from the very beginning: "These are the techniques I have learned, and a little bit is my experience. I will give you the techniques, and I will share my experience. But you are not my disciples; you are just friends in need. I have some understanding, not much, but I can share it with you. Perhaps many of you have your own understanding coming from different areas, different directions. You can also share your experience and make the group richer."

In other words, what I am saying is a totally new concept of therapy. The therapist is only a coordinator. He just tries to make the group more silent, serene; he keeps an eye that nothing goes wrong…more of a guardian than a master. And you have also to make it clear: "I am also learning while I am trying to share my experience. When I am listening to you, it is not only your problems; they are my problems too. And when I am saying something, I am not only saying it, I am listening also."

Emphatically make it clear that you are nobody special. This has to be done at the beginning of the group, and this has to be carried on as the group goes deeper, exploring. You just remain an elder, who has gone a few steps ahead; otherwise you will not be able to help people. They will learn the technique and they will become therapists on their own. And there are enough fools – five billion fools – on the earth; they will find their own followers. It is a human weakness that when people start looking up to you, you start thinking, "There must be something great in me if people are looking up to me." They are in trouble, they are suffering from human frailties. But you are also human, and to err is absolutely human. Without any condemnation, with great love, help them to open themselves – and this is possible only if you open yourself.

I have come to know a strange fact: strangers tell each other things that they can never say to people they know. In a railway train you meet somebody; you don't know his name, you don't know where he is going, from where he is coming, and people start sharing. I have been travelling for twenty years non-stop in the whole country, watching a strange phenomenon – that people give their secrets to strangers, because the stranger is not going to exploit it. Just the next station comes, and the stranger is gone; perhaps you may never see him again. And he is not concerned to destroy your reputation or anything. On the contrary, sharing your secrets, your weaknesses, your vulnerabilities makes others more confident and more loving and more trusting in you. Your trust provokes their trust in you, and when they see you are so innocent and so open and available, they start opening up: it is a chain reaction….

But a therapy group is not the end. It is only the beginning. It is a preparation for meditation, just as meditation is a preparation for enlightenment. If you understand things in their simple arithmetic, you will not find it difficult – and you will enjoy the group more, because the group will be able to go deeper with you. You will not be only a teacher in the group; you will be also a learner. Kahlil Gibran's prophet, al-Mustafa, has a beautiful statement. When somebody asks, "Tell us something about learning." he says, "Because you have asked I will speak. But remember – I am speaking and I am also listening with you...."

Love the people who have become participants in your group. I ove them as they are, not as they should be. They have suffered their whole life from all kinds of religious, political, social, theological, philosophical leaders who would love them if they follow, who would love them if they become just images according to *their* idea. They will love you only when they have killed you completely, demolished you and put you together according to their idea.

All the religions have done that to humanity. Nobody is left undamaged. And these people have been thinking that they are helping, consciously. They were giving you ideals, ideologies, principles, commandments with the certain fixed attitude that they want to help you; otherwise you will go astray. They cannot trust your freedom and they cannot respect your dignity; they have reduced you so badly – and nobody even objects....

I am reminded of one statement of a great doctor who is my friend. I don't know whether he is still alive or not, I have not heard anything about him for these last six years. He was the most prominent doctor in the city where I lived before I moved to Bombay and then to Poona. He said to me, "My whole life's experience is that the function of the physician is not the cure of the patient. The patient cures himself; the physician simply gives a loving atmosphere, promising. The physician simply gives the confidence and revives the longing to live longer. All his medicines are of secondary help." But if the person has lost the desire to live, his whole life's experience was that no medicine, nothing, helps.

The same is the situation for the therapist. The therapist is not the person who is going to cure people's psychological troubles. He can only create a loving atmosphere in which they can open up their repressed, unconscious imaginations, repressions, hallucinations, desires, without any fear that they will be laughed at, with absolute certainty that all will feel compassion and love for them. The whole group should function as a therapeutic situation.

The therapist is only a coordinator. He brings psychologically sick or disturbed people together, and just watches that nothing goes wrong. And if he can support them with some idea, some insight, some observation, he should always make it clear, "This is only my knowledge, not my experience" – unless he has the experience.

If you are sincere and truthful and honest and authentic, you will never fall into the trap of becoming a master, a saviour – which is very simple to fall in. The moment you become a master and a saviour – and you are not – you are not even helping those people, you are simply exploiting those people, their weaknesses, their troubles.

The whole psychoanalysis movement around the world is the most exploitative experiment that is going on. Nobody is helped; everybody is exploited tremendously. And nobody is helped because the psychoanalyst, psychotherapist…, psychology has bifurcated in many branches, but they all do the same work: they reduce you to a patient and they are the physicians.

And the trouble is that they themselves are suffering from the same diseases. Each psychoanalyst goes to another psychoanalyst almost twice a year to be helped. It is a great conspiracy. Listening to all kinds of insanities, unless you are beyond mind and its problems, you are going to be insane yourself. You are going to start suffering from the same problems your patients are suffering from. Rather than making them cured, they are making you sick. But the responsibility is yours.

Bring love, openness, sincerity…. Before they start opening the doors of their heart – they are keeping them tightly closed so that nobody knows their problems – the first function of the psychotherapist is to open *his* heart and let them know that he is also as human as they are. He suffers from the same weaknesses, the same lust, the same desire for power, the same desire for money. He suffers from anguish and anxiety, suffers from the fear of death.

Open your heart totally. That will help others to trust you – that you are not a pretender. The days of saviours and prophets and messengers and *tirthankaras* and *avataras* are completely gone. None of them will be acceptable today. And this time, if any of them reappears, people are not even going to stone him to death, people are just going to make fun of him. People are simply going to tell him, "You are stupid. The very idea that you can save the whole humanity is mad. First save yourself, and we will see your light and we will see your grandeur and we will see your splendour."

And trust comes on its own accord. It is not to be asked. It comes just like a fresh breeze from the mountains, a tidal wave from the oceans. You have to do nothing for it. You have just to be available at the right time, in the right place.

Nobody can save you except yourself. I say unto you: Be a saviour unto yourself. But help is possible, with a condition: that it comes with love, that it comes with the gratitude that, "You trusted me and opened your heart."

The function of a therapist is certainly very complex – and idiots are doing it! The situation is almost as if butchers are doing surgery; they know how to cut, but that does not mean they can become brain surgeons. They can kill buffaloes and cows and all kinds of animals, but their function is in the service of death. The therapist is in the service of life. He has to create life-affirmative values by living them himself, by going to the silences of his heart.

The deeper you are within yourself, the deeper you can reach into the heart of the other. It is exactly the same…because your heart or the other's heart are not very different things. If you understand *your* being, you understand everybody's being. And then you understand you have also been foolish, you have also been ignorant, you have also fallen many times, you have also committed crimes against yourself and against others, and if other people are still doing it there is no need of condemnation. They have to be made aware and left to themselves; you are not to mould them in a certain framework.

Then it is a joy to be a therapist, because you come to know the interiority of human beings — which is one of the most secret hiding places of life. And by knowing others you know yourself more. It is a vicious circle; there is no other word — otherwise I will not use the word 'vicious.' Allow me to coin a word: it is a virtuous circle. You open to your patients, participants, and they open themselves to you. That helps you to open more, and that helps them to open more. Soon there is no therapist and there is no patient, but simply a loving group helping each other.

Unless the therapist is lost in the group, he is not a successful therapist. That's my criterion.

You are saying, "Under your guidance I have learned not to dominate others when I use my capacity to see, but am I still dominating myself?" They are not two things. Domination is domination, whether you dominate others or you dominate yourself. If you are dominating yourself, then in some subtle way you will dominate others too. How can it be otherwise?

The first domination that you have to drop is not over others…because it is not certain that they will accept your domination. The first domination you have to drop is over yourself. Why become a prisoner yourself — with great effort create a prison around yourself — and then carry it wherever you go? First learn the utter joy of freedom, of a bird on the wing in the vast sky. Your very freedom will become a transforming force for others. Domination is so ugly. Leave it to the politicians, who don't have any sense of shame at all. They live in the gutters and they think they are living in palaces. Their whole life is a life in the gutters — they will live there and they will die there. They are prime ministers, they are presidents, they are kings, they are queens….

One of the most significant Egyptian poets was asked once, "How many kings are there in the world?" At that time…he said, "There are only five kings. One is in England, and four are in playing cards." Now it can be changed: there are five queens, one in England and four in playing cards…. But they don't have anything more. They are just trying to achieve more and more power simply to fill their inside which they feel is empty.

Looking from the outside, the inside is empty. Looking from the inside, the whole world is empty. Only your inside is overflowing, but the things that are overflowing are invisible: the fragrance of your being, the love, the blissfulness, the ecstasy, the silence, the compassion – nothing can be seen with eyes. That's why if you look from the outside it seems everything is empty. And then a great urge arises: How to fill it? – with money, with power, with prestige, by becoming a president or prime minister? Do something and fill it! One cannot live with an emptiness inside, a hollowness inside.

But these people have not gone inside; they have looked from outside. And this is the problem: from the outside you can only see objects, and love is not an object, bliss is not an object, enlightenment is not an object, understanding is not an object, wisdom is not an object. All that is great in human existence and life is subjective, not objective. But from the outside you can only see objects. That gives a tremendous urgency to fill your hollow inside with any rubbish. There are people who are filling it with borrowed knowledge; there are people who are filling it with self-imposed torture – they become saints. There are people who are beggars to become the prime minister, to become the president. Everywhere the hollow people are in tremendous need to dominate others. That gives them the feeling that they are not hollow.

A sannyasin begins by inquiring into his subjectivity, from within, and he becomes aware of tremendous treasures, inexhaustible treasures. Only then do you stop dominating yourself, and you stop dominating others. There is no need at all. From that moment your whole effort is to make everybody aware of his individuality, of his freedom, of his immense, inexhaustible sources of bliss, contentment, peace.

To me, if therapy prepares the ground for meditation, therapy is going right... ground for the patients and ground for the therapist, both. Therapy should turn at a certain point into meditation. Meditation turns at a certain point into enlightenment. And to have such tremendous potential and just remain a beggar.... I feel so sad sometimes when I think of others. They are not beggars, but they are behaving like beggars, and they are not ready to drop their begging – because they are afraid that is all they have got. And unless they drop their begging, they will never know that they are emperors and their empire is of the within....

Try to understand yourself as deeply as possible. Therapy comes second. And unless you have refined your being through meditation and silences.... I am not saying, stop the work; I am saying, transform its quality. Make it real work. Open your heart, tell them your weaknesses, tell them your problems, ask their advice – can they help you? And once the participants understand that the therapist is not an egoist, they will come with absolute humbleness, opening their hearts. Then you can help them.

But always and always remember: therapy in itself is incomplete. Even the perfect therapy is just the first step. Without the second step it is meaningless.

So leave the patients on the point from where they start moving towards meditation. Your therapy is complete only when your patients start inquiring about meditation. Create a great longing in their hearts for meditation, and tell them that meditation too is only a step – the second step. In itself that too is not enough, unless it leads you to enlightenment; that is the culmination of the whole effort. And I trust in you, that you are capable of it.

A Jew from Odessa was sitting in the same compartment as a Czarist Russian officer who had a pig with him. To annoy the Jew, the officer kept calling the pig Moishe. "Moishe! Keep still! Moishe! Come here! Moishe! Go there!"

This went on all the way to Kiev. Eventually the Jew got fed up and said, "You know, Captain, it is a great shame your pig has a Jewish name."

"Now why is that, Jew?" smirked the officer.

"Well, otherwise it could have become an officer in the Czar's army."

There is a limit to everything!

Make it a point that the limit of therapy is where meditation begins, and the limit of meditation is where enlightenment begins. Of course, enlightenment is not a step to anything: you simply disappear into the universal consciousness, you become just a dewdrop slipping from the lotus leaf into the ocean. But it is the greatest experience. It makes life finally meaningful, significant. It allows you to become part of the universe from which your ego has separated you.

You just have to move in the right direction. A sense of right direction, and everything can become a stepping stone towards higher states of consciousness. I have been using everything, but the direction is the same. I have used many kinds of meditations. On the periphery they look different. There are one hundred and twelve methods of meditation: they look very different from each other, and you may think, "How can all these different methods lead to meditation?"

But they lead.... Just as a thread running through a garland of flowers is not seen, you see only the flowers, those one hundred and twelve flowers have a running thread: that thread is witnessing, watching, observation, awareness.

So help the patients as much as you can to understand their problems, but make it clear that even if these problems are solved, *you* are the same person. Tomorrow you will start creating the same problems again – perhaps in a different way, with a different colour. So your therapy should become nothing but an opening for meditation. Then your therapy has a tremendous value. Otherwise it is just a mind game.[31]

CHAPTER 5

THE BODY

It seems that after lifetimes of being conditioned to be against the body, to deny and repress its natural urges, to regard caring for it as an irreligious indulgence, man is now more body conscious. On the other hand, some people's care for their physical well-being seems to have gone the other way, and is almost an obsession. Can you talk about a healthy relationship with one's body?

For centuries man has been told all kinds of life-negative things. Even to torture your body has been a spiritual discipline....

You walk, you eat, you drink, and all these things indicate that you are a body and a consciousness as an organic whole. You cannot torture the body and raise your consciousness. The body has to be loved — you have to be a great friend. It is your home, you have to clean it of all junk, and you have to remember that it is in your service continuously, day in, day out. Even when you are asleep, your body is continuously working for you digesting, changing your food into blood, taking out the dead cells from the body, bringing new oxygen, fresh oxygen into the body — and you are fast asleep!

It is doing everything for your survival, for your life, although you are so ungrateful that you have never even thanked your body. On the contrary, your religions have been teaching you to torture it: the body is your enemy and you have to get free from the body, its attachments. I also know that you are more than the body and there is no need to have any attachment. But love is not an attachment, compassion is not an attachment. Love and compassion are absolutely needed for your body and its nourishment. And the better body you have, the more is the possibility for growing consciousness. It is an organic unity.

A totally new kind of education is needed in the world where fundamentally everybody is introduced into the silences of the heart – in other words into meditations – where everybody has to be prepared to be compassionate to one's own body, because unless you are compassionate to your own body, you cannot be compassionate to any other body. It is a living organism, and it has done no harm to you. It has been continuously in service since you were conceived and will be till your death. It will do everything that you would like to do, even the impossible, and it will not be disobedient to you.

It is inconceivable to create such a mechanism which is so obedient and so wise. If you become aware of all the functions of your body, you will be surprised. You have never thought what your body has been doing. It is so miraculous, so mysterious – but you have never looked into it. You have never bothered to be acquainted with your own body and you pretend to love other people. You cannot, because those other people also appear to you as bodies.

The body is the greatest mystery in the whole of existence. This mystery needs to be loved – its mysteries, its functionings to be intimately inquired into.

The religions have unfortunately been absolutely against the body. But it gives a clue, a definite indication that if a man learns the wisdom of the body and the mystery of the body, he will never bother about the priest or about God. He will have found the most mysterious within himself, and within the mystery of the body is the very shrine of your consciousness.

Once you have become aware of your consciousness, of your being, there is no God above you. Only such a person can be respectful towards other human beings, other living beings, because they all are as mysterious as he himself is...different expressions, varieties which make life richer. And once a man has found consciousness in himself, he has found the key to the ultimate. Any education that does not teach you to love your body, does not teach you to be compassionate to your body, does not teach you how to enter into its mysteries, will not be able to teach you how to enter into your own consciousness.

The body is the door – the body is the stepping stone. And any education that does not touch the subject of your body and consciousness is not only absolutely incomplete, it is utterly harmful because it will go on being destructive. It is only the flowering of consciousness within you that prevents you from destruction. And that gives you a tremendous urge to create – to create more beauty in the world, to create more comfort in the world....

Man needs a better body, a healthier body. Man needs a more conscious, alert being. Man needs all kinds of comforts and luxuries that existence is ready to deliver. Existence is ready to give you paradise herenow, but you go on postponing it – it is always after death.

In Sri Lanka one great mystic was dying.... He was worshipped by thousands of people. They gathered around him. He opened his eyes: just a few more breaths would he take on the shore and he would be gone, and gone forever. Everybody was eager to listen to his last words. The old man said, "I have been teaching you for my whole life about blissfulness, ecstasy, meditativeness. Now I am going to the other shore – I will not be available anymore. You have listened to me, but you have never practiced what I have been telling you. You have always been postponing. But now there is no point in postponing, I am going. Is anyone ready to go with me?"

There was a great pindrop silence. People looked at each other thinking that perhaps this man who had been a disciple for forty years, *he* may be ready.... But he was looking at the others – nobody was standing up. Just from the very back a man raised his hand. The great mystic thought, "At least, one person is courageous enough."

But that man said, "Please let me make it clear to you why I am not standing up. I have only raised my hand. I want to know how to reach to the other shore, because today of course I am not ready. There are many things which are incomplete: a guest has come, my young son is getting married, and this day I cannot go – and you say from the other shore, you cannot come back. Some day, one day certainly, I will come and meet you. If you can just explain to us once more – although you have been explaining to us for your whole life – just once more how to reach the other shore? But please keep in mind that I am not ready to go right now. I just want to refresh my memory so that when the right time comes...."

That right time never comes. It is not only a story about that poor man, it is the story of millions of people, of almost all. They are all waiting for the right moment, the right constellation of stars.... They are consulting astrology, going to the palmist...inquiring in different ways what is going to happen tomorrow. Tomorrow does not happen – it never has happened. It is simply a stupid strategy of postponement. What happens is always today.

A right kind of education will teach people to live herenow, to create a paradise on this earth, not to wait for death to come, and not to be miserable till death stops your misery. Let death find you dancing and joyous and loving. It is a strange experience that if a man can live his life as if he is *already* in paradise, death cannot take away anything from that man's experience.

My approach is to teach you that this is the paradise, there is no paradise anywhere else, and no preparation is needed to be happy. No discipline is needed to be loving; just a little alertness, just a little wakefulness, just a little understanding.[32]

Respect your body the same way as you respect your soul. Your body is as sacred as your soul is. In existence everything is sacred because the whole thing is throbbing with the heartbeat of the divine....

You are moving moment to moment, from one stage of consciousness to another stage of consciousness. The body may be fast asleep, but it is also conscious. You know if you are asleep and a mosquito starts disturbing you, you remain asleep and your hand removes the mosquito.... The body has its own consciousness.

The scientists say the body has millions and millions of living cells; each cell has its own life. You have lost the capacity of wonder; otherwise you would wonder first about your own body, how the body turns the bread into blood. We have not been able to find a factory yet where bread can be turned into blood. And not only that, it sorts out what is needed and what is not needed by your body; that which is not needed is thrown out, and that which is needed is needed for different functions.

The body goes on supplying different places, different parts of your body, whatever their need is. You eat the same food for all your needs; out of the same food your bones are made, your blood is made, your skin is made, your eyes are made, your brain is made; and the body knows perfectly well what is needed and where it is needed. The blood is circulating continuously, supplying particular chemicals to particular parts.

Not only that, the body also knows the priority. The first priority is your brain — hence, if there is not enough oxygen, first the body will give the oxygen to the brain. The other parts are tougher and they can wait a little, but the brain cells are not so tough. If they don't get oxygen for six minutes they will die, and once they are dead they cannot be revived.

It is a tremendous work of intelligence to be alert about the different functions. When you have a wound, then the body stops supplying certain parts which can survive, but first the wound has to be healed. Immediately the white cells of the body rush towards the wound to cover it so it is not open. And then inside, the work, the very subtle work, continues.

Medical science knows that we are not yet as wise as the body is. The most prominent physicians have said that we cannot cure the body; the body cures itself — we can only help. At the most our medicines can be of some help, but the basic cure comes from the body itself. It is a wonder how it is being done. It is such a vast work.

I have come to know from one scientist friend, who has been working on the functions of the body, that if we want to do all those functions we will need almost one square mile of factory with many complicated mechanisms, computers. Then, too, we are not certain that we will succeed — and your religions have been condemning the body and telling you that to take care of the body is irreligious....

First, inside become one with your body, then become one with the whole existence. The day your heartbeat has a synchronicity with the universe and its heartbeat you have found religion – not before it. [33]

CHAPTER 6

TENSION AND RELAXATION

? *What is the cause of the tensions that we feel in the body?*

The original source of all tension is becoming. One is always trying to be something; no one is at ease with himself as he is. The being is not accepted, the being is denied, and something else is taken as an ideal to become. So the basic tension is always between that which you are and that which you long to become.

You desire to become something. Tension means that you are not pleased with what you are, and you long to be what you are not. Tension is created between these two. What you desire to become is irrelevant. If you want to become wealthy, famous, powerful, or even if you want to be free, liberated, to be divine, immortal, even if you long for salvation, *moksha,* then too the tension will be there.

Anything that is desired as something to be fulfilled in the future, against you *as you are,* creates tension. The more impossible the ideal is, the more tension there is bound to be. So a person who is a materialist is ordinarily not so tense as one who is religious, because the religious person is longing for the impossible, for the far-off. The distance is so great that only a great tension can fill the gap.

Tension means a gap between what you are and what you want to be. If the gap is great, the tension will be great. If the gap is small, the tension will be small. And if there is no gap at all, it means you are satisfied with what you are. In other words, you do not long to be anything other than what you are. Then your mind exists in the moment. There is nothing to be tense about; you are at ease with yourself. To me, if there is no gap you are religious.

The gap can have many layers. If the longing is physical, the tension will be physical. When you seek a particular body, a particular shape – if you long for something other than what you are on a physical level – then there is tension in your physical body. One wants to be more beautiful. Now your body becomes tense. This tension begins at your first body, the physiological, but if it is insistent, constant, it may go deeper and spread to the other layers of your being.

If you are longing for psychic powers, then the tension begins at the psychic level and spreads. The spreading is just like when you throw a stone in the lake. It drops at a particular point, but the vibrations created by it will go on spreading into the infinite. So tension may start from any one of your seven bodies, but the original source is always the same: the gap between a state that is and a state that is longed for.

If you have a particular type of mind and you want to change it, transform it – if you want to be more clever, more intelligent – then tension is created. Only if we accept ourselves totally is there no tension. This total acceptance is the miracle, the only miracle. To find a person who has accepted himself totally is the only surprising thing.

Existence itself is non-tense. Tension is always because of hypothetical, non-existential possibilities. In the present there is no tension; tension is always future-oriented. It comes from the imagination. You can imagine yourself as something other than you are. This potential that has been imagined will create tension. So the more imaginative a person is, the more tension is a possibility. Then the imagination has become destructive.

Imagination can also become constructive, creative. If your whole capacity to imagine is focused in the present, in the moment, not in the future, then you can begin to see your existence as poetry. Your imagination is not creating a longing; it is being used in living. This living in the present is beyond tension.

Animals are not tense, trees are not tense, because they do not have the capacity to imagine. They are below tension, not beyond it. Their tension is just a potentiality; it has not become actual. They are evolving. A moment will come when tension will explode in their beings and they will begin to long for the future. It is bound to happen. The imagination becomes active.

The first thing the imagination becomes active about is the future. You create images, and because there are no corresponding realities you go on creating more and more images. But as far as the present is concerned, you cannot ordinarily conceive of the imagination in relation to it. How can you be imaginative in the present? There seems to be no need. This point must be understood.

If you can be consciously present in the present, you will not be living in your imagination. Then the imagination will be free to create within the present itself. Only the right focus is needed. If the imagination is focused on the real, it begins to create. The creation may take any form. If you are a poet, it becomes an explosion of poetry. The poetry will not be a longing for the future, but an expression of the present. Or if you are a painter, the explosion will be of painting. The painting will not be of something as you have imagined it, but as you have known it and lived it.

When you are not living in the imagination, the present moment is given to you. You can express it, or you can go into silence.

But the silence, now, is not a dead silence that is practiced. This silence too is an expression of the present moment. The moment is so deep that now it can be expressed only through silence. Not even poetry is adequate; painting is not adequate. No expression is possible. Silence is the only expression. This silence is not something negative but, rather, a positive flowering. Something has flowered within you, the flower of silence, and through this silence all that you are living is expressed.

A second point is also to be understood. This expression of the present through the imagination is neither an imagination of the future nor a reaction against the past. It is not an expression of any experience that has been known. It is the experience of experiencing – as you are living it, as it is happening in you. Not a lived experience, but a living process of experiencing.

Then your experience and experiencing are not two things. They are one and the same. Then there is no painter. The experiencing itself has become the painting; the experiencing itself has expressed itself. You are not a creator. You are creativity, a living energy. You are not a poet; you are poetry. The experience is neither for the future nor for the past; it is neither from the future nor from the past. The moment itself has become eternity, and everything comes from it. It is a flowering....

If you can feel this non-tense moment in your body, you will know a well-being that you have not known before, a positive well-being.... Your body can be non-tense only when you are living a moment-to-moment existence. If you are eating and the moment has become eternity, then there is no past and no future. The very process of eating is all that is. You are not doing something; you have become the doing. There will be no tension; your body will feel fulfilled. Or if you are in sexual communion and the sex is not just a relief from sexual tension but, rather, a positive expression of love – if the moment has become total, whole, and you are in it completely – then you will know a positive well-being in your body.

If you are running, and the running has become the totality of your existence; if you *are* the sensations that are coming to you, not something apart from them but one with them; if there is no future, no goal to this running, running itself is the goal

– then you know a positive well-being. Then your body is non-tense. On the physiological level, you have known a moment of non-tense living.[34]

Bodily tension has been created by those who, in the name of religion, have been preaching anti-body attitudes. In the West, Christianity has been emphatically antagonistic toward the body. A false division, a gulf, has been created between you and your body; then your total attitude becomes tension creating. You cannot eat in a relaxed way, you cannot sleep in a relaxed way; every bodily act becomes a tension. The body is the enemy, but you cannot exist without it. You must remain with it, you must live with your enemy, so there is constant tension; you can never relax.

Body is not your enemy, nor is it in any way unfriendly or even indifferent to you. The very existence of the body is bliss. And the moment you take the body as a gift, as a divine gift, you will come back to the body. You will love it, you will feel it – and subtle are the ways of its feeling.

You cannot feel another's body if you have not felt your own, you cannot love another's body if you have not loved your own; it is impossible. You cannot care for another person's body if you have not cared for your own – and no one cares! You may say that you care, but I insist: no one cares. Even if you seem to care, you do not really care. You are caring for some other reason – for the opinion of others, for the look in someone else's eyes; you never care for your body for yourself. You do not love your body, and if you cannot love it, you cannot be in it.

Love your body and you will feel a relaxation such as you have never felt before. Love is relaxing. When there is love, there is relaxation. If you love someone – if, between you and him or you and her, there is love – then with love comes the music of relaxation. Then relaxation is there.

When you are relaxed with someone, that is the only sign of love. If you cannot be relaxed with someone, you are not in love; the other, the enemy, is always there. That is why Sartre has said, "The other is hell." Hell is there for Sartre, it is bound to be. When there is no love flowing between the two, the other is hell, but if there is love flowing in between, the other is heaven. So whether the other is heaven or hell depends on whether there is love flowing in between.

Whenever you are in love, a silence comes. Language is lost; words become meaningless. You have much to say and nothing to say at the same time. The silence will envelop you, and in that silence, love flowers. You are relaxed. There is no future in love, there is no past; only when love has died is there a past. You only remember a dead love, a living love is never remembered; it is living, there is no gap to remember it; there is no space to remember it. Love is in the present; there is no future and no past.

If you love someone, you do not have to pretend. Then you can be what you are. You can put off your mask and be relaxed. When you are not in love, you have to wear a mask. You are tense every moment because the other is there; you have to pretend, you have to be on guard. You have to be either aggressive or defensive: it is a fight, a battle – you cannot be relaxed.

The bliss of love is more or less the bliss of relaxation. You feel relaxed, you can be what you are, you can be nude in a sense, as you are. You need not be bothered about yourself, you need not pretend. You can be open, vulnerable, and in that opening, you are relaxed.

This same phenomenon happens if you love your body; you become relaxed, you care about it. It is not wrong, it is not narcissistic to be in love with your own body. In fact, it is the first step toward spirituality. [35]

?

Whenever I am under emotional stress my body reacts. I have heard you talk about suchness and taking things as they are, and it was the key to calm down my mind. Do you have another key to calm down my body too?

The golden key of suchness is no ordinary key; it is a master key. It can work for the mind, it can work for the heart, it can work for the body; just the body will take a little longer. When you heard me talking about suchness, first your heart calmed down, felt the cool breeze of suchness, a deep acceptance of existence. But as the heart calms down it starts changing your mind. The mind is going to be number two. It will take a little longer time than the heart.

But the same key will work, and your mind will also cool down. The body will be the third, because this is the position: your being is your centre, and closest to your being is the heart; then is the circle of the mind, and then is the outer circle of the body. The body is the farthest from your being, so things reach there a little late. So lying down in your bed, allow the body also to feel suchness, that if it is suffering from a cold it is okay. A cold is not a disease but a cleansing. The inner mechanism of your body has a layer of mucus. It is a kind of lubricant to make your body function more easily, more smoothly. And just as in any mechanism you need a change of the lubricant once in a while – at least once a year, or twice a year the mucus which has become old and is not as efficient as it used to be has to be thrown out, and the body grows new mucus.

A cold is not a disease – that's why there is no medicine for colds. If it was a disease, a medicine would be possible; hence, the saying, "If you don't take the medicine your cold will last for seven days, and if you take the medicine then your cold will last for one week." Medicine or no medicine, it is not a disease, it is a cleansing. So accept it, and even when there is a certain sickness in the body, don't resist it. Use medicine, but the whole attitude, the whole psychology will be different.

Medicine can be used with two different, almost diametrically opposite viewpoints. One is to destroy the disease. That is a negative attitude. That is the attitude almost everybody lives with. One who understands suchness will not take that attitude. His attitude will be that perhaps this illness is needed at this time. You don't reject it. You are taking medicine only to help your body to accept the disease, to give your body enough strength so that you can live with the disease in suchness. You are not taking medicine against the disease; you are taking medicine to help your vitality, your health, to be strong enough so that you can accept this disease as a friend, and not create any antagonism. And you will be surprised that this idea of suchness helps you in the turmoils of your heart, emotions, feelings, in the confusions of your mind, and in the sicknesses of your body.[36]

? *I have heard you have talked about the value of relaxation. But how to relax when one is working?*

The whole society is geared for work. It is a workaholic society. It does not want you to learn relaxation, so from the very childhood it puts in your mind anti-relaxation ideas.

I am not telling you to relax the whole day. Do your work, but find out some time for yourself, and that can be found only in relaxation. And you will be surprised that if you can relax for an hour or two hours out of each twenty-four hours, it will give you a deeper insight into yourself. It will change your behaviour outwardly – you will become more calm, more quiet. It will change the quality of your work – it will be more artistic and more graceful. You will be committing fewer mistakes than you used to commit before, because now you are more together, more centred. Relaxation has miraculous powers.

It is not laziness. The lazy man may look, from the outside, as if he is not working at anything, but his mind is going as fast as it can; and the relaxed man – his body is relaxed, his mind is relaxed, his heart is relaxed. Just relaxation on all three layers – body, mind, heart – for two hours he is almost absent. In these two hours his body recovers, his heart recovers, his intelligence recovers, and you will see all that recovery in his work.

He will not be a loser – although he will not be frantic anymore, he will not be unnecessarily running hither and thither. He will go directly to the point where he wants to go. And he will do things that are needed to be done; he will not be doing unnecessary trivia. He will say only that which is needed to be said. His words will become telegraphic; his movements will become graceful; his life will become a poetry.

Relaxation can transform you to such beautiful heights – and it is such a simple technique. There is nothing much in it; just for a few days you will find it difficult because of the old habit…. Relaxation is bound to come to you. It will bring new light to your eyes, a new freshness to your being, and it will help you to understand what meditation is. It is just the first steps outside the door of the temple of meditation. With just deeper and deeper relaxation it becomes meditation.[37]

? *Will you say something about relaxation? I am aware of a tension deep at the core of me, and suspect that I have probably never been totally relaxed.*

Total relaxation is the ultimate. That's the moment when one becomes a buddha. That's the moment of realization, enlightenment, Christ-consciousness. You cannot be totally relaxed right now. At the innermost core a tension will persist.

But start relaxing. Start from the circumference – that's where we are, and we can start only from where we are. Relax the circumference of your being – relax your body, relax your behaviour, relax your acts. Walk in a relaxed way, eat in a relaxed way; talk, listen in a relaxed way. Slow down every process. Don't be in a hurry and don't be in haste. Move as if all eternity is available to you – in fact, it *is* available to you. We are here from the beginning and we are going to be here to the very end, if there is a beginning and there is an end. In fact, there is no beginning and no end. We have always been here and we will be here always. Forms go on changing, but not the substance; garments go on changing, but not the soul.

Tension means hurry, fear, doubt. Tension means a constant effort to protect, to be secure, to be safe. Tension means preparing for the tomorrow now, or for the afterlife – afraid tomorrow you will not be able to face the reality, so be prepared. Tension means the past that you have not lived really but only somehow bypassed; it hangs, it is a hangover, it surrounds you.

Remember one very fundamental thing about life: any experience that has not been lived will hang around you, will persist: "Finish me! Live me! Complete me!" There is an intrinsic quality in every experience that it tends and wants to be finished, completed. Once completed, it evaporates; incomplete, it persists, it tortures you, it haunts you, it attracts your attention. It says, "What are you going to do about me? I am still incomplete – fulfill me!"

Your whole past hangs around you with nothing completed because nothing has been lived really, everything somehow bypassed, partially lived, only so-so, in a luke-warm way. There has been no intensity, no passion. You have been moving like a somnambulist, a sleepwalker. So that past hangs, and the future creates fear. And between the past and the future is crushed your present, the only reality.

You will have to relax from the circumference. The first step in relaxing is the body. Remember as many times as possible to look in the body, whether you are carrying some tension in the body somewhere – at the neck, in the head, in the legs. Relax it consciously. Just go to that part of the body, and persuade that part, say to it lovingly "Relax!"

And you will be surprised that if you approach any part of your body, it listens, it follows you – it is *your* body! With closed eyes, go inside the body from the toe to the head searching for any place where there is a tension. And then talk to that part as you talk to a friend; let there be a dialogue between you and your body. Tell it to relax, and tell it, "There is nothing to fear. Don't be afraid. I am here to take care – you can relax." Slowly, slowly, you will learn the knack of it. Then the body becomes relaxed.

Then take another step, a little deeper; tell the mind to relax. And if the body listens, the mind also listens, but you cannot start with the mind – you have to start from the beginning. You cannot start from the middle. Many people start with the mind and they fail; they fail because they start from a wrong place. Everything should be done in the right order.

If you become capable of relaxing the body voluntarily, then you will be able to help your mind relax voluntarily. Mind is a more complex phenomenon. Once you have become confident that the body listens to you, you will have a new trust in yourself. Now even the mind can listen to you. It will take a little longer with the mind, but it happens.

When the mind is relaxed, then start relaxing your heart, the world of your feelings, emotions – which is even more complex, more subtle. But now you will be moving with trust, with great trust in yourself. Now you will know it is possible. If it is possible with the body and possible with the mind, it is possible with the heart too. And then only, when you have gone through these three steps, can you take the fourth. Now you can go to the innermost core of your being – which is beyond body, mind, heart – the very centre of your existence. And you will be able to relax it too. And that relaxation certainly brings the greatest joy possible, the ultimate in ecstasy, acceptance.

You will be full of bliss and rejoicing. Your life will have the quality of dance to it.

The whole of existence is dancing, except man. The whole of existence is in a very relaxed movement – movement there is, certainly, but it is utterly relaxed. Trees are growing and birds are chirping and rivers are flowing, stars are moving: everything is going in a very relaxed way…no hurry, no haste, no worry, and no waste. Except man. Man has fallen a victim of his mind.

Man can rise above gods and fall below animals. Man has a great spectrum. From the lowest to the highest, man is a ladder.

Start from the body, and then go slowly, slowly deeper. And don't start with anything unless you have first solved the primary. If your body is tense, don't start with the mind. Wait. Work on the body. And just small things are of immense help.

You walk at a certain pace; that has become habitual, automatic. Now try to walk slowly. Buddha used to say to his disciples: "Walk very slowly, and take each step very consciously." If you take each step very consciously, you are bound to walk slowly. If you are running, hurrying, you will forget to remember. Hence Buddha walks very slowly.

Just try walking very slowly, and you will be surprised – a new quality of awareness starts happening in the body. Eat slowly, and you will be surprised – there is great relaxation. Do everything slowly…just to change the old pattern, just to come out of old habits.

First the body has to become utterly relaxed, like a small child, then only start with the mind. Move scientifically: first the simplest, then the complex, then the more complex. And then only can you relax at the ultimate core….

Relaxation is one of the most complex phenomena – very rich, multi-dimensional. All these things are part of it: let-go, trust, surrender, love, acceptance, going with the flow, union with existence, egolessness, ecstasy. All these are part of it, and all these start happening if you learn the ways of relaxation.

Your so-called religions have made you very tense, because they have created guilt in you. My effort here is to help you get rid of all guilt and all fear. I would like to tell you: there is no hell and no heaven. So don't be afraid of hell and don't be greedy for heaven. All that exists is *this* moment. You can make this moment a hell or a heaven – that certainly is possible – but there is no heaven or hell somewhere else. Hell is when you are all tense, and heaven is when you are all relaxed. Total relaxation is paradise.[38]

When I work I am a very speedy person, but I feel a lot of stress. People tell me to relax, but it is difficult.
Can you give me some advice?

Canadian psychoanalyst, Doctor Hans Sehye, has been working his whole life on only one problem – that is stress. And he has come to certain very profound conclusions. One is that stress is not always wrong; it can be used in beautiful ways. It is not necessarily negative, but if we think that it is negative, that is not good, then we create problems. Stress in itself can be used as a stepping stone, it can become a creative form. But ordinarily we have been taught down the ages that stress is bad, that when you are in any kind of stress you become afraid. And your fear makes it even more stressful; the situation is not helped by it.

For example, there is some situation in the market that is creating a stress. The moment you feel that there is some tension, some stress, you become afraid that this should not be so: "I have to relax." Now, trying to relax will not help, because you cannot relax; in fact, trying to relax will create a new kind of stress. The stress is there and you are trying to relax and you cannot, so you are complicating the problem.

When stress is there use it as creative energy. First, accept it; there is no need to fight with it. Accept it, it is perfectly okay. It simply says, "The market is not going well, something is going wrong," "You may be a loser"...or something. Stress is simply an indication that the body is getting ready to fight with it. Now you try to relax or you take pain-killers or you take tranquilizers; you are going against the body. The body is getting ready to fight a certain situation, a certain challenge that is there: enjoy the challenge!

Even if sometimes you can't sleep in the night there is no need to be worried. Work it out, use that energy that is coming up: walk up and down, go for a run, go for a long walk, plan what you want to do, what the mind wants to do. Rather than trying to go to sleep, which is not possible, use the situation in a creative way. It simply says that the body is ready to fight with the problem; this is no time to relax. Relaxation can be done later on.

In fact if you have lived your stress totally you will come to a relaxation automatically; you can go on only so far, then the body automatically relaxes. If you want to relax in the middle you create trouble; the body cannot relax in the middle. It is almost as if an Olympic runner is getting ready, just waiting for the whistle, the signal, and he will be off, he will go like the wind. He is full of stress; now that is no time to relax. If he takes a tranquilizer he will never be of any use in the race. Or if he relaxes there and tries to do TM he will lose all. He has to use his stress: the stress is boiling, it is gathering energy. He is becoming more and more vital and potential. Now he has to sit on this stress and use it as energy, as fuel.

Sehye has given a new name for this kind of stress: he calls it 'eustress', like euphoria; it is a positive stress. When the runner has run he will fall into deep sleep;

the problem is solved. Now there is no problem, the stress disappears of its own accord.

So try this too: when there is a stressful situation don't freak out, don't become afraid of it. Go into it, use it to fight with. A man has tremendous energy and the more you use it, the more you have of it.... When it comes and there is a situation, fight, do all that you can do, really go madly into it. Allow it, accept it and welcome it. It is good, it prepares you to fight. And when you have worked it out, you will be surprised: great relaxation comes, and that relaxation is not created by you. Maybe for two, three days you cannot sleep and then for forty-eight hours you can't wake up, and that is okay!

We go on carrying many wrong notions – for example, that every person has to sleep eight hours every day. It depends what the situation is. There are situations when no sleep is needed: your house is on fire, and you are trying to sleep. Now that is not possible and that should *not* be possible; otherwise who is going to put that fire out? And when the house is on fire, all other things are put aside; suddenly your body is ready to fight the fire. You will not feel sleepy. When the fire is gone and everything settled you may fall asleep for a long period, and that will do.

Everybody does not need the same length of sleep either. A few people can do with three hours, two hours, four hours, five hours, six, eight, ten, twelve. People differ, there is no norm. And about stress also people differ.

There are two kinds of people in the world: One can be called the racehorse type and the other is the turtle type. If the racehorse type is not allowed to go fast, to go into things with speed, there will be stress; he has to be given his pace. And you are a racehorse! So forget about relaxation and things like that; they are not for you. Those are for turtles like me! So just be a racehorse, that is natural to you, and don't think of the joys that turtles are enjoying; that is not for you. You have a different kind of joy. If a turtle starts becoming a racehorse he will be in the same trouble...!

So accept your nature. You are a fighter, a warrior; you have to be that way, and that's your joy. Now, no need to be afraid; go into it whole-heartedly. Fight with the market, compete in the market, do all that you really want to do. Don't be afraid of the consequences, accept the stress. Once you accept the stress it will disappear. And not only that, you will feel very happy because you have started using it; it is a kind of energy.

Don't listen to people who say to relax; that is not for you. Your relaxation will come only after you have earned it by hard labour. One has to understand one's type. Once the type is understood there is no problem; then one can follow a clean-cut line. [39]

? *How would you define the state of hypertension?*

Hypertension is a state of mind when you have been become too much focused on rationality and you have forgotten your feelings. Hypertension comes out of an imbalance; too much trust in reason is the basis of all hypertension. People who live in their heads become hypertense. Relaxation comes through the heart. One should be capable of moving easily from the head to the heart, just as you move out of your house and inside your house. One should be fluid between head and heart. These are the two shores of the river that you are. You should not cling to one shore, otherwise life becomes lopsided.

The West suffers very much from hypertension, because it has forgotten the language of the heart, and only the heart knows how to relax because only the heart knows how to love. Only the heart knows how to enjoy, celebrate. Only the heart knows how to dance and sing. The head knows nothing of dance – the head condemns dance as stupid. The head knows nothing of poetry, the head condemns poetry.

Do you know that one of the greatest philosophers, Plato, thinking about his ultimate utopian republic, said that no poet should be allowed there? In his republic, in his ultimate state of society, poets should not be allowed. Why? – because he is afraid of poets. He says: Poets bring fantasies, poets bring dreams, poets bring confusion and mysticism, and we don't want any of it. We want a very clear-cut, logical, prosaic society. That society will be hypertense; everybody will be neurotic. In Plato's republic – if it ever happens, and there is every fear that it can happen – everybody will be a neurotic, and everybody will always be carrying his psychoanalyst with him. Wherever he moves, he will have to carry his psychoanalyst. That is already coming in the West.

I have heard: In a New York street two small boys were talking – as they have always talked down the centuries, but what they said was very new. One boy said to the other, "My psychoanalyst can lick your psychoanalyst any time." Small boys, they have always talked that way: "My father can lick your father," or "My house is bigger than your house," or "My dog is stronger than your dog" – a small child's beginning of the ego. But, "My psychoanalyst can lick your psychoanalyst any time" – this is something new.

Three women were talking about their children. One was saying, "He is the top-most in the class. He always comes first."

98

The second said, "That's nothing. My child is only seven but he can play music like a Mozart, like a Wagner."

The third said, "That's nothing. My child is only five and he goes to his psychoanalyst all alone."

Hypertension is a state where you have lost balance. You cannot bring your heart to function in your life; logic has become all – and logic remains superficial. Logic, when it becomes all, only creates anxiety; it never gives any peace, it goes on bringing new problems. It never solves any problem – it cannot solve, it is not in its power – it only pretends, it only promises. It goes on saying, "I will deliver the goods," but it never delivers them. Then problems go on accumulating and you don't know how to get out of the problems, because you don't know how to get out of the head. You don't know how to play with children, how to love your woman, how to go and have a talk with the trees and sometimes have a dialogue with the stars. You have forgotten all, you are no longer a poet, you are no longer an alive heart.

And whenever any part of the body is repressed, that part takes revenge. If another part of the mind is repressed that part takes revenge. And the heart is the most vital part, the most fundamental part. One can live without the head, but one cannot live without heart. The head is a little superficial, it is a kind of luxury, but the heart is very essential. The head exists only in man, so it cannot be very essential. Animals live without it and live perfectly well in a far more silent and blissful way than man. Trees live without the head, and so do the birds and the children and the mystics.

The head is superficial. It has a certain function – use it, but don't be used by it. Once you are being used by it you will become anxious: anxiety will come and life will become nauseating. It will just be a long, stretched-out pain, and you will not find any oasis anywhere in it; it will be a desert thing. Remember, the essential has not to be repressed. The non-essential has to follow the essential, has to become its shadow. You cannot deny *anything* without getting into trouble. Listen to this anecdote:

One day a flying saucer landed in Elsie Gumtree's garden, right in the middle of her summer bloomers – which could have been quite painful if she had been wearing them. There was a whirring sound, and a strange purple man appeared through the hatch in the side of the saucer. Straight away he headed for Elsie's back door and knocked politely.

Elsie opened the door, and quickly taking in the situation said, "Are you from the flying saucer?"

"Mm," replied the man, as though in pain.

"Are you from Mars?" Elsie asked.

"Mm," went the man again, his face contorted.

"How long did it take you to get here? Ten years?" asked Elsie.

"Mm."

"Twenty years?"

"Mm," said the man, an agonized look on his face.

"Twenty years? You've been all that time in your flying saucer?"

"Mm," nodded the man, furiously.

"What can I do for you?" asked Elsie.

The little man opened his mouth, and with great difficulty said, "Can I use your toilet, please?"

Deny anything and it becomes overpowering. Now, for twenty years he has not been able to find a toilet and you are asking nonsense questions: "Where are you coming from?" and "Who are you?" and "How many...?" How can he answer all these things? His denied part is there with a vengeance.

Your heart has been denied for so many lives that when it erupts it is going to create great chaos in your life. First you suffer from the mind, its tensions, anxieties; and then you can suffer from the explosion of the heart. That's what happens when a man breaks down. First he suffers from the tense state of the mind, and then one day the heart takes its revenge, erupts, and the man goes mad, goes berserk.

Both situations are bad. First the sanity was too much – that created the insanity. A really sane person is one who can live between sanity and insanity in absolute balance. A really sane person always has some insanity in him – he accepts it. A really rational person is one who respects irrationality too, because life is such. If you cannot laugh because of your reason – because "laughter is ridiculous" – then you are bound for trouble, you are destined for trouble. Yes, logic is good, laughter too is good – and laughter brings balance. It is good to be serious, it is good to be non-serious too, and there should be a constant balancing.

Have you seen a tightrope walker? He continuously balances himself. Sometimes he leans to the left with his staff, and then he comes to a point where if he leans a single moment more, he will fall. He immediately changes his balance, goes to the other side – to the right – leans to the right. Then again a moment comes when one single moment more and he will be gone; he again starts leaning to the left. That's how he proceeds: leaning to the left, to the right, he keeps in between. That's the beauty – leaning to the left and to the right, leaning toward both extremes, he keeps in between.

If you want to keep yourself in between you will have to lean toward both sides again and again. You are not to choose. If you choose, you will fall. If you have chosen the head, you will fall; you will become hypertense. If you choose the heart and forget the head completely, you will become mad. And if you want to choose anyhow, if you want to choose, then choose being mad. Choose the heart, because it is more essential.

But I am not saying that you should choose. If you insist and you say, "I *have* to choose," then be mad rather than just dry and sane. Be of the heart. Love, love madly; sing, sing madly; dance, dance madly. That is far better than just becoming calculating, logical, rational, and just suffering nightmares.

But I am not saying…it is not *my* suggestion that you do that. My suggestion is to remain choiceless. 'Choiceless awareness' is the keyword. Remain choiceless, aware, and whenever you see that something is going off-balance, lean to the other side. Bring the balance again, and this is how one moves. Life is like tightrope walking.[40]

CHAPTER 7

DEPRESSION

? *In the olden days it was called melancholia; today it is called depression, and it counts as one of the major psychological problems of developed countries. It is described as a sense of despair or hopelessness, a lack of self-esteem with no enthusiasm or interest in the surroundings. In addition, there are physical symptoms of poor appetite, sleeplessness and a loss of sexual energy. Electroshock treatment has largely been abandoned today, and drugs and talk therapy seem equally effective — or ineffective. Explanations for depression have varied from the chemical to the psychological.*

What is depression? Is it a reaction to a depressing world, a kind of hibernation during 'the winter of our discontent'? Is depression just a reaction to repression — or oppression — or is it just a form of self-repression?

Man has always lived with hope, a future, a paradise somewhere far away. He has never lived in the present — his golden age is still to come. It kept him enthusiastic because greater things were going to happen; all his longings were going to be fulfilled. There was great joy in anticipation. He suffered in the present; he was miserable in the present. But all that was completely forgotten in the dreams that were going to be fulfilled tomorrow. Tomorrow has always been life-giving.

But the situation has changed. The old situation was not good because the tomorrow — the fulfillment of his dreams — never became true. He died hoping. Even in his death he was hoping for a future life — but he never actually experienced any rejoicing, any meaning. But it was tolerable. It was only a question of today: it will pass, and tomorrow is bound to come. The religious prophets, messiahs, saviours were promising him all pleasures – which are condemned here – in paradise. The political leaders, the social ideologists, the utopians were promising him the same thing – not in paradise but here on earth, somewhere far away in the future when the society goes through a total revolution and there is no poverty, no classes, no government and man is absolutely free and has everything that he needs.

Both are basically fulfilling the same psychological need. To those who were materialistic, the ideological, political, sociological utopians were appealing; to those who were not so materialistic, the religious leaders appealed. But the object of appeal was exactly the same: all that you can imagine, can dream of, can long for, will be absolutely fulfilled. With those dreams, the present miseries seemed to be very small.

There was enthusiasm in the world; people were not depressed. Depression is a contemporary phenomenon and it has come into being because now there is no tomorrow. All political ideologies have failed. There is no possibility that man will ever be equal, no possibility that there will be a time when there will be no government, no possibility that all your dreams will be fulfilled.

This has come as a great shock. Simultaneously man has become more mature. He may go to the church, to the mosque, to the synagogue, to the temple – but they are only social conformities, because he does not want, in such a dark and depressed state, to be left alone; he wants to be with the crowd. But basically he knows there is no paradise; he knows that no saviour is going to come.

Hindus have waited five thousand years for Krishna. He promised not only that he would come once, he promised that whenever there was misery, suffering, whenever vice was on top of virtue, whenever nice and simple and innocent people were exploited by the cunning and the hypocritical, he would come. But for five thousand years no sign has been seen of him.

Jesus has promised he will come, and when asked when, he said, "Very soon." I can stretch "Very soon," but not for two thousand years; that is too much.

The idea that our misery, our pain, our anguish will be taken away is no longer appealing. The idea that there is a God who cares for us seems to be simply a joke. Looking at the world, it doesn't seem as if there is anybody who cares.

In fact, in England there are almost thirty thousand people who are devil worshippers – just in England, a small part of the world. And their ideology is worth looking at in reference to your question. They say that the devil is not against God, the devil is God's son. God has abandoned the world, and now the only hope is to persuade the devil to take care as God is not taking care. And thirty thousand people are worshipping the devil as a son of God…and the reason is they feel that God has abandoned the world – he no longer cares about it. Naturally, the only way is to appeal to his son; if somehow he can be persuaded by rituals, by prayer, by worship, perhaps the misery, the darkness, the sickness can be removed. This is a desperate effort.

The reality is that man has always lived in poverty. Poverty has one thing beautiful about it: it never destroys your hope, it never goes against your dreams, it always brings enthusiasm for tomorrow. One is hopeful, believing that things will be better: this dark period is already passing; soon there will be light. But that situation has changed. In the developed countries...and remember, the problem of depression is not in undeveloped countries – in the poor countries, people are still hopeful – it is only in the developed countries, where they have everything that they had always longed for. Now paradise will not do anymore; nor can a classless society help anymore. No utopia is going to be better. They have achieved the goal – and this achievement of the goal is the cause of depression. Now there is no hope: tomorrow is dark, and the day after tomorrow will be even darker.

All these things that they have dreamed of were very beautiful. They had never looked at the implications of them. Now that they have got them, they have got them with the implications. A man is poor, but he has an appetite. A man is rich, but he has no appetite. And it is better to be poor and have an appetite than to be rich and have no appetite. What are you going to do with all your gold, all your silver, all your dollars? You cannot eat them. You have everything, but the appetite has disappeared for which you have been struggling all along. You succeeded – and I have said again and again that nothing fails like success. You have reached a place that you wanted to reach, but you were not aware of the by-products. You have millions of dollars, but you cannot sleep....

When man reaches to the cherished goals, then he becomes aware that there are many things around them. For example, for your whole life you try to earn money, thinking that one day, when you have it, you will live a relaxed life. But you have been tense your whole life – tension has become your discipline – and at the end of life, when you have achieved all the money you wanted, you cannot relax. The whole life disciplined in tension and anguish and worry won't let you relax. So you are not a winner, you are a loser. You lose your appetite, you destroy your health, you destroy your sensibility, your sensitiveness. You destroy your aesthetic sense – because there is no time for all these things which do not produce dollars.

You are running after dollars – who has time to look at the roses, and who has time to look at the birds on the wing, and who has time to look at the beauty of human beings? You postpone all these things so that one day, when you have everything, you will relax and enjoy. But by the time you have everything, you have become a certain kind of disciplined person – who is blind to roses, who is blind to beauty, who cannot enjoy music, who cannot understand dance, who cannot understand poetry, who can only understand dollars. But those dollars give no satisfaction.

This is the cause of depression. That's why it is only in the developed countries and only in the richer class of the developed countries – in the developed countries there are poor people also, but they don't suffer from depression – and now you cannot give a man any more hope to remove his depression because he has all, more than you can promise. His condition is really pitiable. He never thought of implications, he never thought of by-products, he never thought of what he would lose by gaining money. He never thought that he would lose everything that could make him happy just because he has always pushed all those things aside. He had no time, and the competition was tough and he had to be tough. At the end he finds his heart is dead, his life is meaningless. He doesn't see that there is any possibility in the future of any change, because "What more is there…?"

I used to stay in Sagar in a very rich man's house. The old man was very beautiful. He was the greatest *bidi* manufacturer in the whole of India. He had everything that you can imagine, but he was absolutely unable to enjoy anything. Enjoyment is something that has to be nourished. It is a certain discipline, a certain art – how to enjoy – and it takes time to get in contact with the great things in life. But the man who is running after money bypasses everything that is a door to the divine, and he ends up at the end of the road and there is nothing ahead of him except death.

His whole life he was miserable. He tolerated it, ignored it in the hope that things were going to change. Now he cannot ignore it and cannot tolerate it because tomorrow there is only death and nothing else. And the whole life's accumulated misery that he has ignored, the suffering that he has ignored, explodes in his being.

The richest man, in a way, is the poorest man in the world. To be rich and not to be poor is a great art. To be poor and to be rich is the other side of the art. There are poor people whom you will find immensely rich. They don't have anything, but they are rich. Their richness is not in things but in their being, in their multidimensional experiences. And there are rich people who have everything but are absolutely poor and hollow and empty. Deep inside there is just a graveyard.

It is not a depression of the society, because then it would affect the poor too; it is simply natural law, and man now will have to learn it. Up to now there was no need, because nobody had reached to a point where he had everything, while inside there was complete darkness and ignorance.

The first thing in life is to find meaning in the present moment.

The basic flavour of your being should be of love, of rejoicing, of celebration. Then you can do anything; dollars will not destroy it. But you put everything aside and simply run after dollars thinking that dollars can purchase everything. And then one day you find they cannot purchase anything – and you have devoted your whole life to dollars.

This is the cause of depression. And particularly in the West, the depression is going to be very deep. In the East there have been rich people, but there was a certain dimension available. When the road to richness came to an end, they did not remain stuck there; they moved into a new direction. That new direction was in the air, available for centuries. In the East the poor have been in a very good condition, and the rich have been in a tremendously good condition. The poor have learned contentment so they do not bother about running after ambition. And the rich have understood that one day you have to renounce it all and go in search of truth, in search of meaning.

In the West, at the end, the road simply ends. You can go back, but going back will not help your depression. You need a new direction. Gautam Buddha, Mahavira, or Parshvanath – these people were at the peak of richness, and then they saw that it is almost a burden. Something else has to be found before death takes you over – and they were courageous enough to renounce all. Their renunciation has been misunderstood. They renounced it all because they did not want to bother a single second more for money, for power – because they have seen the top, and there is nothing there. They went to the very highest rung of the ladder and found that it leads nowhere; it is just a ladder leading nowhere. While you are somewhere in the middle, or lower than the middle, you have a hope because there are other rungs higher than you. There comes a point when you are on the highest rung and there is only suicide or madness – or hypocrisy: you go on smiling till death finishes you, but deep down you know that you have wasted your life.

In the East, depression has never been a problem. The poor learned to enjoy whatsoever little they had, and the rich learned that having the whole world at your feet means nothing – you have to go in a search for meaning, not for money. And they had precedents: for thousands of years people have gone in search of truth and have found it. There is no need to be in despair, in depression, you just have to move into an unknown dimension. They have never explored it, but as they start exploring the new dimension – it means a journey inwards, a journey to their own self – all that they have lost starts returning.

The West needs a great movement of meditation very urgently; otherwise, this depression is going to kill people. And these people will be the talented ones – because they achieved power, they achieved money, they achieved whatsoever they wanted…the highest degrees in education. These are the talented people, and they are all feeling despair.

This is going to be dangerous because the most talented people are no longer enthusiastic about life, and the untalented are enthusiastic about life but they don't even have the talents to get power, money, education, respectability. They don't have the talents, so they are suffering, feeling handicapped. They are turning into terrorists, they are turning towards unnecessary violence just out of revenge – because they cannot do anything else. But they can destroy. And the rich are almost ready to hang themselves from any tree because there is no reason for them to live. Their hearts have stopped beating long ago. They are just corpses – well decorated, well honoured, but utterly empty and futile.

The West is really in a far worse condition than the East, although to those who don't understand it seems that the West is in a better condition than the East because the East is poor. But poverty is not as big a problem as is the failure of richness; then a man is really poor. An ordinary poor man at least has dreams, hopes, but the rich man has nothing.

What is needed is a great meditation movement reaching to every person.

And in the West these people who are depressed are going to psychoanalysts, therapists and all kinds of charlatans who are themselves depressed, more depressed than their patients – naturally, because the whole day they are hearing about depression, despair, meaninglessness. And seeing so many talented people in such a bad state, they themselves start losing their spirit. They cannot help; they themselves need help.

The function of my school is going to be to prepare people with meditative energy and send them into the world just as examples for those who are depressed. If they can see that there are people who are not depressed – but on the contrary, who are immensely joyous – perhaps a hope may be born into them. Now they can have every-thing and there is no need to worry. They can meditate.

I don't teach renunciation of your wealth or of anything. Let everything be as it is. Just add one thing more to your life. Up to now you have been adding only things to your life. Now add something to your being – and that will do the music, that will do the miracle, that will do the magic, that will create a new thrill, a new youth, a new freshness.

It is not unsolvable. The problem is big, but the solution is very simple.[41]

CHAPTER 8

ADDICTIONS

? *What is the basic cause of addiction, any addiction?*

All around you there are people whose vested interest is that you should not live totally. It is surprising: why are they so interested that people do not live totally? Because their whole exploitation of humanity depends on it.

A man who lives totally will not drink alcohol, or take any other kind of drug. Naturally, the people who are earning millions of dollars out of alcohol and drugs cannot allow you to live totally. To live totally is so joyous that you don't want to destroy your joy by drinking alcohol. Alcohol is needed by miserable people, by people who are troubled, by people who want somehow to forget their problems, their anxieties – at least for a few hours. The alcohol is not going to change anything – but even a rest for a few hours seems to be an absolute necessity for millions of people.

If a man lives totally, his every moment is such a fulfillment that you will not see queues before movie halls – who wants to see somebody else making love? When you yourself can make love, why should you go to the movie house? When your own life is such a mystery and such a tremendous challenge to discover, who is going to be interested in third-class film stories?

The man who lives totally becomes unambitious. Because he is so happy right now, he cannot conceive that there is the possibility of more. The ordinary madness of man's mind – of desiring for more and more – is because you are not living totally.

There is always a gap, something is missing. You know things could have been better. Out of this partial living all ambitions arise, and then the whole game of the society goes on: people want to become rich, people want to become famous, people want to become politicians, people want to become presidents and prime ministers.

Up to now humanity has depended on not allowing man to live totally, creating all kinds of barriers, because the total man will destroy so many vested interests in the world. The total man is the most dangerous man to the vested interests. You cannot enslave a man who is enjoying his life in its fullness, in its wholeness. You cannot force him to go into the army to kill people and to be killed. Your whole structure of society will collapse.

With the total man coming in, there will be a different structure of society: unambitious but immensely joyful – without great men. Perhaps you have never thought about it: great men can exist only because millions of people are not great; otherwise, who is going to remember Gautam Buddha? If there were millions of Gautam Buddhas, millions of Mahaviras, millions of Jesus Christs, who would bother about these people? These few people have become great because millions are not allowed to live totally. Who will go to the churches if people are not miserable…to the temples, to the synagogues, to the mosques? Who is going to be there? Who is going to bother about God, and heaven and hell? A man who is living each moment with such intensity that life itself has become a paradise, that life itself has become divine, need not be a worshipper of dead statues, dead scriptures, rotten ideologies, stupid superstitions.

The total man is the greatest risk in the world to your existing establishment.[42]

? *Do I have to know and understand the roots of my old patterns in order to be able to drop them, or is awareness enough?*

This is the dividing line between Western psychology and Eastern mysticism. Western psychology is an effort to understand the roots of your old patterns, but it does not help anybody to get rid of them. You become more understanding, you become more sober, you become more normal; your mind is no longer a great mess. Things are settled a little better than they ever have been before, but every problem remains the same – it simply goes dormant. You can understand your jealousy, you can understand your anger, your hate, your greed, your ambitions, but all this understanding will remain intellectual. So even the greatest psychologists of the West are far away from the Eastern mystics.

The man who founded Western psychology, Sigmund Freud, was so much afraid of death that even the mention of the word 'death' was enough to throw him into a coma; he would become unconscious, the paranoia of death was so great. It happened three times. He was so much afraid of ghosts that he would not pass by the side of a cemetery. Now, a man like Sigmund Freud who has tremendous intellectual acumen, who knows every root of the mind, who knows every subtle functioning of the mind, still remains confined in the mind.

Awareness leads you beyond the mind. It does not bother to understand the problems of the mind, their roots; it simply leaves the mind aside, it simply gets out of it. That is the reason why there has been no development of psychology in the East. It is strange that for ten thousand years, at least, the East has been consistently and one-pointedly working in the field of human consciousness, but it has not developed any psychology, any psychoanalysis or psychosynthesis. It is a great surprise that for ten thousand years nobody even touched the matter. Rather than understanding the mind, the East developed a totally different approach, and their approach was disidentifying with the mind: "I am not the mind." Once this awareness becomes crystallized in you, the mind becomes impotent.

The whole power of the mind is in your identification with it. So it was found to be useless to unnecessarily go digging for roots, finding causes behind causes, working out through dreams, analyzing dreams, interpreting dreams. And every psychologist finds a different root, finds a different interpretation, finds a different cause. Psychology is not yet a science; it is still fictitious.

If you go to Sigmund Freud, your dream will be interpreted in sexual terms. His mind is obsessed with sex. Bring anything and immediately he will find an interpretation that it is sexual. Go to Alfred Adler – the man who founded another school of psychology, analytical psychology – he is obsessed with another idea: will to power. So whatever you dream will be interpreted according to that idea – it is will to power. Go to Carl Gustav Jung; he interprets every dream as a faraway echo from your past lives. His interpretation is mythological. And there are many other schools.

There has been a great effort made by Assagioli – psychosynthesis – to bring all these schools together, but his psychosynthesis is absolutely useless. At least psychoanalysis has some truth in it, and analytical psychology also has some truth in it; but psychosynthesis is simply a hodge-podge. It has taken one part from one school, another part from another school, and it has joined them together. Assagioli is a great intellectual; he could manage to put the pieces of the jigsaw puzzle in the right places. But what was significant in Sigmund Freud was significant in a certain context; that context is no longer there. He has only taken what appears to be significant, but without the context it loses all meaning. Hence, Assagioli has worked his whole life for some synthesis, but he has not been able to create anything significant. And all these schools have been working hard.

But the East simply bypassed the mind. Rather than finding out the causes and roots and reasons, they found out one thing: from where does the mind get its power? From where does the energy come to feed it? The energy to feed the mind comes from your identification that "I am it." They broke that bridge. That's what awareness is: being aware that "I am not the body, I am not the mind. I am not even the heart – I am simply pure awareness." As this awareness deepens, becomes crystallized, the mind has more and more a shadow existence. Its impact on you loses all force. And when the awareness is a hundred percent settled, mind simply evaporates.

Western psychology still has to figure out why it is not succeeding. Thousands of people are going through psychoanalysis and through other therapeutic methods, but not a single one of them – not even the founder of those schools – can be called enlightened, can be said to be without problems, can be said to be without anxieties, anguishes, fears, paranoia. Everything exists in them as it exists in you.

Sigmund Freud was asked many times by his disciples, "You psychoanalyze all of us; we bring our dreams to you to be interpreted. It will be a great experiment if you allow us to psychoanalyze you. You give us your dreams and we will try to analyze and find out what they mean, from where they come, what they indicate." But Sigmund Freud never agreed to that. That shows an immense weakness in the whole framework of psychoanalysis. He was afraid that they would find the same things in his dreams that he was finding in their dreams. Then his superiority as a founder, as a master, would be lost.

He was not aware at all of people like Gautam Buddha or Mahavira or Nagarjuna. Because these people don't dream, there is nothing to analyze. These people have come so far away from the mind that all connections are cut. They live out of aware- ness, not out of intellect. They respond out of awareness, not out of mind and its memories. And they don't repress anything; hence there is no need for any dreaming.

Dreaming is a by-product of repression. There are aboriginal tribes where people don't dream, or if they dream, they dream only once in a while. They are surprised to know that civilized people dream almost the whole night. In eight hours' sleep, six hours you are dreaming. And the aboriginal is simply sleeping eight hours in deep silence, with no disturbance. Sigmund Freud was aware only of the sick Western people, he was not aware of the men of awareness; otherwise the whole history of Western psychology would have been different.

I will not tell you to make an effort to understand the roots of your mind and its patterns; it is simply a useless wastage of time. Just awareness is enough, more than enough. As you become aware, you come out of the grip of the mind, and the mind remains almost a dead fossil. There is no need to bother from where the greed came, the real question is how to get out of it. The question is not from where the ego arose – these are intellectual questions which are not significant for a seeker.

And then there will be many philosophical standpoints: from where greed arose, from where ego came in; from where your jealousy, from where your hate, from where your cruelty came in – looking for the beginnings of all this. And mind is a vast complex; in fact, life is too small to figure out all the problems of the mind and their origins. Their origins may be of thousands of lives. Slowly Western psychology is coming closer to it – for example, primal therapy.

Janov understood that unless we find the beginnings of the problems – that means to him, being a Christian, believing only in one life, the roots must be found somewhere in childhood. So he started working to remind you of your childhood, and then he stumbled upon a new fact – that in deep hypnosis people not only remember their childhood, they remember their birth. They also remember the nine months in the mother's womb, and a few very sensitive people even remember their previous life.

And then he himself became afraid, that he was going into a tunnel which seemed to be unending. You go into the past life and that will take you again, through the whole long passage, to another life. Your mind is many lives old, so you are not going to be able to find its root in the present. Perhaps you will have to travel backwards through thousands of lives, and it is not an easy thing. And then too, even if you come to understand from where the greed has come, it does not make any change. You will have to then know how to drop it. And there are so many problems that if you start dropping each problem separately you will need millions of lives to be completely finished with the mind. And while you are figuring out about one problem, other problems are growing, gathering more energy, more vitality, more influence. It is a very stupid game.

In the East, not a single person in the whole past – in China, in India, in Japan, in Arabia – has ever bothered about it. It is fighting with shadows. They worked from a very different angle and they succeeded immensely. They simply pulled their awareness out of the mind. They stood outside the mind as a witness and they found a miracle happening: as they became a witness, the mind became impotent, it lost all power over them. And there was no need to understand anything.

Awareness goes on growing higher and the mind goes on growing smaller – in the same proportion. If awareness is fifty percent then mind is cut to fifty percent. If awareness is seventy percent, only thirty percent of the mind remains. The day awareness is a hundred percent, there is no mind to be found at all.

Hence, the whole Eastern approach is to find a state of no-mind – that silence, that purity, that serenity. And mind is no longer there with all its problems, with all its roots; it has simply evaporated the way dewdrops evaporate in the sun in the morning, leaving no trace behind. Hence I will say to you, awareness is not only enough, it is more than enough. You don't need anything else.

Western psychology has no place for meditation in it yet, and that's why it keeps on going round and round, finding no solution. There are people who have been in psychoanalysis for fifteen years. They have wasted fortunes on it – because psychoanalysis is the most highly paid profession. Fifteen years in psychoanalysis and all that has happened is that they have become addicted to psychoanalysis. Now they cannot remain without it. Rather than solving any problem, a new problem has arisen. Now it has become almost like a drug addiction. So when they get fed up with one psychoanalyst, they start with another. If they are not being psychoanalyzed, then they feel something is missing.

But it has not helped anybody. Even they accept that there is not a single man in the whole West who has been completely analyzed. But such is the blindness of people that they cannot see the simple point, why there is not a single person – when there are thousands of psychoanalysts analyzing people – who has been perfectly analyzed and who has gone beyond mind.

Analysis cannot take you beyond. The way beyond is awareness, the way beyond mind is meditation. It is a simple way and it has created thousands of enlightened people in the East. And they were not doing anything with the mind, they were doing something else: they were simply becoming aware, alert, conscious. They were using mind also as an object.

The way you see a tree, the way you see pillars, the way you see other people – they were trying to see the mind also as separate, and they succeeded. And the moment they succeeded in seeing the mind as separate, that was the death of the mind. In its place grows a clarity; intellect disappears, intelligence arises. One does not react anymore, one responds. Reaction is always based on your past experiences, and response is just like a mirror: you come in front of it and it responds, it shows your face. It does not carry any memory. The moment you have moved away, it is again pure, no reflection.

The meditator becomes finally a mirror. Any situation is reflected in him and he responds in the present moment, out of presence. Hence, his every response has a newness, a freshness, a clarity, a beauty, a grace. It is not some old idea that he is repeating. This is something to be understood, that no situation is ever exactly the same as any other situation that you have encountered before. So if you are reacting out of the past, you are not able to tackle the situation; you are lagging far behind.

That is the cause of your failure. You don't see the situation, you are more concerned with your response; you are blind to the situation. The man of meditation is simply open, with his eyes available to see the situation and let the situation provoke the response in him. He is not carrying a ready-made answer to it.

A beautiful story about Gautam Buddha.... One morning a man asked him, "Is there a God?" Buddha looked at the man, looked into his eyes and said, "No, there is no God."

That very day, in the afternoon, another man asked, "What do you think about God? Is there a God?" Again he looked at the man and into his eyes and said, "Yes, there is a God."

Ananda, who was with him, became very much puzzled, but he was always very careful not to interfere in anything. He had his time when everybody had left in the night and Buddha was going to sleep; if he had to ask anything, he would ask at that time.

But by the evening, as the sun was setting, a third man came with almost the same question, formulated differently. He said, "There are people who believe in God, there are people who don't believe in God. I myself don't know with whom I should stand. Help me."

Ananda was very intensely listening now to what Buddha says. He had given two absolutely contradictory answers in the same day, and now the third opportunity has arisen – and there is no third answer. But Buddha gave him the third answer. He did not speak, he closed his eyes. It was a beautiful evening. The birds had settled in their trees – Buddha was staying in a mango grove – the sun had set, a cool breeze had started blowing. The man, seeing Buddha sitting with closed eyes, thought that perhaps this is his answer, so he also sat with closed eyes with him.

An hour passed, the man opened his eyes, touched the feet of Buddha and said, "Your compassion is great. You have given me the answer. I will always remain obliged to you."

Ananda could not believe it, because Buddha had not spoken a single word. And as the man went away, perfectly satisfied and contented, Ananda asked Buddha, "This is too much! You should think of me – you will drive me mad. I am just on the verge of a nervous breakdown. To one man you say there is no God, to another man you say there is a God, and to the third you don't answer. And that strange fellow says that he has received the answer and he is perfectly satisfied and obliged, and touches your feet. What is going on?"

Buddha said, "Ananda, the first thing you have to remember is, those were not your questions, those answers were not given to you. Why did you get unnecessarily concerned with other people's problems? First solve your own problems."

Ananda said, "That's true, they were not my questions and the answers were not given to me. But what can I do? I have ears and I hear, and I have heard and I have seen, and now my whole being is puzzled – what is right?"

Buddha said, "Right? Right is awareness. The first man was a theist. He wanted my support – he already believed in God. He had come with an answer, ready-made, just to solicit my support so that he can go around and say, 'I am right, even Buddha thinks so.' I had to say no to him, just to disturb his belief, because belief is not knowing. The second man was an atheist. He had also come with a ready-made answer, that there is no God, and he wanted my support to strengthen his disbelief and so he can go on proclaiming around that I agree with him. I had to say to him, 'Yes, God exists.' But my purpose was the same.

"If you see my purpose, there is no contradiction. I was disturbing the first man's preconceived belief, I was disturbing the second person's preconceived disbelief. Belief is positive, disbelief is negative, but both are the same. Neither of them was a knower and neither of them was a humble seeker; they were already carrying a prejudice.

"The third man was a seeker. He had no prejudice, he had opened his heart. He told me, 'There are people who believe, there are people who don't believe. I myself don't know whether God exists or not. Help me.' And the only help I could give was to teach him a lesson of silent awareness; words were useless. And as I closed my eyes he understood the hint. He was a man of certain intelligence – open, vulnerable. He closed his eyes.

"As I moved deeper into silence, as he became part of the field of my silence and my presence, he started moving into silence, moving into awareness. When one hour had passed, it seemed as if only a few minutes had passed. He had not received any answer in words, but he had received the authentic answer in silence: don't be bothered about God; it does not matter whether God exists or does not exist. What matters is whether silence exists, awareness exists or not. If you are silent and aware, you yourself are a god. God is not something far away from you; either you are a mind or you are a god. In silence and awareness mind melts and disappears and reveals your divineness to you. Although I have not said anything to him, he has received the answer, and received it in a perfectly right way."

Awareness brings you to a point where you are able to see with your own eyes the ultimate reality of yourself and the universe...and a miraculous experience that you and the universe are not separate, that you are part of the whole. To me this is the only meaning of holy.

You have been trained for analysis, for understanding, for intellectual gymnastics. Those things are not going to help anybody; they have never helped anybody. That's why the West lacks one most precious dimension – that of enlightenment, awakening. All its richness is nothing in comparison to the richness that comes from enlightenment, from achieving the state of no-mind.

So don't get entangled with the mind; rather, become a watcher by the side of the road and let the mind pass on the road. Soon the road will be empty. The mind lives as a parasite. You are identified with it; that is its life. Your awareness cuts the connection, it becomes its death.

The ancient scriptures of the East say that the master is a death – a very strange statement, but of immense meaning. The master is a death because meditation is the death of the mind, meditation is the death of the ego. Meditation is the death of your personality and the birth and the resurrection of your essential being. And to know that essential being is to know all.

Becky Goldberg phoned down to the hotel manager. "I am up here in room five hundred and ten," she shouted angrily, "and I want you to know there is a man walking around the room across the way stark naked, and his blinds are up."

"I will be up right away," said the manager. He entered Becky's room, peered through the window and said, "You are right, Madam, the man does appear to be naked. But his window still covers him from the waist down, no matter where he is in the room."

"Ah, yes," yelled Becky. "Just stand on the bed, just stand on the bed!"

Mind is a strange fellow. Where there is no problem, it creates a problem. Why should you stand on the bed? Just to find that somebody is naked in his room? One has to be aware of all these stupidities of the mind. I don't agree with the theory of evolution of Charles Darwin, but I have a certain respect for the theory, because it may not be historically true that the monkeys became men, but it is certainly psychologically true – because man's mind is just like a monkey...stupid in every way.

There is no point in digging deep into the rubbish of the mind. It is not your being, it is not you; it is just the dust that you have gathered through many, many lives around you.

A young woman went to the doctor, afraid that she had gangrene because of two small spots, one on each of her thighs. The doctor examined her carefully and then told her it was not gangrene and she had nothing to worry about. "But by the way," he asked the girl as she was leaving, "is your boyfriend a gypsy?"

"Yes," replied the girl, "as a matter of fact he is."

"Well," said the doctor, "tell him that his earrings are not gold."

These are mind's functionings – it is a great discoverer.

The old definition of a philosopher is that he is blind, in a dark night, in a dark house where there is no light, and he is searching for a black cat which is not there. But this is not all: he finds her! And he writes great treatises, theses, systems, proves logically the existence of the black cat.

Beware of the mind: it is blind. It has never known anything but it is a great pretender. It pretends to know everything.

Socrates has categorized humanity into two classes. One class he calls the knowledgeably ignorant: the people who think they know and they are basically ignorant; that is the work of the mind. And the second category he calls the ignorant knowers: the people who think, "We don't know." In their humbleness, in their innocence, descends knowing.

So there are pretenders of knowledge – that is the function of the mind – and there are humble people who say, "We don't know." In their innocence there is knowledge, and that is the work of meditation and awareness.[43]

? *I have always felt the need for little rewards at the end of the day: a few beers, cigarettes or drugs. Now none of these things bring any satisfaction, yet the desire for something, some form of gratification, continues. What is this longing and what will satisfy it?*

Nothing will satisfy it. There is a subtle mechanism of desire to be understood. Desire functions in this way: desire places a condition on your happiness. "I will be happy if I can get this car, this woman, this house." Fulfillment of the desire removes that condition on your happiness. In your relief you feel good. Actually all you have done is remove a quite unnecessary obstruction to your happiness, but it is not long before you find yourself thinking, "If I can create that obstruction again, then remove it all over again, the relief I felt in removing it the last time will feel as good as it did then." And so it is that desires, even when we fulfill them, lead again and again to the creation of new desires.

Do you follow it? First you make a condition. You say, "Unless I get this woman I am not going to be happy. I can be happy only with this woman." Now you start striving to get this woman. The more difficult it is, the more you become enthusiastic, feverish.

The more difficult it is, the more you are challenged. The more difficult it is, the more you put all your being at stake; you are ready to gamble. And of course more hope arises and more desire to possess the woman. It is so hard, it is so difficult. It must be something great; that's why it is so hard, that's why it is so difficult. You chase and chase and chase and one day you get the woman. The day you get the woman the condition is removed: "If I get the woman then I will be happy" – you had put that condition in the first place. Now you get the woman, you feel relief. Now there is no more chasing, you have arrived, the result is in your hands, you feel good – good because of the relief.

One day I saw Mulla Nasruddin walking, swearing, and in great pain. I asked him, "What is the matter? Is your stomach aching or do you have a headache or something? What is the matter? You look in such agony."

He said, "Nothing. The shoes that I am wearing are too small."

"But then why are you wearing them?"

He said, "This is the only relief that I get at the end of the day – when I take my shoes off. This is the only joy I have, so I cannot leave these shoes. They are one size too small, it is really hell, but in the evening it gives heaven. When I go home and I take my shoes off and I fall on my sofa, I say I have arrived. It's so beautiful."

That's what you are doing. You create pain, you create anguish, chasing, fever, and then one day you come home and take the shoes off and you say, "Great, this is great! So I have arrived." But how long can it last? The relief lasts only a few moments. Then again you are hankering.

Now this woman is useless because you have got her. You cannot make a condition again. You can never say again, "If I get this woman I will be happy," because she is already with you. Now you start looking around at somebody else's woman: "If I get that woman…." Now you know one trick – that first you have to put a condition on your happiness, then you have to follow the condition desperately, then one day relief comes. Now this is futile.

A man of understanding will see that there is no need to put any condition. You can be unconditionally happy. Why go on walking in small shoes and suffer just to get relief in the end? Why not have the relief all the time? But then you will not feel it – that is the problem. To feel it, you need contrast. You will be happy but you will not feel it.

And that is the definition of a really happy man: a really happy man is one who does not know anything about happiness, who has never heard about it; who is so happy, so unconditionally happy, how can he know that he is happy? Only unhappy people say, "I am happy, things are going great." These are unhappy people. A happy person knows nothing about happiness. It is simply there, it is always there. It is like breathing.

You don't feel very happy about breathing. Then just do one thing: close your nose. Do some yoga exercises and repress your breath inside and go on repressing and go on repressing. Now the agony arises. And you go on repressing. Be a real yoga disciple – go on repressing. And then it bursts forth and there is such great joy. But this is foolish – but this is what everybody is doing. That's why you wait for the result in the evening.

Happiness is herenow; it needs no condition. Happiness is natural. Just see the point of it. Don't make conditions on your happiness. Remain happy for no reason at all. There is no reason to find some cause to be happy. Just be happy.

If you cannot be happy, then don't make such impossible conditions that it is difficult. Then Mulla is right – such a small thing. I understand. He is far more intelligent than you understand him to be. Such a simple device – wearing one size smaller shoes – such a small device, nobody can prevent you from doing it, and by the evening time you are happy. Just small devices, create small devices, and be as happy as you want.

But you say, "I will be happy only when this great house is mine." Now you are making a big condition. It may take years, and you will be tired and exhausted, and by the time you reach the palace of your desires, you may be close to death. That's what happens. You wasted your whole life and your great house will become your grave. You say, "Unless I have a million dollars, I am not going to be happy." And then you have to work and waste your whole life. Mulla Nasruddin is far more intelligent: make small conditions and have as much happiness as you want.

And if you understand, then there is no need to put any conditions. Just see the point of it – that conditions don't create happiness, they only give relief. But the relief cannot be permanent; no relief can ever be permanent. It lasts only for a few moments.

Have you not watched it again and again? You wanted to purchase a car; the car is in your porch and you are standing there, very, very happy. How long does it last? Tomorrow it is this old car, one day old. Two days after, it is two days old, and all the neighbourhood has seen it and they all have appreciated it, and finished! Now nobody talks about it. That's why car companies have to go on putting out new models every year, so that you can have new conditions.

People go on hankering after things just to get relief, and relief is available. Have you heard the story?

A beggar was sitting under a tree and a rich man's car broke down. The driver was fixing it and the rich man came out and the beggar was having a good rest under the tree. It was breezy and sunny and beautiful, and the rich man also came and he sat by the side of the beggar and he said, "Why don't you work?"

The beggar asked, "For what?"

The rich man felt a little annoyed and he said, "When you have money you can have a big balance in the bank."

But the beggar again asked, "For what?"

The rich man was even more annoyed. He said, "For what? Then you can retire in your old age and rest."

"But," the beggar said, "I am resting now! Why wait for old age? And do all this nonsense? – earn money and make a bank balance and then finally rest. And can't you see? – I am resting now! Why wait?"

Why wait for the evening? And why wait for the beer? Why not drink water and enjoy it while you are drinking it?

You have heard Jesus' story that he turned water into wine? Christians have missed it. They think he really turned it into wine. That is not true. He must have taught a secret that I am teaching you, to his disciples. He must have told them. "Drink it so joyously that water becomes wine."

You can drink water so joyously that it almost intoxicates you. Try! Just water can intoxicate you. It depends on you. It does not depend on the beer or the wine. And if you don't understand it, ask some hypnotist – he knows. Even if water is given to somebody who has been hypnotized and told under hypnosis that this is wine, he will become intoxicated – with water.

Now doctors know about placebos, and sometimes the results are very puzzling. In one hospital they were doing some experiments. To one group of twenty patients of the same disease medicine was given, and to the other twenty with the same disease, just water was given – just to see whether water can work. Neither the doctors nor the patients know which is water and which is medicine, because if the doctor knows, then even his behaviour will change. Giving water, he will not give it that seriously and that will make some suspicion arise in the patient. So neither the doctor nor the patient – nobody knows. The knowledge is kept in a vault, locked.

And the miracle is that the same number of patients are helped by water as are helped by medicine. Out of twenty, seventeen persons are healthy by the second week, from both the groups. And the more miraculous thing is, those who were kept on water remained healthy longer than those who were kept on medicine. The people who were kept on real medicine started coming back soon, after a few weeks.

What happened? Why did water help so much? The idea that it is medicine helps, not medicine. And because water is pure water, it cannot harm; medicine will harm. That's why the people who had been given real medicine started coming back. They started creating some new desire, some new disease, some new problems…because no medicine can go without affecting your system in some way or other. It will have its reactions. Water cannot have any reaction. This is pure hypnosis.

You can drink water with such zest, with such prayer, that it becomes wine. You see the Zen people drinking tea with such ceremony and ritual, with such awareness. Then even tea becomes something phenomenal. Ordinary tea is transformed. Ordinary acts can be transformed – a morning walk can be intoxicating. And if a morning walk cannot be intoxicating then something is wrong with you. Just watching a rose flower can be intoxicating. And if it cannot intoxicate you, then nothing can intoxicate you. Just looking in the eyes of a child can be intoxicating.

Learn how to live the moment joyously. Don't look for results; there are none. Life is not going anywhere, it has no ends. Life is not a means to any end. Life is just herenow. Live it. Live it totally, live it consciously, live it joyously – and you will be fulfilled.

Fulfillment should not be postponed, otherwise you will never be fulfilled. Fulfillment has to be now – now or never.[44]

? *Can a chain-smoker become meditative? I have smoked for twenty-five years, and I feel that in smoking I stop going deeply into meditation. Still, I can't stop smoking. Can you tell me something about it?*

A meditator cannot smoke, for the simple reason that he never feels nervous, in anxiety, in tension.

Smoking helps – on a momentary basis – to forget about your anxieties, your tensions, your nervousness. Other things can do the same; chewing gum can do the same, but smoking does it the best.

In your deep unconscious, smoking is related with sucking milk from your mother's breast. And as civilization has grown, no woman wants the child to be brought up by breast-feeding – naturally; he will destroy the breast. The breast will lose its roundness, its beauty. The child has different needs. The child does not need a round breast, because with a round breast the child will die. If the breast is really round, while he is sucking the milk he cannot breathe; his nose will be stopped by the breast. He will get suffocated.

The child's needs are different from a painter's need, from a poet's need, from that of a man of aesthetic sensibility. The child needs a long breast so his nose is free and he can do both – he can breathe and also feed himself. So every child will try to make the breast according to his needs. And no woman wants the breast to be destroyed. It is part of her beauty, her body, her shape.

So as civilization has grown, children are taken away from the breast of the mother sooner and sooner. The longing to drink from the breast goes on in their minds, and whenever people are in some nervous state, in tension, in anxiety, the cigarette helps. It helps them to become a child again, relaxed in their mother's lap. The cigarette is very symbolic. It is just like the nipple of the mother, and the smoke that goes through it is warm, just as the milk is warm. So it has a certain symmetry, and you become engaged in it, and for the moment you are reduced to a child who has no anxieties, no problems, no responsibilities.

You say that for thirty years you have been smoking, a chain-smoker; you want to stop it but you cannot stop it. You cannot – because you have to change the causes that have produced it.

I have been successful with many of my sannyasins. First they laughed when I suggested to them…they could not believe that such a simple solution could help them. I said to them, "Don't try to stop smoking, but rather bring a milk bottle that is used for small children. And in the night when nobody can see you, under your blanket enjoy the milk, the warm milk. It is not going to do any harm at least."

They said, "But how is it going to help?"

I said, "You forget about it – how and why – you just do it. It will give you good food before you go to sleep, and there is no harm. And my feeling is that the next day you will not feel so much need for cigarettes. So you count." And they were surprised…slowly, slowly the cigarettes were disappearing, because their basic need which had remained hanging in the middle was fulfilled: they are no longer children, they are maturing, and the cigarette disappears. You cannot stop it. You have to do something which is not harmful, which is healthier, as a substitute for the time being so that you grow up and the cigarettes stop themselves.

Small children know this – I have learned the secret from them. If a child is crying or weeping and is hungry, and the mother is far away, then he will put his thumb in his mouth and start sucking it. He will forget all about hunger and crying and weeping, and will fall asleep. He has found a substitute – although that substitute is not going to give him food, at least it gives a sense that something similar is happening. It relaxes him. I have suggested to a few of my sannyasins, even sucking the thumb. If you are too afraid to bring a bottle and fill it with milk, and if your wife comes to know about it, or your children see you doing it, then the best way is: you go to sleep with the thumb in the mouth. Suck it and enjoy it.

They have always laughed but they have always come back and said, "It helps, and the number of cigarettes next day is less and it goes on becoming less." Perhaps it will take a few weeks, then the cigarettes will disappear. And once they have disappeared without your stopping them.... Your stopping is repression, and anything repressed will try to come up again with greater force, with vengeance.

Never stop anything. Find the basic cause of it and try to work out some substitute which is not harmful. So the basic cause disappears – the cigarette is only a symptom. So the first thing is, stop stopping it. The second thing is, get a good bottle, and don't be embarrassed. If you are embarrassed then use your own thumb. Your own thumb will not be that great, but it will help. And I have never seen anybody failing who has used what I am saying. One day suddenly he cannot believe that he was unnecessarily destroying his health rather than having pure and clean air, smoking dirty smoke and destroying his lungs.

And this is going to become a problem more and more because as the women's liberation movement grows children will not be breast-fed. I am not saying that they *should* be breast-fed; but they should be given some substitute breast so that their unconscious does not carry some wound that will create problems for them – chewing gum and cigarettes and cigars.... These are all symptoms. In different countries they are different. In India they go on chewing *pan* leaves, or there are many people who use snuff. These are all the same. The snuff looks far away, but it is not that far away. The people who are nervous, tense, in anxiety, will take a dose of snuff. It gives a good sneeze, clears their mind, shakes their whole being, and it feels good. But those anxieties will come back. The snuff cannot destroy them. You have to destroy the very base of your being nervous. Why should you be nervous?

Many journalists have told me, "With you one of the greatest difficulties is that we feel nervous." And they have said, "This is strange because we interview politicians – they feel nervous, we make them nervous. You make *us* nervous, and immediately the desire to smoke arises. Then you prevent us smoking: 'You cannot smoke here.' You are allergic.

"You have a great strategy! – we cannot smoke, and you are making us nervous and tense, and this allergy you have which prevents us from smoking... so you have no way out for us." But why should they feel nervous in front of me? Those politicians are powerful people – if they feel nervous in front of them, it can be understood. But the reality is those powerful people are just hollow inside, and that power is borrowed from others, and they are afraid for their respectability. Each word they have to speak, they have to think twice. They are nervous that these journalists may create a situation in which their influence over people is destroyed. Their image that they have created has to become better and better. That is their fear. Because of that fear, the journalist – any journalist, who has no power – can make them nervous.

To me there is no problem. I have no desire for respectability. I am notorious enough – they cannot make me more notorious. I have done everything that could have made me nervous; I have managed already. What can they do to me? — I don't have any power to lose, and I can say anything that I want because I am not worried about being contradictory, inconsistent. On the contrary, I enjoy being contradictory, inconsistent. *They* start feeling nervous, and the nervousness immediately brings the idea to do something, to get engaged, so nobody feels that they are nervous. Just watch: when you start feeling that you need a cigarette, just watch why you need it. There is something that is making you nervous, and you don't want to be caught. I am reminded:

One day in a New York church, as the bishop entered he saw a strange man, a perfect hippie-type. But he made the bishop nervous, because that man looked into his eyes, and said, "Do you know who I am? I am Lord Jesus Christ."

The bishop phoned Rome: "What am I supposed to do?" he asked the pope, "…a hippie-looking man, but he also looks like Jesus Christ. I am alone here, early in the morning and he has come here. I have never been told what we have to do when Jesus Christ comes, so I want instruction, clearly, so I don't commit any mistake."

The pope himself was nervous. He said, "Do only one thing: look busy! What else can be done? Meanwhile make a phone call to the police station, and look busy so that man cannot see your nervousness."

Cigarettes help you to look busy; your nervousness is covered by it. So don't try to stop it; otherwise you will feel nervous and then you will fall back to the old pattern. The desire is there because something is left incomplete in you. Complete it — and there are simple methods to complete it. Just a baby's milk bottle will do. It will give you good food, it will make you healthier and it will take away all your desire for looking busy![45]

A man came to me. He had been suffering from chain-smoking for thirty years; he was ill and the doctors said, "You will never be healthy if you don't stop smoking." But he was a chronic smoker; he could not help it. He had tried — not that he had not tried, he had tried hard, and he had suffered much in trying; but only for one day or two days, and then again the urge would come so tremendously, it would simply take him away. Again he would fall into the same pattern. Because of this smoking he had lost all self-confidence: he knew he could not do a small thing; he could not stop smoking. He had become worthless in his own eyes; he thought himself just the most worthless person in the world. He had no respect for himself. He came to me. He said, "What can I do? How can I stop smoking?"

I said, "Nobody can stop smoking. You have to understand. Smoking is not only a question of your decision now. It has entered into your world of habits; it has taken root. Thirty years is a long time. It has taken root in your body, in your chemistry; it has spread all over. It is not just a question of your head deciding; your head cannot do anything. The head is impotent; it can start things, but it cannot stop them so easily. Once you have started and once you have practiced so long...you are a great yogi – thirty years' practising smoking! It has become autonomous; you will have to de-automatize it."

He said, "What do you mean by 'de-automatization'?"

And that's what meditation is all about, de-automatization.

I said, "You do one thing: forget about stopping. There is no need either. For thirty years you have smoked and lived; of course it was a suffering, but you have become accustomed to that too. And what does it matter if you die a few hours earlier than you would have died without smoking? What are you going to do here? What have you done? So what is the point – whether you die Monday or Tuesday or Sunday, this year, that year – what does it matter?"

He said, "Yes, that is true, it doesn't matter."

Then I said, "Forget about it; we are not going to stop it at all. Rather, we are going to understand it. So next time, you make it a meditation."

He said, "A meditation out of smoking?"

I said, "Yes. If Zen people can make a meditation out of drinking tea and can make it ceremony, why not? Smoking can be as beautiful a meditation."

He looked thrilled. He said, "What are you saying?" He became alive! He said, "Meditation? Just tell me – I can't wait!"

I gave him the meditation. I said, "Do one thing. When you are taking the packet of cigarettes out of your pocket, move slowly. Enjoy it, there is no hurry. Be conscious, alert, aware; take it out slowly, with full awareness. Then take the cigarette out of the packet with full awareness, slowly – not in the old hurried way, unconscious way, mechanical way. Then start tapping the cigarette on your packet – but very alertly. Listen to the sound, just as Zen people do when the samovar starts singing and the tea starts boiling...and the aroma. Then smell the cigarette and the beauty of it...."

He said, "What are you saying? The beauty?"

"Yes, it is beautiful. Tobacco is as divine as anything.... Smell it; it is God's smell."

He looked a little surprised. He said, "What! Are you joking?"

"No. I am not joking." Even when I joke, I don't joke. I am very serious. "Then put it in your mouth, with full awareness, light it with full awareness. Enjoy every act, every small act, and divide it into as many small acts as possible, so you can become more and more aware.

"Then have the first puff: God in the form of smoke. Hindus say, 'Annam Brahma' – Food is God'. Why not smoke? All is God. Fill your lungs deeply – this is a *pranayam*. I am giving you the new yoga for the new age! Then release the smoke, relax, another puff – and go very slowly.

"If you can do it, you will be surprised; soon you will see the whole stupidity of it – not because others have said that it is stupid, not because others have said that it is bad. You will see it, and the seeing will not just be intellectual. It will be from your total being; it will be a vision of your totality. And then one day, if it drops, it drops; if it continues, it continues. You need not worry about it."

After three months he came and he said, "But it dropped!"

"Now," I said, "try it on other things too."

This is the secret: de-automatize. Walking, walk slowly, watchfully. Looking, look watchfully, and you will see trees are greener than they have ever been, and roses are rosier than they have ever been. Listen! Somebody is talking, gossiping: listen, listen attentively. When you are talking, talk attentively. Let your whole waking activity become de-automatized.[46]

? *I would like you to comment on the drug problem.*

It is nothing new, it is as ancient as man. There has never been a time when man was not in search of escape. The most ancient book in the world is the *Rig Veda*, and it is full of drug use. The name of the drug is *soma*. Since those ancient times all the religions have tried to get people not to use drugs. All the governments have been against drugs. Yet drugs have proved more powerful than governments or religions, because nobody has looked into the very psychology of the drug user. Man is miserable. He lives in anxiety, anguish and frustration. There seems to be no way out except drugs. The only way to prevent the use of drugs will be to make man joyful, happy, blissful.

I am also against drugs, for the simple reason that it helps you to forget your misery for a time. It does not prepare you to fight misery and suffering, rather it weakens you.

But the reasons of religions and governments for being against drugs and my reasons for being against drugs are totally different. They want man to remain miserable and frustrated, because the man in suffering is never rebellious; he is tortured in his own being, he is falling apart. He cannot conceive of a better society, of a better culture, of a better man. Because of his misery he becomes an easy victim of the priests because they console him, because they say to him, "Blessed are the poor, blessed are the meek, blessed are those who suffer, because they shall inherit the kingdom of God."

The suffering humanity is also in the hands of the politicians, because the suffering humanity needs some hope – hope of a classless society somewhere in the future, hope of a society where there will be no poverty, no hunger, no misery. In short, they can manage and be patient with their sufferings if they have a utopia just close to the horizon. And you must note down the meaning of the word utopia. It means that which never happens. It is just like the horizon; it is so close that you think you can run and meet the place where earth and sky meet. But you can go on running your whole life and never meet the place, because there is no such place. It is an hallucination.

The politician lives on promise, the priest lives on promise. In the last ten thousand years nobody has delivered the goods. Their reason for being against drugs is that drugs destroy their whole business. If people start taking opium, hashish, LSD, they don't care about communism, and they don't care about what is going to happen tomorrow; they don't care about life after death, they don't care about God, paradise. They are fulfilled in the moment.

Here my reasons are different. I am also against drugs, not because they will cut the roots of religions and the politicians, but because they destroy your inner growth towards spirituality. They prevent you from reaching the promised land. You remain hanging around the hallucinations, while you are capable of reaching the real. They give you a toy.

But since drugs are not going to disappear, I would like every government, every scientific lab, to purify drugs, to make them healthier, without any side effects, which is possible now. We can create a drug like the one which Aldous Huxley, in the memory of the *Rig Veda*, called soma, which will be without any bad effects, which will not be addictive, which will be a joy, a happiness, a dance, a song. If we cannot provide for everybody to become a Gautam Buddha, we have no right to prevent people at least having illusory glimpses of the aesthetic state which Gautam Buddha must have had. Perhaps these small experiences will lead the person to explore more. Sooner or later he is going to be fed up with the drug, because it will go on repeating the same scene again and again. Howsoever beautiful a scene is, repetition makes it a boredom.

So first purify the drug of all bad effects. Second, let people who want to enjoy, enjoy. They will become bored by it. And then their only path will be to seek some method of meditation to find the ultimate bliss.

Your question is basically concerned with the New Age people. The generation gap is the world's very latest phenomenon, it never used to exist. In the past, children of six and seven started using their hands, their minds, with their fathers in their traditional professions. By the time they were fourteen they were already craftsmen, workers, they were married, they had responsibilities. By the time they were twenty or twenty-four they had their own children, so there was never a gap between the generations. Each generation overlapped the other generation.

For the first time in the history of humanity, the generation gap has happened. It is of tremendous importance. Now, for the first time, up to the age of twenty-five or twenty-six when you come back from the university you have no responsibility, no children, no worries, and you have the whole world before you to dream about – how to better it, how to make it richer, how to create a race of supermen. And these are the days, between fourteen and twenty-four, when a person is a dreamer, because his sexuality is maturing, and with sexuality dreams are maturing. His sexuality is repressed by the schools and colleges, so his whole energy is available to dream. He becomes a communist, he becomes a socialist, he becomes a Fabian, all sorts of things. And this is the time when he starts feeling frustrated, because the way the world works, the bureaucracy, the government, the politicians, the society, the religion, it does not seem that he will be able to create a reality out of his dream.

He comes home from the university full of ideas, and every idea is going to be crushed by the society. Soon he forgets about the new man and the new age. He cannot even find employment, he cannot feed himself. How can he think of a classless society where there will be no rich and no poor? It is this moment when he turns towards drugs; they give him a temporary relief. But all drugs as they are right now are addictive, so you have to go on increasing the dose. And they are destructive to the body, to the brain; soon you are absolutely helpless. You cannot live without drugs, and with drugs there is no space in life for you. But I don't say that the younger people are responsible for it; and to punish them and to put them in jail is sheer stupidity. They are not criminals, they are victims....

The people who are in power go on doing idiotic things – prohibition, punishment. They know that for ten thousand years we have been prohibiting, and we have not succeeded. If you prohibit alcohol more people become alcoholic, and a dangerous kind of alcohol becomes available. Thousands of people die by poisoning, and who is responsible? Now they are punishing young people for years in jail without even understanding that if a person has taken a drug or has been addicted to a drug he needs treatment, not punishment. He should be sent to a psychiatric home where he can be taken care of, where he can be taught meditation, and slowly, slowly can be directed from the drugs towards something better.

Instead they are forcing them into jails – ten years in jail. They don't value human life at all. If you give ten years in jail to a young man of twenty you have wasted his most precious time and without any benefit, because in jail every drug is more easily available than anywhere else. The inmates are all highly skilled drug users, who become teachers for those who are amateurs. After ten years the person will come out perfectly trained. One thing only your jails teach: anything you do is not wrong unless you are caught – just don't be caught. And there are masters who can teach you how not to be caught again.

So this whole thing is absolutely absurd. I am also against drugs, but in a totally different way. I think you have got the point.[47]

? *Can LSD be used as a help in meditation?*

LSD can be used as a help, but the help is very dangerous. It is not so easy. If you use a mantra, even that can become difficult to throw, but if you use acid it will be even more difficult to throw.

The moment you are on an LSD trip you are not in control. Chemistry takes control and you are not the master. And once you are not the master, it is difficult to regain that position. The chemical is not the slave, now *you* are the slave. Now how to control it is not going to be your choice. Once you take LSD as a help you are making a slave of the master, and your whole body chemistry will be affected by it. Your body will begin to crave LSD. Now the craving will not just be of the mind as it is when you get attached to a mantra. When you use acid as a help, the craving becomes part of the body; the LSD goes to the very cells of the body. It changes them, your inner chemical structure becomes different. Then all the body cells begin to crave acid and it will be difficult to drop it.

LSD can be used to bring you to meditation only if your body has been prepared for it. So if you ask if it can be used in the West, I will say that it is not for the West at all. It can be used only in the East – if the body is totally prepared for it. Yoga has used it, Tantra has used it – there are schools of Tantra and Yoga that have used LSD as a help – but then they prepare your body first. There is a long process of purification of the body. Your body becomes so pure and you become such a great master of it that even chemistry cannot become your master now. So Yoga allows it, but in a very specific way.

First your body must be purified chemically. Then you will be in such control of the body that even your body chemistry can be controlled. For example, there are certain yogic exercises.... If you take poison, through a particular yogic exercise you can order your blood not to mix with it and the poison will pass through the body and come out in the urine without having mixed with the blood at all. If you can do this, if you can control your body chemistry, then you can use *anything* because you have remained the master.

In Tantra, particular in 'leftist' Tantra, they use alcohol to help meditation. It looks absurd; it is not. The seeker will take alcohol in a particular quantity and then will try to be alert. Consciousness must not be lost. By and by the quantity of alcohol will be raised, but the consciousness must remain alert. The person has taken alcohol, it has been absorbed in the body, but the mind remains above it. Consciousness is not lost. Then the quantity of alcohol is raised higher and higher. Through this practice a point comes when any amount of alcohol can be given and the mind remains alert. Only then can LSD be a help.

In the West there are no practices to purify the body or to increase consciousness through changes in body chemistry. Acid is taken without any preparation in the West. It is not going to help. Rather, on the contrary, it may destroy the whole mind.

There are many problems. Once you have been on an LSD trip you have a glimpse of something you have never known, something you have never felt. If you begin to practice meditation it is a long process, but LSD is not a process. You take it, and the process is over. Then the body begins to work. Meditation is a long process – you have to do it for years; only then will the results be forthcoming – and when you have experienced a shortcut it will be difficult to follow a long process. The mind will crave to return to using the drugs. So it is difficult to meditate once you have known a glimpse through chemistry. To undertake something that is a long process will be difficult. Meditation needs more stamina, more faith, more waiting, and it will be difficult because now you can compare.

Secondly, any method is bad if you are not in control all the time. When you are meditating, you can stop at any moment. If you want to stop, you can stop this very moment. You can come out of it. You cannot stop an LSD trip: once you have taken LSD you have to complete the circle. Now you are not the master.

Anything that makes a slave of you is ultimately not going to help spiritually, because spirituality basically means to be the master of oneself. So I wouldn't suggest shortcuts. I am not against LSD, I may sometimes be for it, but then a long preliminary preparation is necessary. Then you will be the master.

But then LSD is not a shortcut. It will take even longer than meditation. Hatha Yoga takes years to prepare a body. Twenty years, twenty-five years – then a body is ready. Now you can use any chemical help and it will not be destructive to your being.

But then the process is far longer. Then LSD can be used; I am in favour of it then. If you are prepared to take twenty years to prepare the body in order to take LSD then it is not destructive, but the same thing can be done in two years with meditation. Because the body is more gross, mastery is more difficult. The mind is more subtle so mastery is easier. The body is further away from your being, so there is a greater gap; with the mind the gap is shorter.

In India, the primitive method to prepare the body to be ready for meditation was Hatha Yoga. It took so long a time to prepare the body that sometimes Hatha Yoga had to invent methods to prolong life so that Hatha Yoga could be continued. It was such a long process that sixty years might not be enough, seventy years might not be enough. And there is a problem: if the mastery is not achieved in this life then in the next life you have to begin from ABC because you have a new body. The whole effort has been lost. You do not have a new mind in your next life so whatever is attained through the mind remains with you, but whatever is attained through the body is lost with every death. So Hatha Yoga had to invent methods to prolong life for two hundred to three hundred years so that mastery could be attained.

If the mastery is of the mind then you can change the body, but the preparedness of the body belongs to the body alone. Hatha Yoga invented many methods so that the process could be completed, but then even greater methods were discovered: how to control the mind directly – Raja Yoga. With these methods the body can be a little helpful, but there is no need to be too concerned with it. So Hatha Yoga adepts have said that LSD can be used, but Raja Yoga cannot say LSD can be used because Raja Yoga has no methodology to prepare the body. Direct meditation is used.

Sometimes it happens – only sometimes, rarely – that if you have a glimpse through LSD and do not become addicted to it, that glimpse may become a thirst in you to seek something further. So to try it once is good, but it becomes difficult to know where to stop and how to stop. The first trip is good, to be on it once is good – you become aware of a different world and then you begin to seek, you begin to search, because of it – but then it becomes difficult to stop. This is the problem. If you can stop, then to take LSD once is good. But that 'if' is a great one.

Mulla Nasruddin used to say that he never took more than one glass of wine. Many friends objected to his statement because they had seen him taking one glass after another. He said, "The second glass is taken by the first; 'I' take only one. The second is taken by the first and the third by the second. Then I am not the master. I am master only for the first, so how can I say that I take more than one? 'I' take only one – always only one!"

With the first you are the master; with the second you are not. The first will try to take a second and then it will go on continuously. Then it is no longer in your hands. To begin anything is easy because you are the master, but to end anything is difficult because then you are not the master. So I am not against LSD...and if I *am* against it, it is conditional. This is the condition: if you can remain the master, then okay. Use anything, but remain the master. And if you cannot remain the master, then do not enter into a dangerous road at all. Do not enter at all. It will be better.[48]

CHAPTER 9
FOOD

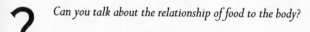

? *Can you talk about the relationship of food to the body?*

Accoording to the mystic traditions of the East, all that you think you are is nothing but food. Your body is food, your mind is food, your soul is food. Beyond the soul there is certainly something which is not food. That something is known as *anatta,* no-self. It is utter emptiness. Buddha calls is *shunya,* the void. It is pure space. It contains nothing but itself; it is contentless consciousness.

While the content persists, the food persists. By food is meant that which is ingested from the outside. The body needs physical food; without it, it will start withering away. This is how it survives; it contains nothing but physical food.

Your mind contains memories, thoughts, desires, jealousies, power trips, and a thousand and one things. All that is also food; it is food on a little more subtle plane. Thought is food. Hence when you have nourishing thoughts your chest expands, when you have thoughts which give you energy you feel good. Somebody says something good about you, a compliment, and look what happens to you: you are nourished. And somebody says something wrong about you, and watch: it is as if something has been snatched away from you, you are weaker than you were before.

The mind is food in a subtle form. The mind is nothing but the inner side of the body; hence what you eat affects your mind. If you eat non-vegetarian food you will have a particular kind of mind; if you eat vegetarian food you will certainly have a different kind of mind.

Do you know this immensely important fact about Indian history? India never attacked any country in its whole history of ten thousand years. Never – not a single aggressive act. How was it possible? Why? The same humanity exists here as exists everywhere else. But it is just that a different kind of body created a different mind.

You can watch it yourself. Eat something and watch, eat something else and watch. Keep notes, and you will become aware and surprised to find that each thing that you digest is not only physical, it has a psychological part to it. It makes your mind vulnerable to certain ideas, to certain desires. Hence, down the ages, there has been a search for a kind of food that will not strengthen the mind but will help it to finally dissolve; a kind of food which, instead of strengthening the mind, will strengthen meditation, no-mind. No fixed and certain rules can be given, because people are different and each one has to decide for himself.

And watch what you allow into your mind. People are completely unaware; they go on reading everything and anything, they go on looking at the TV, any silly, stupid thing. They go on listening to the radio, they go on chit-chatting, chattering with people, and they are all pouring rubbish into each other's heads. Rubbish is all that they have.

Avoid such situations in which you are unnecessarily burdened with rubbish. You already have too much as it is; you need to be unburdened of it. And you go on collecting it as if it is something precious. Talk less, listen only to the essential, be telegraphic in talking and listening. If you talk less, if you listen less, slowly, slowly you will see that a cleanliness, a feeling of purity, as if you have just taken a bath, will start arising within you. That becomes the necessary soil for meditation to arise. Don't go on reading all kinds of nonsense.

Once I used to live in a house where the neighbour was a madman who was very much interested in newspapers. He would come every day to collect all the newspapers from me. If sometimes he was ill or I was not at home, then he would come later on. Once it happened, for ten days I was away. And when I came back he came again to collect all the newspapers. I said to him, "But these are old now – ten days old."

He said, "What does it matter? It is the same rubbish! Only the dates change."

It must have been a very sane moment in that madman's life. Yes, there are insane moments in so-called sane people's lives, and vice versa. He was telling the truth, saying, "It is the same old nonsense. What does it matter? I have time, and I have to remain occupied."

I asked him, "What did you do for these ten days?" He said, "I was reading the old newspapers – reading them again and again and again."

Leave a few gaps in your mind unoccupied. Those moments of unoccupied consciousness are the first glimpses of meditation, the first penetrations of the beyond, the first flashes of no-mind. And then if you can manage to do this, the other thing is to choose physical food which does not help aggression and violence, which is not poisonous.

Now even scientists agree with this, that when you kill an animal, out of fear he releases all kinds of poisons. Death is not easy. When you are killing an animal, out of fear a great trembling arises inside. The animal wants to survive: all kinds of poisons are released.

When you are in fear you also release poisons in the body. Those poisons are helpful: they help you to either fight or take flight. Sometimes it happens that in anger you can do things which you could never have imagined yourself doing. You can move a rock which ordinarily you could not have even shaken, but anger is there and poison is released. In fear, people can run so fast that even Olympic runners will be left behind. Just think of yourself running if somebody is behind you with a dagger to kill you. You will do the best you can do, your whole body will be geared to function at its optimum.

When you kill an animal there is anger, there is anxiety, there is fear. Death is facing him: all the glands of the animal release many kinds of poisons. Hence the modern idea is that before killing an animal, make him unconscious, give him anaesthesia. In modern butcheries, anaesthesia is being used. But that does not make much difference, only a very superficial difference, because at the deepest core where no anaesthesia can ever reach, death has to be encountered. It may not be conscious, the animal may not be aware of what is happening, but it is happening as if in a dream. He is passing through a nightmare. And to eat meat is to eat poisoned food.

Avoid anything that is poisoned on the physical plane, avoid anything that is poisoned on the mental plane. And on the mental plane things are more complicated. If you think you are a Hindu, you are poisoned; if you think you are a Mohammedan, you are poisoned. If you think you are a Christian, a Jaina, a Buddhist, you are poisoned. And you have been poisoned slowly – so slowly that you have become attuned to it. You are addicted to it. You have been spoon-fed since the very first day; from your mother's breast, you have been poisoned. All kinds of conditionings are poisons. To think of oneself as a Hindu is to think of oneself opposed to humanity. To think of oneself as German, as Chinese, is to think of oneself opposed to humanity; is to think in terms of enmity, not friendship.

Think of yourself only a human being. If you have any intelligence, think of yourself only as a simple human being. And when your intelligence grows a little more you will drop even the adjective 'human'. You will think of yourself only as a being. And the being includes all – the trees and the mountains and the rivers and the stars and the birds and the animals.

Become bigger, become huge. Why are you living in tunnels? Why are you creeping into small dark black holes? But you think you are living in great ideological systems. You are not living in great ideological systems, because there *are* no great ideological systems. No idea is great enough to contain a human being; being-hood cannot be contained by any concept. All concepts cripple and paralyze.

Don't be a Catholic and don't be a communist – just be a human being – these are all poisons, these are all prejudices. And down the ages you have been hypnotized into these prejudices. They have become part of your blood, your bones, your very marrow. You will have to be very alert to get rid of all this poisoning.

Your body is not poisoned as much as your mind is. The body is a simple phenomenon, it can be easily cleaned. If you have been eating non-vegetarian foods it can be stopped, it is not such a big deal. And if you stop eating meat, within three months your body will be completely free of all the poisons created by non-vegetarian foods. It is simple. Physiology is not very complicated. But the problem arises with psychology. A Jaina monk never eats any poisoned food, never eats anything non-vegetarian. But his mind is polluted and poisoned by Jainism as nobody else's is.

The real freedom is freedom from any ideology. Can't you simply live without any ideology? Is an ideology needed? Why is an ideology needed so much? It is needed because it helps you to remain stupid, it is needed because it helps you to remain unintelligent. It is needed because it supplies you ready-made answers and you need not find them on your own.

The real man of intelligence will not cling to any ideology – for what? He will not carry a load of ready-made answers. He knows that he has enough intelligence so that whatever situation arises, he will be able to respond to it. Why carry an unnecessary load from the past? What is the point of carrying it…?

If you change your poisonous foods you will be surprised: a new intelligence will be released in you. And this new intelligence will make it possible not to go on stuffing yourself with nonsense. This new intelligence will make you capable of dropping the past and its memories, of dropping unnecessary desires and dreams, dropping jealousies, angers, traumas and all kinds of psychological wounds.

Because you cannot drop psychological wounds, you become victims of psycho-fraud. The world is full of psychoanalysts of many kinds, they come in all shapes and sizes. The world is full of all kinds of psychotherapies. But why are so many psychotherapies needed? They are needed because you are not intelligent enough to heal your own wounds. Instead of healing them, instead of opening them to the winds and to the sun, you go on hiding them. You need psychotherapists to help you to open your wounds to the sun so that they can be healed, so that they can be allowed to heal. But it is very difficult to find a real psychotherapist. Out of a hundred psychotherapists, ninety-nine are psycho-frauds, not psychotherapists.

You will be surprised to know that more psychotherapists and psychoanalysts commit suicide than people in any other profession. The number is almost double. Now, what kind of people are these? And how were they going to help others? What were they doing their whole lives helping people? More psychoanalysts go mad, insane, than people in any other profession of the world. The number is almost double. Why? And they were helping other people towards sanity, when they themselves were insane. There is every possibility that they became interested in psychotherapy because of their insanity. It was an effort to find a cure for themselves. And you will be surprised to know that psychotherapists of one kind go for psychotherapy to psychotherapists of another kind. The Freudian goes to the Jungian, the Jungian goes to the Freudian, and so on and so forth. This is a very strange situation.

If intelligence is released in you, you will be able to do all that is needed. You will be able to heal your own wounds, you will be able to see your own traumas, you need not go to a primal therapist.

I am allowing all kinds of therapies in this commune. In fact, in no other place in the world are so many psychotherapies available — sixty in all. Why am I allowing these therapies? Just because of you, because you are not yet ready to release your intelligence. As the commune goes deeper and deeper into inner realizations, therapies can be dropped. When the commune has really bloomed, there will be no need of any therapy. Then love is therapy, intelligence is therapy. Then living day to day, moment to moment, aware and alert, is therapy. Then all kinds of things that you do during the day, cleaning and cooking and washing, they are all therapy.

Therapies are here only for the time being. The day I become convinced that now the major part of you has gone beyond therapies, therapies will disappear, because then the major part will be able to pull the minor part into intelligence also.

We are trying to create an intelligent kind of life. I am not much of a religious person, I am not a saint, I have nothing to do with spirituality. All those categories are irrelevant about me. You cannot categorize me, you cannot pigeonhole me. But one thing can be said, that my whole effort is to help you release the energy called love-intelligence. If love-intelligence is released, you are healed.

And the third kind of poisoned food is spiritual. That's what the self is. The self needs continuous attention: it feeds on attention, attention is its food. It is not only the politician who hankers for attention, more and more attention from more and more people — your so-called saints are doing the same. There is no difference between saints and politicians and actors, no difference at all. Their basic need is the same – attention: "More people should pay attention to me, more people should look up to me." That becomes food for the ego, and it is the subtlest kind of poisoned food....

Physical, psychological, spiritual.... Let your physiological body be pure of all poisons and toxins, and your mind be unburdened of all kinds of rubbish and junk. And let your soul be free from the idea of the self. When the soul is free from the idea of "I" you have arrived at that inner space called no-self, *anatta*. That is freedom, that is nirvana, that is enlightenment. You have come home. Now there is nowhere to go; now you can settle, rest and relax. Now you can enjoy the millions of joys that are being showered upon you by existence.

When these three poisoned foods are dropped, you become empty. But this emptiness is not a negative kind of emptiness. You are empty in the sense that all poisons, all contents, are gone. But you are full – full of something which cannot be named, full of something which devotees call 'God.'[49]

There are two types of food. One is that which you like, which you have a fancy for, about which you fantasize. There is nothing wrong in it, but you will have to learn a small trick about it. There are foods which have a tremendous appeal. The appeal is not because you see that the food is available. You go into a hotel, into a restaurant, and you see certain foods – the smell coming from the back room, the colour and the aroma of the food. You were not thinking about the food and suddenly you are interested in it – this is not going to help. This is not your real desire. You can eat this thing – it will not satisfy you. You will eat and eat and nothing will come out of it; no satisfaction will come out of it. And satisfaction is the most important thing. It is the dissatisfaction that creates the obsession.

Simply meditate every day before you take food. Close your eyes and just feel what your body needs – whatsoever it is! You have not seen any food – no food is available; you are simply feeling your own being, what your body needs, what you feel like, what you hanker for.

Dr. Leonard Pearson calls this 'humming food' – food that hums to you. Go and eat as much of it as you want, but stick to it. The other food he calls 'beckoning food': when it becomes available, you become interested in it. Then it is a mind thing and it is not your need. If you listen to your humming food, you can eat as much as you want and you will never suffer, because it will satisfy you. The body simply desires that which it needs; it never desires anything else. That will be satisfactory, and once there is satisfaction, one never eats more. The problem arises only if you are eating foods which are beckoning foods: you see them available and you become interested and you eat. They cannot satisfy you because there is no need in the body for them.

When they don't satisfy you, you feel unsatisfied. Feeling unsatisfied, you eat more, but howsoever much you eat, it is not going to satisfy because there is no need in the first place.

The first type of desire has to be fulfilled, then the second will disappear. What people are doing is that they never listen to the first, so the second becomes a problem. If you listen to the humming food, the beckoning food will disappear. The second is a problem only because you have completely forgotten that you have to listen to your inner desire, and people have been taught not to listen to it. They have been taught, "Eat this, don't eat that" – fixed rules. The body knows no fixed rules.

They have found that if small children are left alone with food, they will eat only that which is needed for their body; and they were surprised. Many psychological findings are available now; they were simply surprised. If a child is suffering from some disease, and if apple is good for that disease, the child will choose the apple. All other foods are available but the child will go to the apple.

That's what all animals are doing; only man has forgotten the language. You bring a buffalo and leave her in the garden. The whole garden is there – all the greenery is available; she will not bother. The flowers and the trees may be beckoning but she won't bother with them. She will go to the grass that hums to her, and she will choose only certain grass that is her need. You cannot deceive a buffalo; you can only deceive man.

Man has fallen even below buffaloes. You cannot befool a donkey – he will eat his food. Man is befooled. Everywhere through advertisements, coloured pictures, TV, movies, you are being attracted and distracted from your humming body. Some company is interested in selling something to you. That is in the favour of the company, it is beneficial to the company, not to you.

Some Cola company is interested in selling Cola to you. It has nothing to do with your body; it allures you. Wherever you go, there is Cola; Cola seems to be one of the most universal things. Even in Soviet Russia – nothing else American is allowed, but Cola is there. From everywhere the bottle is calling you, beckoning, "Come here." And suddenly you start feeling thirsty. That thirst is false. I'm not saying don't drink Cola – but let it hum; make it a point.

It will take a few days, even a few weeks for you to come to feel what appeals to you. Eat as much as you want of what appeals to you. Don't bother about what others say. If ice-cream appeals to you, eat ice-cream. Eat to your satisfaction, to your heart's desire, and then suddenly you will see that there is satisfaction. And when you feel satisfied, the desire to stuff disappears. It is an unsatisfied state that makes you stuff yourself more and more and still to no purpose. You feel full and still unsatisfied, so the problem arises.

So first start learning something which is natural and which will come because we have only forgotten; it is there in the body. When you are going to take your breakfast, close your eyes and see what you want; what your desire really is. Don't think about what is available; simply think what your desire is, and then go and find that thing and eat it. Eat as much as you want. For a few days just go with it. By and by you will see that now no food beckons you.

The second thing: when you eat, chew it well. Don't swallow it in a hurry, because if it is oral, you enjoy it in the mouth, so why not chew it more? If you take ten bites of something you can enjoy one bite, chew it ten times more. It will almost be like taking ten bites if your enjoyment is only of the taste.

It happened once that a man drank some hot coffee somewhere in Japan and he burned his throat inside. Some complication arose and his throat was completely cut from inside; the passage had to be closed otherwise the man was going to die. The doctors fixed a pipe into his stomach so he had to chew the food, throw it into the pipe, and the pipe would take it into the stomach.

The man was surprised because he continued to enjoy his food as much as before. And even the doctors were surprised. They were at first feeling very sympathetic towards him because the poor man would no longer enjoy his food. But the man continued to enjoy it. In fact he started to enjoy it more because now he would chew it and if he did not want to take it into the stomach, he would simply throw it out. Now he could eat as much as he wanted. There was no need to take it into the stomach; the mouth and the stomach were completely separate.

So whenever you are eating, chew more, because the enjoyment is just above the throat. Below the throat there is no taste – nothing of the sort – so why be in a hurry? Just chew it more, taste it more. And to make this taste more intense, do all that can be done. When you are eating something, first smell it. Enjoy the smell of it because half the taste consists of smell.

Many experiments have been done. If your nose is completely closed and then something is given to you, you cannot taste it. Then you will understand that the food was more smell than taste. If your eyes are closed, you cannot taste it even that much, because the colour, the appeal to the eyes, is no longer there. They have done beautiful experiments: eyes closed, nose completely closed, and then they give you something; you cannot even tell what it is. They may give you onion and you cannot say that it is onion because much depends on the smell. That's why when you have a cold you cannot enjoy food, because the smell is not there, the taste is not there. When people are suffering from a cold they start eating spicy food because only then can they feel a little tingling.

So smell the food, look at the food. There is no hurry...take time. Make it a meditation. Even if people think you have gone mad, don't be worried. Just look at it from all sides. Touch it with closed eyes, touch it with your cheek. Feel it in every way; smell it again and again. Then take a small bite and chew it, enjoy it; let it be a meditation. A very small quantity of food will be enough and will give you more satisfaction.[50]

? *How does fasting help the body's well-being?*

Whenever you are on a fast the body has no more work of digestion. In that period the body can work in throwing out dead cells, toxins. It is just as one day, Sunday or Saturday, you are on a holiday and you come home and you clean the whole day. The whole week you were so engaged and so busy you couldn't clean the house. When the body has nothing to digest, you have not eaten anything, the body starts a self-cleaning. A process starts spontaneously and the body starts throwing out all that is not needed, which is like a load. Fasting is a method of purification. Once in a while a fast is beautiful – not doing anything, not eating, just resting. Take as much liquid as possible and just rest, and the body will be cleaned.

Sometimes, if you feel that a longer fast is needed, you can do a longer fast also – but be deep in love with the body. And if you feel the fast is harming the body in any way, stop it. If the fast is helping the body, you will feel more energetic; you will feel more alive; you will feel rejuvenated, vitalized. This should be the criterion: if you start feeling that you are getting weaker, if you start feeling that a subtle trembling is coming into the body, then be aware – now the thing is no longer a purification, it has become destructive. Stop it.

But one should learn the whole science of it. In fact one should do fasting near somebody who has been fasting for long and who knows the whole path very well, who knows all the symptoms: if it becomes destructive what will start happening; if it is not destructive then what will happen. After a real, purifying fast you will feel new, younger, cleaner, weightless, happier; and the body will be functioning better because now it is unloaded. But fasting comes only if you have been eating wrongly. If you have not been eating wrongly there is no need for fasting. Fasting is needed only when you have already done the wrong with the body – and we all have been eating wrongly.[51]

? *Do you recommend any particular kind of food or eating regimes?*

The first thing: I am not a believer in fasting, I believe in feasting. My whole approach is that of celebration. I am not against your pleasures – they are not all, one should go beyond them, but in themselves they are beautiful. A man should not deny anything, because the denied part will take revenge. The moment you start denying you go against Tao. Tao is to be natural – a feast and not a fast. A fast can be used only when it comes naturally.

Sometimes animals fast. Sometimes you may have observed your dog fasting: you put the food down and he will not eat. But he is not a Jaina, he is not a believer in fasting; he does not feel like eating. It is not a question of principle, it is not a philosophy. He is ill, his whole being is against eating – rather than eat, he would like to vomit. He will go and eat grass and vomit. He would like to relieve himself, his stomach is not in a condition to digest any more. But he is not a faster. It is natural.

So, if sometimes you feel that the fast comes naturally – not as a law, not as a principle, not as a philosophy to be followed, as a discipline to be imposed, but out of your natural feel for it – good. Then, too, remember always that your fast is in the service of feasting, so that you can eat well again. The purpose of fasting is as a means, never as an end; and that will happen rarely, once in a while. And if you are perfectly aware while you are eating, and enjoying it, you will never eat too much.

My insistence is not on dieting but on awareness. Eat well, enjoy it tremendously. Remember, the rule is: If you don't enjoy your food you will have to eat more to compensate. If you enjoy your food you will eat less, there will be no need to compensate. If you eat slowly, tasting every bit of it, chewing well, you are completely absorbed in it. Eating should be a meditation.

I am not against taste because I am not against the senses. To be sensitive is to be intelligent, to be sensitive is to be alive. Your so-called religions have tried to de-sensitize you, to make you dull. They are against taste, they would like you to make your tongue absolutely dull so you don't taste anything. But that is not a state of health; the tongue becomes dull only in illness. When you have a fever, the tongue becomes dull. When you are healthy the tongue is sensitive, alive, throbbing, pulsates with energy. I am not against taste, I am for taste. Eat well, taste well; the taste is divine.

And so, exactly like taste, you have to look at beauty and enjoy; you have to listen to music and enjoy; you have to touch the rocks and leaves and human beings – the warmth, the texture – and enjoy. Use all your senses, use them to their optimum, then you will really live and your life will be aflame. It will not be dull, it will be aflame with energy and vitality. I am not for those people who have been teaching you to kill your senses; they are against the body.

And remember, the body is your temple, the body is a divine gift. It is so delicate and it is so beautiful and it is so wonderful – to kill it is to be ungrateful to God. God has given you taste; you have not created it, it is not anything to do with you. God has given you eyes and God has made this psychedelic world so colourful, and he has given you eyes. Let there be a great communion between the eye and the colour of the world.... Everything is in a tremendous harmony. Don't break this harmony.

These so-called *mahatmas* are just on ego-trips, and the best way to feel that you are great is to be against the body. Children do it. The child feels that the motion is coming; he holds it, he feels powerful because he feels his will: he will not yield to the body. His bladder is full and he holds it. He wants to show the body "I'm not your servant, I'm your master." But these are destructive habits.

Listen to the body. The body is not your enemy, and when the body is saying something, do accordingly, because the body has a wisdom of its own. Don't disturb it, don't go on a mind-trip. That's why I don't teach you any dieting, I teach you only awareness. Eat with full awareness, eat meditatively, and then you will never eat more and you will never eat less. More is as bad as less. Too much eating is bad, just like too much fasting; these are extremes. Nature wants you to be balanced, to be in a sort of equilibrium, to be in the middle, neither less nor more. Don't go to the extreme.

To go to the extreme is to be neurotic. So there are two types of neurotics about food: those who go on eating, not listening to the body – the body goes on crying and screaming "Stop!" and they go on. These are neurotic people. And then there is the other variety: the body goes on screaming "I am hungry!" and they are on a fast. Neither is religious, both are neurotic, both are pathological – they need treatment, they need to be hospitalized. A religious person is one who is balanced: in whatsoever he is doing, he is always in the middle. He never goes to the extreme because all extremes will create tensions, anxieties. When you eat too much there is anxiety because the body is burdened. When you don't eat enough there is anxiety because the body is hungry. A religious person is one who knows where to stop; and that should come out of your awareness, not out of a certain teaching.

If I tell you how much to eat, that is going to be dangerous because that will be just an average. Somebody is very thin and somebody is very fat, and if I tell you how much to eat – "three *chappatis*" – then for somebody it may be too much and for somebody it may be nothing. So I don't teach rigid rules, I simply give you a sense of awareness. Listen to your body: you have a different body. And then there are different types of energies, different types of involvement. Somebody is a professor in a university; he does not exert much energy as far as his body is concerned. He will not need much food, and he will need a different kind of food. Somebody is a labourer; he will need much food, and a different kind of food. Now a rigid principle is going to be dangerous. No rule can be given as a universal rule.

George Bernard Shaw has said that there is only one golden rule, that there are no golden rules. Remember it, there is no golden rule – there cannot be, because each individual is so unique that nobody can prescribe. So I simply give you a sense.... And my sense is not of principles, of laws; my approach is of awareness, because today you may need more food and tomorrow you may not need that much food. It is not only a question of you being different from others – every day of your life is different from every other day. The whole day you have rested, you may not need much food. The whole day you have been in the garden digging a hole, you may need much food. One should be just alert and one should be capable of listening to what the body is saying. Go according to the body.

Neither is the body the master, nor is the body the slave; the body is your friend – befriend your body. The one who goes on eating too much and the one who goes on dieting are both in the same trap. They are both deaf; they don't listen to what the body is saying....

Eat for the joy of it; then you are man, human, a higher being. Love for the joy of love; then you are man, a higher being. Listen for the joy of listening and you will be freed from the confinement of instincts.

I am not against happiness, I am all for it. I am a hedonist, and this is my understanding: all the great spiritual people of the world have always been hedonists. If somebody is not a hedonist and pretends to be a spiritual person, he is not – then he is a psychopath, because happiness is the very goal, the very source, the very end of all things. God is seeking happiness through you, in millions of forms. Allow him all the happiness that is possible and help him to go to higher peaks, higher reaches, of happiness. Then you are religious, and then your temples will become places of celebration and your churches will not be so sad and ugly, so somber, so dead, like graveyards. Then there will be laughter and there will be song and there will be dance and there will be great rejoicing.

Religion has suffered very much because of these people who have been teaching self-torture. Religion has to be freed from all this nonsense. Great rubbish has become attached to religion. The essential religion is nothing but joy. So whatsoever gives you joy is virtuous; whatsoever makes you sad, unhappy, miserable is a sin. Let that be the criterion.

And I don't give you rigid rules because I know how the human mind functions. Once a rigid rule is given, you forget awareness and you start following the rigid rule.

A rigid rule is not the question – you can follow the rule and you will never grow. Listen to a few anecdotes:

Benny arrived home to find the kitchen a mess of broken crockery.

"What happened?" he asked his wife.

"There's something wrong with this cookbook," she explained. "It says that an old cup without a handle will do for the measuring – and it's taken me eleven tries to get a handle off without breaking the cup."

Now if the cookbook says that, it has to be done. Human mind is foolish – remember it. Once you have a rigid rule, you follow it.

The mob was meeting the big guy, and what the big guy said, went. The buzzer rang and the servant went over to answer the door. He peeked through the slot in the frame, and, recognizing the visitor, allowed the panel to swing back.

"Leave your umbrella at the door," the servant told the visitor.

"I ain't got one," answered the visitor.

"Then get back home and get one. The boss told me everyone must leave their umbrella at the door. Otherwise I am not going to allow you in."

A rule is a rule....

It was a desperate chase but the police-car was catching up to the bank-robbers when suddenly it swerved into a gas station, from which point the cop driving phoned his chief.

"Did you catch them?" the chief asked excitedly.

"They were lucky," replied the cop. "We were closing the gap, only half a mile away, when I noticed our five hundred miles were up and we had to stop and change our oil."

What can you do when the oil has to be changed after each five hundred miles and five hundred miles are up? You have to change the oil first.

I never give you rigid rules because I know how stupid human mind is and can be. I simply give you a feel, a sense of direction. Be aware and live through awareness.

Ordinarily you are living a very unconscious life. You eat too much because you are unconscious – you don't know what you are doing. You become jealous, you become possessive, because you are unconscious and you don't know what you are doing. You get mad in anger, you become almost possessed of the devil when you are in a rage, and you do things which you don't know that you are doing.

Jesus said on the cross – the last of his words, but of tremendous import – he said: "Father forgive these people because they don't know what they are doing." Now Christianity has never interpreted these tremendous words rightly. Jesus' message is simple. He is saying: These people are unconscious people. They don't know awareness at all, so they cannot be responsible. Whatsoever they are doing, they are doing in sleep; they are somnambulists, sleep-walkers. Please forgive them. They cannot be held responsible.

So when you eat too much, I pray to God, "Father, forgive this man. He does not know what he is doing." When you fast, I again have to pray to God, "Forgive this man because he does not know what he is doing." The real question is not of doing but of bringing an awareness into your being, and that awareness will change everything. You are like drunkards.

I have heard: Mike told Pat he was going to a wake, and Pat offered to tag along. On the way Pat suggested a nip or two and they both got well sloshed. As a result Mike couldn't remember the address of the wake. "Where is your friend's house?" Pat asked.

"I forgot the number, but I'm sure this is the street."

They had walked along for a few minutes when Mike squinted at a house that he thought was it. So they staggered in but the hall was dark. They opened the door and discovered a living room, which was also dark except for the faint glimmer of candles sitting on the piano. They went down in front of the piano, knelt and prayed. Pat stopped long enough to look at the piano. "Mike," he said "I don't know your friend, but he sure had a fine set of teeth."

This is the situation. This is how man is. The only thing that I would like to give to you is a taste of awareness. That will change your whole life. It is not a question of disciplining you, it is a question of making you luminous from within.[52]

 What is the relationship between food and our emotions?

You may have observed it: if you are in a very loving and flowing relationship you will not eat too much, you will never need to diet. Love fills you so much that there is no need to go on stuffing yourself with all kinds of junk. If there is no love you feel so empty. That emptiness hurts, you want to fill it with something. And why do you choose food? — because love and food are associated psychologically.

The child got both food and love from the mother's breast simultaneously. Whenever the mother was loving she was willing to give her breast to him, and whenever she was not loving, angry, she used to pull the breast away from him. And the mother's breast was the first contact with another's body.

It is not strange that all the painters, sculptors, poets, are so obsessed with the female breast. It seems absolutely unbelievable that for millions of years painters have been painting the female breast, sculptors have been wasting their whole life cutting stones, marble.... If you have been to Indian temples like Khajuraho, you cannot believe it.

Thirty temples are still there. There must have been hundreds more because there are ruins. But even these thirty temples...just one temple is unbelievable; to think of thirty will make you giddy. In just one temple, if you start counting how many naked women are sculpted, you will be at a loss. You will have to start again and again because thousands are on each pillar, on each wall, everywhere; not a single inch is left unsculpted. And such huge breasts, which are just imagination – such huge breasts don't exist, cannot exist. The woman has to stand up with that much weight! And Khajuraho is not the only place. In India there are thousands of temples all around: Puri, Konarak, Ellora – beautiful sculpture, but from a sick mind.

Why do all these painters, great painters of the world, go on painting the breast? Somewhere they have been deprived, somewhere the mother was not loving. And more or less every child has been taken off the breast before his time. Only in aboriginal societies is the child given the mother's breast as long as he wants; and those are the only societies where nobody is obsessed with breasts. They don't have any paintings of breasts, they don't have any sculptures of breasts, they don't have any poetry, no songs, nothing. The breast does not enter their imagination at all.

Because of the breast, love and food become associated deep down in the mind. So whenever you are not being loved you start eating, stuffing yourself. When you are loved that stuffing disappears by itself, there is no need. Love is such a nourishment, such a subtle, invisible nourishment, that who bothers about chewing gum?

I cannot believe that human beings are chewing gum. Has the whole earth gone mad? Chewing gum cannot give you any nourishment, but it must be doing something, something psychological. Perhaps it is a breast substitute, that you go on using your mouth.[53]

No animal eats like man; every animal has its chosen food. If you bring buffaloes in the garden and leave them, they will eat only a particular grass. They will not go on eating everything and anything – they are very choosy. They have a certain feeling about their food. Man is completely lost, has no feeling about his food. He goes on eating everything and anything. In fact you cannot find anything which is not eaten somewhere or other by man. In some places, ants are eaten. In some places, snakes are eaten. In some places, dogs are eaten. Man has eaten everything. Man is simply mad. He does not know what is in resonance with his body and what is not. He is completely confused.

Man, naturally, should be a vegetarian, because the whole body is made for vegetarian food. Even scientists concede to the fact that the whole structure of the human body shows that man should not be a non-vegetarian. Man comes from the monkeys. Monkeys are vegetarians – absolute vegetarians. If Darwin is true then man should be a vegetarian. Now there are ways to judge whether a certain species of animal is vegetarian or non-vegetarian: it depends on the intestine, the length of the intestine. Non-vegetarian animals have a very small intestine. Tigers, lions – they have a very small intestine, because meat is already a digested food. It does not need a long intestine to digest it. The work of digestion has been done by the animal. Now you are eating the animal's meat. It is already digested – no long intestine is needed. Man has one of the longest intestines: that means man is a vegetarian. A long digestion is needed, and much excreta will be there which has to be thrown out.

If man is not a non-vegetarian and he goes on eating meat, the body is burdened. In the East, all the great meditators – Buddha, Mahavira – they have emphasized the fact, not because of any concept of nonviolence, that is a secondary thing, but because if you really want to move in deep meditation, your body needs to be weightless, natural flowing. Your body needs to be unloaded; and a non-vegetarian's body is very much loaded.

Just watch what happens when you eat meat: when you kill an animal what happens to the animal when he is killed? Of course, nobody wants to be killed. Life wants to prolong itself; the animal is not dying willingly. If somebody kills you, you will not die willingly. If a lion jumps on you and kills you, what will happen to your mind? The same happens when you kill a lion. Agony, fear, death, anguish, anxiety, anger, violence, sadness – all these things happen to the animal. All over his body violence, anguish, agony spreads. The whole body becomes full of toxins, poisons. All the body glands release poisons because the animal is dying very unwillingly. And then you eat the meat – that meat carries all the poisons that the animal has released. The whole energy is poisonous, then those poisons are carried in your body.

And that meat which you are eating belonged to an animal body. It had a specific purpose there. A specific type of consciousness existed in the animal's body. You are on a higher plane than the animal's consciousness, and when you eat the animal's meat your body goes to the lowest plane, to the lower plane of the animal. Then there exists a gap between your consciousness and your body, and a tension arises, an anxiety arises.

One should eat things which are natural – natural for you. Fruits, nuts, vegetables – eat as much as you can. And the beauty is that you cannot eat these things more than is needed. Whatsoever is natural always gives you a satisfaction, because it satiates your body, saturates you. You feel fulfilled. If something is unnatural it never gives you a feeling of fulfillment. Go on eating ice cream: you never feel that you are satiated. In fact the more you eat, the more you feel like eating. It is not a food. Your mind is being tricked. Now you are not eating according to the body need, you are eating just to taste it. The tongue has become the controller.

The tongue should not be the controller. It does not know anything about the stomach. It does not know anything about the body. The tongue has a specific purpose to fulfill: to taste food. Naturally, the tongue has to judge, that is the only thing, which food is for the body – for my body – and which food is not for my body. It is just a watchman on the door; it is not the master. And if the watchman on the door becomes the master, then everything will be confused.

Now advertisers know well that the tongue can be tricked, the nose can be tricked. And they are not the masters. You may not be aware: much food research goes on in the world, and they say if your nose is closed completely and your eyes closed, and then you are given an onion to eat, you cannot tell what you are eating. You cannot tell onion from apple if the nose is closed completely because half of the taste comes from the smell, is decided by the nose, and half is decided by the tongue – and these two have become the controllers. Now they know: whether ice cream is nutritious or not is not the point. It can carry a flavour, it can carry some chemicals which fulfill the tongue but are not needed for the body.

Man is confused – more confused than buffaloes. You can not convince buffaloes to eat ice-cream. Try!

A natural food…and when I say 'natural' I mean that which your body needs. The need of a tiger is different; he has to be very violent. If you eat the meat of a tiger you will be violent, but where will your violence be expressed? You have to live in human society, not in a jungle. Then you will have to suppress the violence. Then a vicious circle starts. When you suppress violence, what happens? When you feel angry, violent, a certain poisonous energy is released, because that poison creates a situation where you can be really violent and kill somebody. The energy moves towards your hands; the energy moves towards your teeth – these are the two places from where animals become violent. Man is part of the animal kingdom.

When you are angry, energy is released – it comes to the hands and to the teeth, to the jaw – but you live in a human society and it is not always profitable to be angry. You live in a civilized world, and you cannot behave like an animal. If you behave like an animal, you will have to pay too much for it – and you are not ready to pay that much. Then what do you do? You suppress the anger in the hand; you suppress the anger in your teeth – you go on smiling a false smile, and your teeth go on accumulating anger.

I have rarely come to see people with a natural jaw. It is not natural – blocked, stiff – because too much anger is there. If you press the jaw of a person, the anger can be released. Hands become ugly. They lose grace, they lose flexibility, because too much anger is suppressed there. People who have been working on deep massage, they have come to know that when you touch the hands deeply, massage the hands, the person starts becoming angry. There is no reason. You are massaging the man and suddenly he starts feeling angry. If you press the jaw, persons become angry again. They carry accumulated anger.

These are the impurities in the body: they have to be released. If you don't release them the body will remain heavy. Yoga exercises exist to release all sorts of accumulated poisons in the body. Yoga movements release them; and a yogi's body has a suppleness of its own. Yoga exercises are totally different from other exercises. They don't make your body strong; they make your body more flexible. And when your body is more flexible, you are strong in a very different sense: you are younger. They make your body more liquid, more flowing – no blocks in the body. The whole body exists as an organic unity, in a deep rhythm of its own. It is not like noise in the market, it is like an orchestra. A deep rhythm inside, no blocks, then the body is pure. Yoga exercises can be tremendously helpful.

Everybody is carrying much rubbish in the stomach, because that is the only space in the body where you can suppress things. There is no other space. If you want to suppress anything it has to be suppressed in the stomach. If you want to cry – your wife has died, your beloved has died, your friend has died – but it doesn't look good, looks as if you are a weakling, crying for a woman, you suppress it. Where will you put that crying? Naturally, you have to suppress it in the stomach. That is the only space available in the body, the only hollow place, where you can force it.

If you suppress in the stomach...and everybody has suppressed many sorts of emotions: of love, of sexuality, of anger, of sadness, of weeping – even of laughter. You cannot laugh a belly laugh. It looks rude, looks vulgar – you are not cultured then. You have suppressed everything. Because of this suppression, you cannot breathe deeply, you have to breathe shallowly. If you breathed deeply then those wounds of suppression, they would release their energy. You are afraid. Everybody is afraid to move in the stomach.

Every child, when born, breathes through the belly. Look at a child sleeping: the belly goes up and down – never the chest. No child breathes from the chest; they breathe from the belly. They are completely free now, nothing is suppressed. Their stomachs are empty, and that emptiness has a beauty in the body. Once the stomach has too much suppression in it, the body is divided in two parts, the lower and the higher. Then you are not one; you are two. The lower part is the discarded part. The unity is lost; a duality has entered into your being. Now you cannot be beautiful, you cannot be graceful. You are carrying two bodies instead of one – and there will always remain a gap between the two. You cannot walk beautifully. Somehow you have to carry your legs. In fact, if the body is one, your legs will carry you. If the body is divided in two then you have to carry your legs.

You have to drag your body. It is like a burden – you cannot enjoy it. You cannot enjoy a good walk, you cannot enjoy a good swim, you cannot enjoy a fast run – because the body is not one. For all these movements, and to enjoy them, the body needs to be reunited. A unison has to be created again: the stomach will have to be cleansed completely.

For the cleansing of the stomach very deep breathing is needed, because when you inhale deeply and exhale deeply, the stomach throws all that it is carrying. In exhalations, the stomach releases itself. Hence the importance of *pranayam,* of deep rhythmic breathing. The emphasis should be on the exhalation so that everything that the stomach has been unnecessarily carrying is released. And when the stomach is not carrying emotions inside, if you have constipation it will suddenly disappear. When you are suppressing emotions in the stomach there will be constipation because the stomach is not free to have its movements. You are controlling it deeply; you can't allow it freedom. So if emotions are suppressed, there will be constipation. Constipation is more a mental disease than a physical one. It belongs to the mind more than it belongs to the body.

But remember, I am not dividing mind and body in two. They are two aspects of the same phenomenon. Mind and body are not two things. In fact to say 'mind and body' is not good: 'mind-body' will be the right expression. Your body is a psychosomatic phenomenon. Mind is the subtlest part of the body, and body is the grossest part of the mind. And they both affect each other; they run parallel. If you are suppressing something in the mind, the body will start a suppressing journey. If the mind releases everything, the body also releases everything. That's why I emphasize catharsis very much. Catharsis is a cleansing process.

These are all austerities: fasting; natural eating; deep, rhythmic breathing; yoga exercises; living a more and more natural, flexible, supple life; creating less and less suppressed attitudes; allowing the body to have its own say, following the wisdom of the body....

When the body is pure, you will see tremendous new energies arising, new dimensions opening before you, new doors suddenly opening, new possibilities. The body has much hidden power. Once it is released, you will not be able to believe it, that the body carried so many things in it, and so close.[54]

? *I am a compulsive overeater. Any suggestions to help me?*

While hungry, why not meditate a little? – there is no hurry. While hungry just close your eyes and meditate on the hunger, on how the body is feeling. You have lost contact, because our hunger is less bodily, more mental. You eat every day at one o'clock. You look at the watch; it is one – so then you feel hunger. And the clock may not be right. If somebody says, "That clock has stopped at midnight – it is not functioning. It is only eleven o'clock," the hunger disappears. This hunger is false, this hunger is just habitual, because the mind creates it, not the body. Mind says, "One o'clock – you are hungry." You have to be hungry. You have always been hungry at one o'clock, so you are hungry.

Our hunger is almost ninety-nine percent habitual. Go on a fast for a few days to feel real hunger, and you will be surprised. For the first three or four days you will feel very hungry. On the fourth or fifth day you will not feel so hungry. This is illogical, because as the fast grows, you should feel more and more hungry. But after the third day you will feel less hungry, and after the seventh day you may completely forget hunger. After the eleventh day almost everybody forgets hunger completely and the body feels absolutely okay. Why? And if you continue the fast.... Those who have done much work on fasting say that only after the twenty-first day will real hunger happen again.

So it means that for three days your mind was insisting that you were hungry because you had not taken food, but it was not hunger. Within three days the mind gets fed up with telling you; you are not listening, you are so indifferent. On the fourth day the mind doesn't say anything; the body doesn't feel hunger. For three weeks you will not feel hunger, because you have accumulated so much fat – that fat will do. You will feel hunger only after the third week. And this is for normal bodies.

If you have too much fat accumulated, you may not feel hungry even after the third week. And there is a possibility to accumulate enough fat to live on for three months – ninety days. When the body is finished with the accumulated fat, then for the first time real hunger will be felt. But it will be difficult. You can try with thirst; that will be easy. For one day don't take water, and wait. Don't drink out of habit. Just wait and see what thirst means; what thirst would mean if you were in a desert....

You know only by your tongue, and that tongue is very deceptive. That tongue has been serving the mind so long it is no longer serving the body. The tongue can deceive you; it has become a slave of the mind. It can go on saying, "Go on eating – it is very beautiful." It is not serving the body anymore; otherwise the tongue would say, "Stop!" The tongue would say, "Whatsoever you are eating is useless. Don't eat!" Even the tongues of cows and buffaloes are more body-rooted than your tongue. You cannot force a buffalo to eat any type of grass – she chooses. You cannot force your dog to eat when he is ill – he will immediately go out, eat some grass, and vomit. He is more in contact with his body.

First one has to become deeply aware of this phenomenon of the body. A revival of the body, a resurrection, is needed – you are carrying a dead body. Then only will you feel, by and by, that the whole body with all its desires, thirsts, and hungers, is revolving around the heart. Then the beating heart is not only a mechanism, it is the beating life, it is the very pulsation of life. That pulsation gives contentment and bliss. [55]

?

Several sannyasins have told me that you do not approve of macrobiotics. Is this so? I wonder whether your criticisms were directed at obsessive attitudes toward diet rather than at the principles of macrobiotics.

Macrobiotics is pure Taoism. There are no rules and no prohibitions. Its emphasis is on awareness, freedom, sensitivity and flexibility. It has nothing at all to do with food fads, rigid diets or obsessive attitudes. Brown rice is mistakenly regarded by some as the basis of macrobiotics, but it is only one element and can be used or discarded, recognized or ignored. Could you please comment?

The first thing: I am against all fads. Irrespective of what the fad is, I am against all fads, because fads attract obsessive people. Fads become hiding-places for insane people. People who are abnormal, they hide themselves behind fads, and they create systems, theories, dogmas, to rationalize.

I used to live with a woman. She was a very lovely woman, but almost crazy about cleanliness. The whole day she was cleaning the house, the whole day she was decorating – for no purpose, because she never allowed anybody in the house. If guests would come she would meet them on the lawn.

I asked her, "You continuously go on decorating and cleaning your house, but I see that nobody is ever allowed in."

She said, "Those people, they may make everything dirty."

"Then what is the purpose of it?"

She said, "Cleanliness is next to God."

Now, this woman is mad. Cleanliness has become just a hiding-place. It has become a ritual. Now, cleaning the whole day, she remains occupied. Cleaning the whole day has become her whole life – it is a sheer wastage. But you cannot say that cleanliness is bad; cleanliness is good. So she has a reason. She is mad with a perfect rationality. Even her husband was not allowed to come into the drawing room. And she never allowed herself to have any children, because children are dirty and they would create trouble and they would make things messy. Her whole life was sacrificed at the altar of cleanliness.

I said, "Of course, you have proved that cleanliness is second to God. You have made it an altar of God and you are sacrificing your whole life to it."

But she would say, "Am I wrong?"

You cannot say she is wrong. Cleanliness is good, hygienic – but there is a limit to it. The faddist always goes beyond the limit. He is deep down very troubled. I told the woman, "You do one thing: for three days don't clean the house. If you can remain sane for three days without cleaning the house, I will also join you and I will also clean your house the whole day."

She said, "Three days without cleaning? That is impossible – I will go mad." She is already mad!

So whenever there is someone who is hiding behind a fad, whatsoever the fad is – it may be macrobiotics or something else – I am against it. I am against the attitude of obsessiveness.

Let me tell you one anecdote: A man came home from the match. His wife looked up from the paper and said, "Look here, Fred, there's a report in the paper about a man who's just given his wife to a friend in return for a football season-ticket. You're a keen fan but you wouldn't do a thing like that, would you?"

Fred said, "Of course I wouldn't. It is ridiculous and criminal – the season is half over!"

This is the mind of a fan, of a faddist. But these people can go on hiding behind beautiful reasons.

Mahatma Gandhi was continuously concerned about his bowel movements. He was almost obsessive about it. Sometimes when your stomach is disturbed, you can think about it, but continuously pondering and meditating and brooding over it is nonsense. But he was continuously brooding – as if that was the greatest subject in the world to think about. He would do his prayer, or he was going to see the viceroy, or he was going to take part in the round-table conference which was going to decide the fate of India and its freedom, but first he would take an enema. You would be surprised: in his diary, the enema is as much referred to as God. The enema seems to be a second god.

But if you argued with him, he would look perfectly clear about it: the stomach has to be completely clean, because without a clean stomach the whole body gets toxins, this and that, and only with a clean stomach can the mind be clean. How can the mind be healthy without a healthy body? Then he would go on and on, arguing about it, thinking about it. But in fact it is a fad and a sort of illness. And it doesn't show a healthy mind, it shows an unhealthy mind.

This type of attitude I am against. I have said to many sannyasins…because they come to me with their fads. One young man came and he said he had come to me to learn how to live only on water! I told him, "You will make me a criminal. If I tell you how to live on water, you will die!" He was lean and thin, almost on the verge of collapse, but he had a fad that purity is possible only through water. Only water is pure and everything else is impure. His eyes were becoming yellow, ill. He was not eating well, his body was starved, and by and by his brain would start getting feverish. And the more feverish he would become, the more he would make efforts to purify himself. I have to tell such people that they are moving in a very, very dangerous direction.

Macrobiotics addicts come to me…. I am not against anything in particular, because I am not in favour of anything in particular. I am just in favour of life, life in its tremendous richness….

You say: "Macrobiotics is pure Taoism." No principle, no theory, can be pure Taoism. Even Taoism is not pure Taoism. Lao Tzu resisted for his whole life…he denied his disciples, he rejected all appeals to him to make a theory about his whole principle, because he said, "Once Tao is said, it is no longer Tao. Truth cannot be said, cannot be theorized." Only in the end he wrote something, and that too under pressure. He was leaving China. It seems he was coming to India. Everybody has to come finally to India. India is not a geographical point, it is the very source of all human consciousness. Everyone who wants to be reoriented has to come to the orient. Orient simply means orientation.

Lao Tzu…of course, Chinese scholars never say that he was going to India; that offends their ego. They say he was going to the south, but India is the south. They say he moved towards the south, but India is the south for China. And, of course, it seems meaningful – Lao Tzu coming back to India. That seems absolutely relevant. Everybody has to come. India is everybody's home.

He was caught on the boundaries of China by the government officials and they said, "We will not allow you to go out of the country with your treasure. You have to leave the treasure."

He asked, "What do you mean?"

They said, "You have to write a book before you leave our country. You know something: you have to write it down and hand it over to the government. Then you can leave."

So he was forced on the boundary by these officials. In three days he went and quickly wrote the whole *Tao Teh Ching*. But in the first line he says, "Tao cannot be uttered, and the Tao that is uttered is no longer Tao." So even Taoism is not pure Tao – the 'ism' makes it impure. So forget about macrobiotics – that it can be pure Taoism. It is a theory, an hypothesis.

There are no rules and no prohibitions. If there are no rules and no prohibitions, then why be unnecessarily worried about macrobiotics? Then what is the point of calling yourself a follower of macrobiotics if there are no rules and no regulations? There are....

"Macrobiotics has nothing to do with brown rice." They are mad about brown rice! They think brown rice is God, and unless you live on brown rice you will miss out. But you say: "Brown rice is mistakenly regarded by some as the basis of macrobiotics but it is only one element and can be used or discarded, recognized or ignored." But then what remains? If even brown rice is discarded, ignored, and there are no principles and no regulations and it is pure Taoism, then what remains? Nothing remains. Then I can happily say, "Yes, be a macrobiotic follower – no problem!"

I am against fads. I am against a disciplined life. I am not against discipline; I am against disciplined life. Discipline should come moment to moment from your inner being. It should be an inner light, not imposed from the outside. One should move in deep response to life. One should not follow any doctrine, because if you follow a doctrine then you already have a conclusion with you. You live through that conclusion. You live from a centre which is already fixed. Then you are not free. You cannot be flexible; your principle, your idea, your centre, your conclusion, will not allow you to be flexible. You will react according to your conclusion. But if you are free and each moment decides its own conclusion, it is not carried over from the past, then it is perfectly okay. Then you have a discipline – real discipline – but you don't have a disciplined life.

Any man who is really alive has no character, cannot have a character. Character is always dead – a dead structure around you, carried over from the past, the past experience. If you act out of your character, you don't act at all; you simply react. You don't respond. Response is immediate: life creates a situation, a challenge, and you respond. You respond out of your being, with no centre, with no conclusion. Not through the past; herenow comes the response – pure, virgin.

That discipline I appreciate. That discipline I love. But any other discipline that you force yourself into, that you practice, is dangerous. That is going to kill you. That's how many people are already dead – their discipline has killed them.[56]

? *I hate being overweight but can't lose any weight for very long in spite of all the diets I have tried.*

You have a very perfectionistic idea about how the body should be, how you should be. You have a very clear-cut goal, and because of that clear-cut goal you fall short and you cannot accept yourself, you go on rejecting. And out of that rejection, you feel miserable.

Just destroy those goals and ideals: those ideals and goals that you are keeping in your mind of how things should be, how you should be. Drop them! And there is nothing missing, nothing is lacking; your energy can start flowing. Once you are in the moment, your body will start losing weight. It is continuous antagonism with the body that is making it fat, because when you are continuously against the body the body feels insecure, and out of insecurity it goes on eating.

It is like a child who cannot trust its mother. If the child cannot trust the mother, once he has the mother's breast he will not leave it because he cannot trust; he does not know when he will get the breast again. It is not certain, he cannot remain secure in it – so he will grab. He will go on drinking as much as he can. He will stuff himself because the future is uncertain. When the child knows the mother loves him and knows the mother will be available – whenever she is needed she will be available – he does not bother to stuff himself. He can rest, he can eat as much as he needs in that moment, there is no need to hoard.

In fact fat is a hoarding; for some uncertain future one goes on hoarding. A man can live three months without food, one can gather that much fat. It is an old, ancient habit, biological. There were times, thousands of years back, when man was a hunter and the food was not certain. One day it was there, and in abundance, and for days together it was not there at all. Man carries that biological habit. That is associated with insecurity. Now there is no problem – at least not in America: you have enough food. For the first time society has enough food. Americans should not be fat at all. Indians can be allowed to be fat because the food is not certain.

What I am saying is that now food is available, good food, good nourishment, there is no physical need to eat more, but now psychological insecurity triggers the mechanism of the body, and the body starts feeling insecure. It knows only one way of how to avoid insecurity, and that is to eat more, to go on eating and stuff itself. It becomes an occupation.

Drop the ideals! There is nothing that you have to improve; you are perfectly beautiful as you are. And start living! Rather than thinking that you will live in the future when you are perfect, when you are like this, like that, you will live when you have attained a certain standard according to your mind.... But life is herenow and slipping out of our hands. Tomorrow there is death – only today there is life... it is always today.

Start living and start enjoying. The more you enjoy, the less you will eat. A really happy person does not eat much. It is out of misery, out of pain, out of emptiness, out of a meaninglessness that one wants to grab on to something – at least food, something.[57]

The body has accumulated much wisdom, the body is very wise. If you eat too much the body says, "Stop!" The mind is not so wise. The mind says, "The taste is beautiful – a little more." And if you listen to the mind, then the mind becomes destructive to the body, this way or that. If you listen to the mind, first it will say, "Go on eating," because mind is foolish, a child. He does not know what he is saying. He is a new arrival, he has no learning. He is not wise, he is still a fool. Listen to the body. When the body says, "Hungry" – eat. When the body says, "Stop" – stop.

If you listen to the mind, it is as if a small child is leading an old man – they will both fall in a pit. If you listen to the mind, then first you will be in the senses too much; and then you will get fed up. And every sense will bring you misery, every sense will bring you more anxiety, conflict, pain. If you eat too much there will be pain and there will be vomiting, and the whole body will be disturbed. Then the mind says, "Eating is bad, so go on a fast." And a fast is also dangerous. If you listen to the body it will never overeat, it will never undereat – it will simply follow the Tao.

A few scientists have been working on this problem and they have discovered a very beautiful phenomenon: small children eat whenever they feel hungry, they go to sleep whenever they feel that sleep is coming – they listen to their bodies. But parents disturb them, they go on forcing: "It is dinnertime, or lunchtime, or this and that, or sleeping-time – go!" They don't allow their bodies. So one experimenter tried leaving children on their own. He was working with twenty-five children. They were not forced to go to sleep, they were not forced to get up. They were not forced at all for six months. And a very deep understanding came.

They slept well. They had less dreams – no nightmares, because nightmares were coming from the parents who were forcing them. They ate well, but never too much – never less than necessary, never more than necessary. They enjoyed eating and sometimes they would not eat at all. When the body was not feeling well they would not eat, and they never fell ill because of eating. And one more thing which no one ever suspected came to be understood, and it was miraculous. Only Sosan can understand, or Lao Tzu or Chuang Tzu, because they are the masters of Tao. This was such a discovery: they came to understand that if a child was ill, then he would not eat particular foods. Then they tried to understand why he was not eating those foods. The foods were analyzed and it was found that for that disease, those foods were dangerous. How did the child decide? – just the body.

When the child was growing he would eat more of whatsoever was needed for his growth. Then they analyzed and they found that these ingredients were helpful and the food would change, because the needs changed. One day a child would eat something and the next day the same child would not eat it. And the scientists felt that there is a body-wisdom.

If you allow the body to have its say, you are moving on the right path, the great way. And this is so not only with food – this is so with the whole life. Your sex goes wrong because of your mind, your stomach goes wrong because of your mind. You interfere with the body. Don't interfere! Even if you can do it for three months – don't interfere, and suddenly you will become so healthy, and a well-being will descend on you.[58]

CHAPTER 10

PSYCHOLOGY

? *You have often talked about psychoanalysis and related therapies. Would you please comment on more recent developments like Fritz Perls' Gestalt therapy and – the latest fashion – Voice Dialogue? Can these therapies help a person who is already meditating to see himself and his games more clearly?*

In the first place, psychotherapies like Fritz Perls' Gestalt therapy and others are already old, they are not new. The only new thing which is the latest fashion is Voice Dialogue – but they are all just mind games.

They cannot contribute anything to a man who is already meditating – no psychotherapy has the quality of meditation, because no psychotherapy has produced a single enlightened being. Their founders were not enlightened and the enlightened beings in the East never bothered about any psychotherapy. They have not even bothered about psychology or mind itself, because for them the question was not to solve the problems of the mind, for them the question was how to get out of the mind, which is easier. Then the problems are all finished, because once you are out of the mind, the mind has no nourishment to go on creating problems; otherwise it is an unending process. You get psychoanalyzed, whether old or new fashions it doesn't matter; they are just variations of the same theme. Your mind feels a little fresh and good after a psychological session because you have unburdened yourself. A little understanding of mind also comes – that keeps you normal.

In fact, all psychotherapies are in the service of the establishment; their function is not to let people go abnormal. Somebody is going outside the herd and the norms of the herd and doing things which it is not supposed that you should do…. They may be harmless but the society cannot tolerate such people. They have to be brought to the normal, to the average standard.

The psychotherapist's work is to clean your mind. It is a kind of lubricating your mechanism – it functions a little better and you start becoming a little more understanding about the functionings of the mind, although that does not make any revolutionary change. And it is possible you may solve one problem, but you have not removed the cause. Mind itself is the problem. So *you* can remove one problem, *mind* will create another problem.... It is just like pruning the trees: you prune one leaf and just out of self-respect and dignity the tree will grow three leaves in the place where there used to be one. That's why gardeners go on pruning; that gives trees more foliage, more leaves.

The same is the situation with the mind: you can remove one problem by understanding it – and it is costly – but the mind is still there which has created the problem, and psychoanalysis does not go beyond the boundaries of the mind. The mind will create a new problem, more complicated than the one that you have solved. Naturally, because the mind understands you can solve that kind of problem, it creates something new, more complicated, more foliage.

Meditation is a totally different thing than psychoanalysis or any therapies which are confined to the mind. It is simply a jumping out of the mind: "You have your problems – I'm going home." Because mind is a parasite it does not have its own existence. It needs you inside in it, so it can go on eating you, your head. Once you jump out of it, the mind is just a graveyard. All those problems that were too big drop, they simply drop dead.

Meditation is a totally different dimension: you simply watch the mind and in watching you come out of it. And slowly, mind with all its problems disappears; otherwise the mind is going to create strange problems....

Mind is your only problem – all other problems are just offshoots of the mind. Meditation cuts the mind from the very roots. And all these therapies – Gestalt and Voice Dialogue and Fritz Perls – we can use them for those who have not yet entered into meditation just to have a little understanding of the mind so they can find the door from where to get out. We are using all kinds of therapies which are helpful, but not for the meditators. They are only helpful in the beginning when you have not yet become accustomed to meditation. Once you are meditative you don't need any therapy, no therapy is helpful then. But in the beginning, it can be helpful, and particularly for the Western sannyasins....

Sigmund Freud is right only about the Western mind and its tradition. When he says that every girl hates her mother because she loves the father, the whole thing is based on their understanding of sex, that one loves the opposite sex. So girls love the fathers, the boys love the mother. But the girls cannot express their love, particularly they cannot be sexually related with the father, and the mother *is* related sexually. So they become jealous of the mother – the mother is their enemy. The boys become enemies of the father and because of that the boy cannot make love to the mother. The Japanese cannot even think of this; even Indians cannot think of this – just a totally different upbringing. Sigmund Freud or Jung or Adler or Assagioli or Fritz Perls have no idea. Not even in their dreams have they thought that people can be different from the Western people....

In the East, psychoanalysis is not of much help. For the Westerners, I like them to go through groups just to clean the mind. With a clean mind, to enter into meditation is easier. But if you don't enter meditation and you simply depend on cleaning the mind, then you will be cleaning the mind for your whole life and you will not go anywhere else. Because of its different orientation the East should find seats in the universities for meditation, not for psychoanalysis....

In the East for centuries the problem has been how to get beyond the mind – the only problem, the single problem. But for the Western mind, because it has developed in a different way it has never thought about transcending mind. I have looked into Jewish sources, into Christian sources; there is not a single statement in the whole history of the West where somebody has made an effort to go beyond the mind. They have used the mind to pray, they have used the mind to believe in God; they have used the mind to become religious, virtuous, but they have never even thought that there is a possibility of going beyond the mind.

In the East that has been the only, single search. The whole genius of the East has been working for one thing, no other problems: how to go beyond the mind, because if you can solve your problems wholesale just by going beyond, then why go for retail solving of problems? The mind will go on creating; it is a very creative force. You solve one problem, another problem arises. You solve that problem, another problem arises. It is a good business for the psychoanalyst, because he knows you are never going to be cured. You are not going to be cured of the mind; he cures your specific problems. Your mind is there, the source. He never cuts the roots, he only cuts leaves, branches at the most, but they go on growing again – the roots are there.

Meditation is cutting the very roots of problems. I repeat: the mind is the only problem, and unless you go beyond the mind, you will never go beyond problems. It is strange that even today, the Western psychologists have not even pondered over the fact that the East has created so many enlightened people. None of them has bothered about the analysis of the mind.... Hundreds of methods have been found which can help you to transcend the mind, and once you are beyond the mind all its problems look as if they are somebody else's problems. You attain to a state of a watcher on the hills, and all the problems are in the valleys. And they don't have any impact on you; you have gone beyond them.

The West has remained utterly mind-centered. In the West the only thing they have thought about is matter and mind. And matter is the reality and mind is only a by-product; beyond mind there is nothing. In the East matter is illusory, mind is a by-product of all your illusions, projections, dreams. Your reality is beyond matter and mind, both. So we divide reality in the East into three parts: matter, the outermost; the soul, the innermost; the mind is in between the two. Matter has a relative reality; it is not absolutely real, just relatively real. The mind is absolutely unreal, and the soul is absolutely real.

This is a totally different categorization of humanity. In the West the categories are simple: matter is real, mind is just a by-product, and there is nothing beyond mind. So remember, if you are meditating then nothing else is needed. If you are not meditating, then these psychotherapies may be helpful as a stepping stone for meditation…. The West is being exploited by all kinds of frauds for the simple reason that the West has not looked into the matter of meditation itself. So any idiot goes and says anything, and gathers followers because they don't know what meditation is. Neither will chanting a mantra nor hopping nor levitation…. These things have nothing to do with meditation. Meditation has only one meaning, and that is going beyond the mind and becoming a witness. In your witnessing is the miracle – the whole mystery of life.[59]

 Can you please say something about the difference between the spiritual question, "Who am I?" and the psychological trauma of, "Who am I?"?

It is the difference between the ego and the self.

The ego is your false idea of who you are; it is just a fabrication of the mind. It is your own homemade mind-manufactured concept, but it has no corresponding reality to it. It is perfectly good as far as the world is concerned, because there you are dealing with other egos. The moment you go beyond your mind, you also go beyond your ego, and suddenly you realize that you are not what you have always thought yourself to be – that your reality is totally different, that it does not consist of your body or of your mind, that in fact you don't have any word to express it. But it is still not the ultimate reality; it is just in between, between the ultimate reality and the ultimate falsehood. It is better than the false, but it is lower than the really real.

You are still carrying a certain idea of separation from existence. That separation keeps you unavailable to all the blessings which are your birthright. If you can drop those walls and open yourself to the immensity of reality, you will disappear as a separate entity. But this is only one side. On the other side you will appear as the eternal, the immense, the vast reality – the oceanic experience, which is the only experience of enlightenment or liberation.

You have to get rid of the ego first. That is your psychological trauma, or better, your psychological drama. There are religions which have accepted the false ego as the end of all, there is nothing beyond it. That is the religion of all the atheists of different trends, a communist. Or, the atheist may not be a communist, but the atheist in any form stops himself at the ego; that is his ultimate reality. He is the poorest man in the world. All other religions except atheism...because I take atheism also as a sort of religion, a lower form of religion than other religions. Christianity, Judaism, Mohammedanism, go a step further. They all insist to drop the ego and to recognize your authentic reality, your real self. But there are religions like Zen which go to the very end of the road. They are not satisfied just by dropping the ego. They are satisfied only when there is nothing left to drop – even the self is gone – when the house is absolutely empty, when you can say, "I am not." This nothingness is creating the space for the ultimate to blossom. It does not come from anywhere else. It has always been there, just cluttered with rotten furniture, with unnecessary things.

As you remove all those things and your subjectivity becomes empty – just as a room becomes empty as you remove everything from it – in this emptiness of your subjectivity, blossoms the flower of ultimate experience – you are no more. Naturally, you cannot have your old miseries, your old traumas and dramas. You cannot have any connection with your own past; you have abruptly cut yourself away from all that you used to be. Suddenly a new, totally fresh opening...in a way, you disappear. In a way your authentic essence has the first opportunity to come into its full glory, into its absolute splendour.

This is what enlightenment is. It is a negative process: negate the ego, the psychological; negate the self, the spiritual. Go on negating until nothing remains to negate – and the explosion! Suddenly you have arrived home, with the revelation that you have never been out of your home. You have always been there, your eyes were just focused on objects. Now all those objects have disappeared. Only a witnessing, pure awareness, has remained. This witnessing is the end of all your misery and all your hell. It is also the beginning of the golden gate – the doors are open for the first time....

People have forgotten completely to live. Who has time? Everybody is training everybody else in how to be – and nobody seems to be satisfactory, never. If one wants to live, one should learn one thing, to accept things as they are, and to accept yourself as you are. Start living. Don't start training for a life sometime in the future. All the misery in the world is created because you have completely forgotten to live; you have become engaged in an activity which has nothing to do with life.

The moment you are married to a man, you start training him to be faithful. Live while he is faithful – it will not be more than two weeks; two weeks is the human limit! Live as deeply as possible – perhaps your living and loving deeply may help him to remain faithful the third week also. And never project too much; three weeks is enough. My own experience is that if you have lived three weeks lovingly, the fourth week will follow. But you start disturbing things from the first moment. Before you start living, training is needed; you spoil the time by training, and a man who could have loved you for at least two weeks becomes bored within two days.

One woman never married. And when she was dying, a friend asked, "Why have you never married? You are so beautiful." She said, "What is the need? As far as training is concerned I train my dog, and he never learns! Every day I am training and he still comes home late in the night. I have a parrot who tells me everything a husband is expected to say. In the morning he says, "Hello darling!" I have a servant who steals, who continuously lies. What need have I for a husband? Everything is being fulfilled." A husband is needed for these things?

A wife is needed, not to have an experience of intimacy and love, but to make an exhibition of her; just to show around the neighbourhood and make everybody jealous that you have such a beautiful woman. Load her with all the ornaments and make everybody jealous of your richness; otherwise, how are you going to show your richness? A wife is a show-window; she shows your achievements, your power. Naturally, you have to train her how to become more social, how to help you in your businesses. The saying seems to be perfect that behind the success of every great man there is a woman – in many different senses. Sometimes just to escape from her, one becomes madly engaged in earning money.

When Henry Ford was asked, "Why did you go on earning and earning, when you have earned so much? It was time to enjoy and relax." He said, "That was not the reason for earning. I was engaged in earning first to escape from my wife, and secondly, I became interested in whether I can earn more or she can spend more." A competition, a lifelong competition! People get involved in strange dramas. Very few people live authentically – they just act.

A man is sitting in a cinema, and the wife is continually reminding him how the hero is showing his love so deeply to his wife. Finally, the husband said, "Stop all this nonsense! You don't know how much he's paid for it! And moreover, it is only acting; it is not reality. I will certainly say he is a good actor."

The wife said, "Perhaps you are not aware that in actual life also they are wife and husband."

He said, "My God! If that is true, then he is the greatest actor I have ever seen; otherwise, even on the stage, to show so much love to your own wife is simply beyond human capacity. He is almost a genius as far as acting is concerned."

...You are here to live. You are here to dance. You are here to experience life. Others are doing it for you. On your behalf people are loving, people are playing, people are doing all kinds of things. And what is left for you? – just to watch. Death will not be able to take much from you – only your television, because you don't have anything else. This is the false ego that has created a false life pattern and lifestyle.

Drop everything false. Be authentic and true; that is the first step. And once you are authentic and true, you will see how beautiful it is. And that will create the longing to go beyond, in search of the ultimate truth, the final statement and the final experience, beyond which nothing else exists.

People are almost crazy – a tremendous cleansing is needed – and most of their insanity is because of their false life; it is not satisfying. False food cannot be nourishment, false water cannot quench your thirst, and false ego cannot give you real life. It is simple arithmetic.[60]

?

In Newsweek I read a joke within an article on so-called quick-fix therapy. A middle-aged man had been the despair of his family for years because of his compulsive habits of tearing papers to bits and scattering the pieces all over the ground wherever he went. His family dragged him to famous Freudians, Jungians, and Adlerians at great expense but with frustrating results. Trying to shed light into the dismal abyss of his unconscious, where the habit must have its home, failed.

Finally his relatives took him to an obscure but innovative new psychotherapist. This magician took a little walk with his new patient up and down his office, whispering something in his ear. Then he declared to the surprised family, "You can take him home; he's cured."

A year later the habit hadn't returned and the grateful family asked the doctor what he had told his patient. He said, shrugging his shoulders, "Don't tear paper." Would you like to comment?

The secrets of life are very simple, but the mind tries to make them complex. Mind loves complexity, for the simple reason that mind is needed only if there is something complex. If there is nothing complex, the very necessity for mind's existence disappears. Mind does not want to let go of his mastery over you. He is only a servant but he has managed to become the master, and things have become upside down in your life.

The joke simply indicates a very obvious fact. The man was tearing up bits of paper and throwing them all over; naturally everybody thought something has gone wrong: he needs psychoanalysis, he needs some great person who understands the ways of the mind so that he can be fixed up. Nobody even bothered to tell him, "Don't do this."

It was obvious that the man was getting insane, so they went to the Freudians, the Adlerians, the Jungians, to great psychoanalysts. And all those psychoanalysts must have worked hard, for hours, for years, analyzing the dreams of the man to find out why he tears up bits of paper and throws them all over the place. But nobody succeeded. As a last resort they took him to a magician, and he cured the man.

But *Newsweek* is a snobbish magazine, so the joke is not complete. That's why you don't see what is so great about the joke.

The magician walked up and down the staircase and then whispered in the ear of the man, "You stop tearing papers; otherwise I will kick you down from the top." And he was a strong man. "So take heed, because I don't believe in psychoanalysis or anything, I simply believe in kicking. And I kick people from this place. Then they go rolling down hundreds of steps to the road. Now you can go home; just remember that I have only one trick. When any kind of mentally sick person is brought to me, I cure him. That's why I have been walking with you up and down these steps, to show you what it means when I kick you. So now just go home and remember it. Next time I will not say anything, I will simply do it." And the man understood it; anybody would have understood it.

They have left that part out of the joke and destroyed the beauty of it. That man must have been enjoying just a childish thing, tearing papers into bits, into pieces, and throwing them all over the place. And it became an enjoyment because everybody was puzzled. It was simply a childish phenomenon. The man was retarded; he did not need any psychoanalysis. He needed a good kick – that was the language that he understood immediately.

In many ways we go on thinking about simple things in complex ways. Our problems are mostly very simple, but the mind confuses you. And there are people to exploit you. They make your problem even more complex.

Once a boy was brought to me. He must have been sixteen or seventeen years old, and his family was puzzled, harassed, although there was no need for anybody to be harassed. The boy went on saying that two flies have entered into his belly, and they go on moving around inside his body – now they are in the head, now they have come in the hand.

He was taken to doctors, physicians, and they said, "It is not a disease." He was X-rayed, and there were no flies or anything. They tried saying, "You don't have any flies."

But he said, "How can I believe you? They are moving all around inside my body. Should I believe my experience or your explanation?"

Just by chance somebody suggested me to the parents, so they brought the boy. I heard the whole story. The boy was looking very reluctant, stubborn, because he was getting tired of this doctor, that doctor, and they all were saying, "There are no flies."

I said, "You have brought him to the right man. I can see the flies. The poor boy is suffering, and you have been telling him that he is stupid." The boy relaxed. I was favourable – for the first time, a man who has accepted his idea of the flies.

I said, "I know how they have entered. He must be sleeping with an open mouth."

The boy said, "Yes."

I said, "It is such a simple thing. When you sleep with an open mouth, anything can enter. You are fortunate that only flies have entered. I have seen people…rats have entered…"

He said, "My God, rats?"

I said, "Not only rats, but behind rats, cats also."

He said, "Those people must be in great trouble."

I said, "They are. You are nothing, your case is very simple – just two flies. You just lie down here, and I will take them out."

He said, "You are the first man who has shown understanding to a poor boy. Nobody listens to me. I am insistently saying that they are there. I show them the place…they are here, now they have moved here…and they all laugh, and they make me look foolish."

I said, "They are all fools. They have not come across such cases, but this is my special expertise. I deal only with people who sleep with an open mouth."

He said, "I know you understand, because immediately you recognized that they are there – exactly where they were."

I told his parents to stay out of the house and leave him for fifteen minutes with me. I told him to lie down. I blindfolded his eyes and told him to keep his mouth open.

But he said, "If more flies go in…?"

I said, "You don't be worried; this is air-conditioned, and there are no flies. You just lie down with your mouth open and I will try and persuade the flies to come out."

I left him there and ran around the house to catch two flies somehow – for the first time, because I had never done that. But somehow I managed, and I brought two flies in a small bottle. And while I was keeping the bottle by his mouth I removed his blindfold and said, "Look!"

He said, "These two small flies…but what a turmoil they were creating! My whole life was ruined. Now can you give me these flies?"

I said, "I can, yes." I closed the bottle and gave it to him.

I asked him, "What are you going to do?"

He said, "I am going to go to all those doctors and physicians who have been taking fees and doing nothing and just telling me, 'There are no flies.' Anybody who has told me that…I am going to show them that these are the flies."

He was cured. His mind just got stuck with an idea. But if you go to the psycho-analyst, he will make a mountain out of a molehill – so many theories, explanations… and it takes years and still the problem will remain, because the problem has not been touched. He has been philosophizing about it and he is trying his philosophy out on this poor patient.

But most of the diseases of the mind – and seventy percent of diseases are of the mind – can be easily cured. The most basic thing is to accept; don't deny, because your denial is against the pride of the man. The more you deny, the more he is going to insist: it is a simple logic. You are denying his understanding, you are denying his feeling, you are denying his humanity, his dignity. You are saying, "You don't know anything" – about his own body!

The first step is to accept: "You are right. Those who have denied you were wrong." And immediately half of the ground is covered. Now there is a sympathetic relationship with the person. Those who suffer from any mental sickness need sympathy; they need approval, not denial. They don't want you to reduce them to a mad, insane person. Just give them sympathy, give them understanding, be loving.

Let them come close to you and then find a simple way. Don't go roundabout with Freudian scriptures – they are almost holy scriptures, and the literature of psychoanalysis goes on increasing, goes on becoming bigger and bigger. And you start trying all those ideas on the poor man, and he has nothing much.

My own understanding is that every man needs love, and every man also needs to love. Every man needs friendship, friendliness, sympathy – and every man wants to give it, too.

I am reminded: it happened when George Bernard Shaw was almost eighty years old. His doctor was ninety years old – his personal physician – and both were great friends.

Once in the middle of the night Bernard Shaw felt a sudden pain in the heart, and he became afraid: perhaps it was a heart attack. He phoned the doctor and said, "Come immediately because I may not see the sunrise again."

The doctor said, "Hold on. I am coming, don't be worried." The doctor came. He had to come up three flights of stairs – a ninety-year-old man carrying his own bag, perspiring.

He came and put his bag on the floor and sat in the chair and closed his eyes. Bernard Shaw asked, "What is the matter?" The doctor put his hand on his heart, and Bernard Shaw said, "My God, you have got a heart attack!" And he could see…a ninety-year-old man, three flights of stairs, in the middle of the night, and he was perspiring.

Bernard Shaw got up, started waving a fan, washing his face with cold water, gave him some brandy to drink because the night was cold, and tried in every way… covered him with blankets and completely forgot about his own heart attack, for which the doctor was called.

After half an hour the doctor was feeling better and he said, "Now I am okay. This was a great heart attack. This has happened for the third time and I was thinking this is the last, but you helped me immensely. Now give me my fees."

Bernard Shaw said, "Your fees? – and I have been running and bringing things and serving you. You should give me fees."

The doctor said, "Nonsense. This was all acting. I do it with every heart patient – and it always works. They forget their heart attack and they start looking after me – a ninety-year-old man. You just give me my fees. Half the night has passed and I have to go home" – and he took his fee.

And Bernard Shaw said, "This is something. I used to think that I am a joker, but this doctor is a practical joker. He really treated me." He tried his heart, it was perfectly okay. He had completely forgotten it. It was just a small pain that his mind had multiplied…his fear of heart attack, the idea of heart attack, the idea of death became magnified.

But the doctor was really good. He got Bernard Shaw up, got all the services, had a good drink, and finally took his fees and walked down the stairs. And Bernard Shaw simply looked completely mystified. "This man says that he has been doing this with every heart case, and he has always been successful. Just because of his age he manages beautifully. Anybody will forget…. Any other doctor would start making it a complex phenomenon, with injections and medicines and rest, or a change of climate, or a twenty-four-hour nurse. But that man did it quick, fast, without any complexity."

I have seen all kinds of cases concerned with the mind. All that they need is a very sympathetic, friendly, loving approach, and in every case a unique treatment – because whatever has been done to the man is ordinary, common, and slowly, slowly the patient starts feeling that he has been successful in defeating all kinds of doctors – allopathic, homoeopathic, naturopathic, ayurvedic, acupuncturists, acupressurists – all kinds of people, and yet nobody can cure him. He starts having a certain ego about it, that his sickness is something very special. He wants it to be accepted as special. It is a substitute.

This has to be understood: everybody wants to be special, extraordinary – a great musician, a great dancer, a great poet – but everybody cannot manage. It needs a long, arduous discipline to become a great musician....

Everybody seems to be closed. Nobody's heart is with open windows. And nobody's doors are open to welcome a guest. This whole situation creates strange things. The real needs of the human mind are not fulfilled; it starts behaving strangely.

Perhaps that was the only cause of that man tearing up papers and throwing bits here and there – just to make it known, "I am here, and I am different from everybody else. I am doing something that nobody else does." Perhaps he was not accepted, not received, not loved. And the cure that he got is worse than the disease. That was really the disease – that nobody loved him – and now the magician gives him the cure: "If you do it again I will give you such a kick that you will roll down all these hundred stairs, and at the end you may just burst into pieces on the road." But he stopped doing it – that shows that rather than getting love, he got more fear. Fear can also change your behaviour, but it is not a change for the better, it is a change for the worse. And while love is available – and it costs nothing – why not use it?

I don't see that there is any other psychotherapy than love. If the psychotherapist can shower his love, the disease will disappear without any analysis.

All analysis is just bunk. The psychotherapist is avoiding love himself. He is avoiding seeing the patient face to face. He is afraid to recognize the reality. All psychoanalysts of the Freudian camp, which is the biggest camp and the most important, don't sit in front of the patient. The patient lies down on a couch, and behind the couch sits the psychoanalyst. The patient talks, lying down on the couch, to no one, and the psychoanalyst is just sitting there. No human touch – he cannot even hold the hand of the patient, he cannot look in the eyes of the patient.

In the East nothing like psychoanalysis has ever happened for the simple reason that there were thousands of masters, deep in meditation, and anybody who came to

171

them…just their love, their sympathy, the way they looked into the eyes of the patient was enough. People were cured. It was not that without psychoanalysis…. In the East, what happened to neurotics, to psychotics, was that they were instantly changed. All that they needed was an immense love which asks nothing – a man of peace and silence, whose very presence is medicine. A man who has meditated for a long time becomes an immense source. He radiates something that is not visible to the eyes, but the heart catches it. Something reaches to your innermost being and changes you.

Problems are simple. Solutions are simple. Just one has to get out of the mind to see the simplicity. And then whatsoever is done by a man in silence, in peace, in joy, will be medicinal, will be distributing health. It will be a healing force.[61]

? *What is the psychology of the buddhas? It sounds like a science only for enlightened beings who need to pull, push, seduce, hit or kiss their disciples at the right moment, so that they don't wobble, get stuck or fall into traps. Can you please reveal some of your findings of the past thirty years?*

The question you have asked is fundamentally unanswerable. But a few indications, a few hints can certainly be made available to you – with absolute certainty that you will not be able to get the point. But that is not my problem. I will try my best. On your part, if you can be just a passive, silent mind, simply listening as if you are listening to the sound of the birds, not interpreting them, perhaps a certain door may open for you. It all depends on you. The process is not very difficult. It is just an old addiction – we cannot simply listen the way we listen to music; we immediately start reacting, interpreting, trying to find the meaning of it. We get lost in our own minds and the music passes by.

The first thing: I have used the term 'the psychology of the buddhas' not to mean what it means. The man of enlightenment has gone beyond mind. In fact, the mind has faded just like dreams fade away. All the psychologies in the West are concerned with figuring out the functioning of the mind, how it works, why it sometimes works right and sometimes wrong. They have accepted one basic hypothesis which is not true: the hypothesis is that you are no more than mind; you are a structure of body-mind. Naturally, physiology looks into your body and its functioning and psychology looks into your mind and its functioning.

The first point to be noted is about those who have come to know a different space in themselves which cannot be confined by the mind and which cannot be defined as part of the functioning of it. That silent space with no thoughts, no ripples, is the beginning of the psychology of the buddhas.

The word 'psychology' is being used all over the world absolutely wrongly, but when something becomes conventional we forget. Even the very word 'psychology' indicates not something about the mind but about the psyche. The root meaning of psychology is the science of the soul. It is not the science of the mind. And if people are honest they should change the name, because it is a wrong name and takes people on wrong paths. There exists no psychology in the world in the sense of a science of the soul.

You are, for arbitrary reasons – just to be able to understand – divided into three parts. But remember, the division is only arbitrary. You are an indivisible unit.

The body is your outer part. It is an immensely valuable instrument that existence has given to you. You have never thanked existence for your body. You are not even aware what it goes on doing for you, for seventy years, eighty years, in some places one hundred and fifty years – and in a few faraway parts of the Soviet Union, even up to one hundred and eighty years. That leads me to make the statement that the ordinary conception that the body dies at the age of seventy is not a fact but a fiction that has become so prevalent that the body simply follows it.

It happened: Before George Bernard Shaw reached the age of ninety years – his friends were very much puzzled – he started looking for a place outside London, where he had lived his whole life. They asked, "What is the point? You have a beautiful house, all the facilities; why are you looking for a new place to live? And in a very strange way – a few people think you have gone senile" ...because he would go around to the villages, not into the towns but into the cemeteries, and he would read what was written on the stones of the graves. Finally he decided to live in a village where he found a gravestone where it was written: "This man died a very untimely death – he was only one hundred and twelve."

He said to his friends, "As far as I am concerned, it is a worldwide hypnosis: because the idea of seventy years has been insisted on for so many thousands of years, man's body simply follows it. If there is a village where a man dies at a hundred and twelve and the villagers think he died 'very untimely', that this was not the time for him to die...." George Bernard Shaw lived in that village during his last years, and he completed the century.

In Kashmir, the part that is being occupied by Pakistan, people live up to a hundred and fifty without any problem. It is just that the idea of seventy years has not poisoned their minds. In Azerbaijan, in Uzbekistan, faraway corners of the Soviet Union, people live at least one hundred and eighty years, and not just a few people – thousands of people have reached to that point and they are still young. They are still not retired, they are working in the fields, in the gardens.

I had told this to one of my professors – he did not believe me. He said, "I am a professor of philosophy and psychology, and I cannot agree with your idea that the whole humanity is dying because of a psychological conditioning."

I said, "I will show you."

He said, "What do you mean?"

I said, "Just wait a few days, because no argument will prove it — you will need evidence."

He used to live almost one mile away from the philosophy department in the university campus. He was perfectly healthy; he used to walk every day to the department and back to his home. One day I went to his wife and told her, "You have to do me a favour. Next morning when Professor S.S. Roy wakes up you just say, 'What happened? Could you not sleep well? You look so pale, do you have some fever?'"

And he simply refused to listen. "What kind of nonsense are you talking? I am perfectly okay. There is no fever and I have slept well. I am feeling perfectly well." I had told his wife to write down exactly what he said, in a note, and later on I would collect those notes.

I told his gardener, "When he comes out you simply say, 'What has happened to you? You look so sick.' And remember to write down what he says." And to the gardener he said, "It seems that I could not sleep well in the night."

After his house was the post office, which he had to pass. The postmaster was a friend to him, and I told the postmaster, "You have to do this…"

He said, "But what are you trying to do?"

I said, "It is an argument between me and Professor S.S. Roy, and I am going to prove something to him. I will tell you later on, the whole story. You just do one thing: when Professor Roy passes the post office, you come out. Just hold him and tell him, 'You are wobbly, don't go to the university today. I will inform the vice-chancellor that you are not well.'"

And the professor said, "I was also thinking not to go. Something certainly seems to be wrong with the body."

Finally I had to persuade the peon of the philosophy department, because he used to sit in front of the department. It was very difficult to convince him, but he knew that Professor S.S. Roy loved me so much, I could not mean any harm. I told him, "The moment he comes, you simply jump up — take hold of him. Even if he resists, don't bother; make him lie down on the bench and tell him, 'This is not the time for you to walk a mile, you are absolutely sick.'"

He said, "But I am a peon, a poor man…."

I said, "You don't be worried. For that I give the guarantee that you will not be disturbed. Just remember to write what he says, and remember also whether he resists or not."

He did not resist. He simply followed the peon's idea, lay down on the bench and told the peon, "If you can bring the departmental car and tell the driver to take me home...because I don't think I will be able to manage walking one long mile again. I am utterly sick."

Then I collected all those notes. S.S. Roy was lying down on a couch like the ones psychoanalysts use for patients, looking as if he had been sick for months. Even his voice showed that he could only whisper. I told him, "You are certainly very sick, but how have you managed just in one night to be so sick that you look as if you have been sick for months? Just last evening when I left you, you were perfectly okay."

He said, "I am also puzzled."

I said, "There is no need to be puzzled – read these notes!"

Reading the notes – from the wife to the peon – he suddenly became perfectly okay. He said, "You are such a fellow that it is better not to get in an argument with you! You could have killed me. I was already thinking to make my will."

I said, "This is the answer to what I have been talking about with you a few days ago – that the body follows the ideas the mind gets."

Seventy years has become a fixed point, almost all over the world. But it is not the truth of the body. It is a corruption of the body by the mind. And strangely enough, all the religions are against the body – and the body is your life, the body is your communion with existence.

It is the body that breathes, it is the body that keeps you alive, it is the body that does almost miracles. Do you have any idea how to change a loaf of bread into blood and sort it out into its different constituents and send those constituents where they are needed? How much oxygen your brain needs – have you any idea? In just six minutes, if your brain does not get oxygen you will fall into a coma. For such a long time the body continues to supply the exact amount of oxygen to your brain.

How do you explain the process of breathing? Certainly *you* are not breathing, it is the body that goes on breathing. If *you* were breathing, you would not have been here. There are so many worries, you could have forgotten to breathe, and particularly in the night – either you can breathe or you can sleep. And it is not a simple process, because the air the body takes in consists of many elements which are dangerous to you. It sorts out only those which are nourishing to life and breathes out all that is dangerous to you, particularly carbon dioxide.

The wisdom of the body has not been appreciated by any religion of the world. Your wisest people were no wiser than your body. Its functioning is so perfect – its understanding has been kept completely out of your control because your control could have been destructive.

So the first part of your life and being is your body. The body is real, authentic, sincere. There is no way to corrupt it, although all the religions have been trying to corrupt it. They teach you fasting which is against nature and against the needs of the body, and a man who can fast longer becomes a great saint. I will call him the greatest fool who has been dominated by the foolishness of the crowd. The religions have been teaching you to be celibate, without understanding the mechanism of the body. You eat food, you drink water, you breathe oxygen. Just as blood is created in you, your sexual energy is also created – it is beyond you. There has not been a single celibate in the whole world. And I challenge all the religions who pretend that their monks are celibates to have them examined by scientists. They will find that they have the same glands and they have the same energy as anybody else.

Celibacy is a crime – it creates perversions – just as fasting is a crime. Eating too much is a crime; not eating enough is also a crime. If you listen to the body and simply follow the body, you don't need Gautam Buddhas to teach you, or Mahaviras or Jesus Christs to teach you what you have to do with the body. The body has an inbuilt program, and that inbuilt program you cannot change. You can pervert it....

So I teach you, first, a deep respect, love and gratitude for your body. That will be the fundamental of the psychology of the buddhas, of the psychology of the awakened ones.

The second thing after the body is your mind. Mind is simply a fiction. It has been used, in fact used too much, by all kinds of parasites. These are the people who will teach you to be against the body and for the mind. There is a mechanism called the brain. The brain is part of the body, but the brain has no inbuilt program. Nature is so compassionate – leaving your brain without any inbuilt program means existence is giving you freedom. Whatever you want to make of your brain, you can make. But what was compassionate on the part of nature has been exploited by your priests, your politicians, your so-called great men. They found a great opportunity to stuff the mind with all kinds of nonsense.

Mind is a clean slate – whatever you write on the mind becomes your theology, your religion, your political ideology. And every parent, every society is so alert not to leave your brain in your own hands, they immediately start writing the holy *Koran*, the *Holy Bible*, the *Bhagavadgita* – and by the time they call you adult, capable to participate in the affairs of the world, you are no longer yourself.

This is so cunning, so criminal, that I am surprised that nobody has pointed it out. No parent has the right to force the child to be a Catholic or a Hindu or a Jaina. The children are born through you but they don't belong to you. You cannot be the possessors of living beings. You can love them, and if you really love them you will give them freedom to grow according to their own nature, without any persuasion, without any punishment, without any effort by anybody else. The brain is perfectly right – it is the freedom given by nature to you, a space to grow. But the society, before you can grow that space, stuffs it with all kinds of nonsense.

There was a man I knew, Professor Rungar – he lived in Mahatma Gandhi's ashram. It is not much of an ashram, just a few widows and a few weirdoes, and not more than twenty. But free food, free clothing, free shelter, and all they have to do are some stupid things. They call it worship, they call it prayer.

Professor Rungar was an educated man, but it does not matter; before your education you are already contaminated, polluted. He went on eating cow dung for six months, drinking cow's urine – that was his whole food, and this made him a great saint. Even Mahatma Gandhi declared that he had attained enlightenment. If enlightenment is to be attained by eating cow dung, then better enlightenment will be attained by eating bullshit, obviously! And when Mahatma Gandhi says about him that he has become enlightened, the whole country simply believes it. I have not found a single man criticizing it.

I told Professor Rungar, "As far as I am concerned, you are the *most* stupid man in this country." It is a very difficult competition, but look at all your religions, what they have stuffed in your mind....

Every Hindu, when he goes to urinate...he has a thread around his body: that thread ceremony is almost like Jews circumcising their children. And would you believe that I have come across a statement by a rabbi that the reason Jews are so intelligent is because of the circumcision. Mohammedans do the same but at a later age.

Jews have their own baptism. Hindus have their way of introducing the child into the Hindu society with a thread ceremony. Just a thread is put around his neck, and he is surrounded by people chanting from holy scriptures. And every Hindu is expected, when he goes to urinate, to take the thread out of his shirt and wrap the thread around his ear. I have seen professors, vice-chancellors doing the same stupid act.

One vice-chancellor, Dr. Tripathi – I caught him red-handed. I threatened him, "Either you take this thread off your ear, or I will not allow you to urinate."

"But," he said, "it is my religion" – and he was a well-educated man.

I said, "Can you give me any rationalization for it?"

He said, "Certainly. If you put the thread around your ear, it keeps you away from sexual ideas, sexual dreams. It protects your celibacy."

I said, "You are a man, perfectly educated in the West" – and he had been teaching in the West – "you will have to come with me to the medical centre."

He said, "What do you mean?"

I said, "I want it to be confirmed by medical scientists that putting the thread around the ear protects a person from becoming sexual."

He said, "You always come with strange ideas."

The simple proof was that he had thirteen children. I said, "With this thread, you have produced thirteen children; without the thread you would have threatened the whole of humanity! And still you have the nerve to say that it protects your celibacy?"

But you will find the same kind of ideas everywhere forced into the brain. I want it to be clearly understood: the brain is natural; mind is what is stuffed into the brain. So the brain is not Christian, but the mind can be; the brain is not Hindu, but the mind can be. The mind is the creation of the society, not a gift of nature. The first thing the psychology of the buddhas will do is to take away this whole junk that you call mind and leave your brain silent, pure, innocent, the way you were born.

Modern psychology all around the world is doing something stupid: analyzing the brain, analyzing all the thoughts which constitute your mind. In the East we have looked into the innermost parts of humanity and our understanding is, the mind needs no analysis. It is analyzing junk. It needs simply to be erased. The moment the mind is erased – and the method is meditation – you are left with a body which is absolutely beautiful, you are left with a silent brain with no noise. The moment the brain is freed from the mind, the innocence of the brain becomes aware of a new space which we have called the soul.

Once you have found your soul, you have found your home. You have found your love, you have found your inexhaustible ecstasy, you have found that the whole existence is ready for you to dance, to rejoice, to sing – to live intensely and die blissfully. These things happen on their own accord.[62]

CHAPTER 11

BODYWORK

? *Will you talk on the art of massage?*

Massage is something that you can start learning but you never finish. It goes on and on, and the experience becomes continuously deeper and deeper, and higher and higher. Massage is one of the most subtle arts – and it is not only a question of expertise. It is more a question of love.

Learn the technique – then forget it. Then just feel, and move by feeling. When you learn deeply, ninety percent of the work is done by love, ten percent by the technique. By just the very touch, a loving touch, something relaxes in the body.

If you love and feel compassion for the other person, and feel the ultimate value of him; if you don't treat him as if he is a mechanism to be put right, but an energy of tremendous value; if you are grateful that he trusts you and allows you to play with his energy – then by and by you will feel as if you are playing on an organ. The whole body becomes the keys of the organ and you can feel that a harmony is created inside the body. Not only will the person be helped, but you also.

Massage is needed in the world because love has disappeared. Once the very touch of lovers was enough. A mother touched the child, played with his body, and it was massage. The husband played with the body of his woman and it was massage; it was enough, more than enough. It was deep relaxation and part of love. But that has disappeared from the world. By and by we have forgotten where to touch, how to touch, how deep to touch. In fact touch is one of the most forgotten languages. We have become almost awkward in touching, because the very word has been corrupted by so-called religious people. They have given it a sexual colour. The word has become sexual and people have become afraid. Everybody is on guard not to be touched unless he allows it. Now in the West the other extreme has come. Touch and massage have become sexual. Now massage is just a cover, a blanket, for sexuality. In fact neither touch nor massage are sexual. They are functions of love. When love falls from its height it becomes sex, and then it becomes ugly.

So be prayerful. When you touch the body of a person be prayerful – as if God himself is there, and you are just serving him. Flow with total energy. And whenever you see the body flowing and the energy creating a new pattern of harmony, you will feel a delight that you have never felt before. You will fall into deep meditation.

While massaging, just massage. Don't think of other things because those are distractions. Be in your fingers and your hands as if your whole being, your whole soul is there. Don't let it be just a touch of the body. Your whole soul enters into the body of the other, penetrates it, relaxes the deepest complexes. And make it a play. Don't do it as a job; make it a game and take it as fun. Laugh and let the other laugh too.[63]

M assage is to come to a rapport with the energy of somebody else's body and to feel where it is missing, to feel where the body is fragmentary and to make it whole…to help the energy of the body so it is no longer fragmentary, no longer contradictory. When the energies of the body are falling into line and becoming an orchestra, then you succeed.

So be very respectful about a human body. It is the very shrine of God, the temple of God. So with deep reverence, prayer, learn your art. It is one of the greatest things to learn.[64]

 What is a healing touch?

J ust lay your hands on the needed part of the person. If the person has a headache, lay your hands on his head, close your eyes, start feeling energies pouring, and you will have a tingling sensation in the hands, they will become electrified. Or if the person has some trouble with the stomach, put your hands on the stomach. The needed part has to be touched. If it can be touched bare, without clothes, it is better, it will be more effective. But don't touch the needed part for more than one minute. If you touch the needed part for more than one minute, then sometimes the disease can start flowing towards you.

Energy is a rhythm: one minute it goes outwards, another minute it comes inwards. So make it a point that when you put your hands on somebody's body, exhale; it synchronizes with inhalation, exhalation. When you put your hands on them, exhale, and go on exhaling; and when you see that you cannot exhale any more, take your hands off and then inhale. If you inhale while laying your hands on, you can be affected by the illness. The person may be healed but you will suffer, and that is meaningless. Just lay your hands with exhalation, and the moment inhalation starts, withdraw.[65]

? *How to heal a person who is afraid to be touched?*

When you are healing a person, so much energy is pouring out that if you touch, it will be almost as if you are touching him with a live wire, a live electric wire. He will become so afraid that his doors will close – and if the doors are closed, you can go on showering and nothing will happen. Healing is possible not only because of your energy – it is possible only when your energy enters the other person and becomes his energy. If it comes up to the door and returns, no healing happens.

That's why if a person does not trust you, never try healing – never try, because it is not possible. If a person has doubts about you, forget about him. It is possible only in deep trust, and if you try on persons who won't trust you, you will become unconfident about your own energy. If you fail many times, then by and by you will think, "Nothing is happening. I don't have the energy." In fact every person has the energy to heal. It is something natural. It is not that a few people are healers and others are not, no. Every person born is a healer but has forgotten the capacity, or has never used it, or has used it in wrong associations and has come to feel that it never works.

So never try it on somebody who challenges you. It is not a challenge. If somebody is ready to participate, to go with you, then it is a beautiful experience. So in the beginning never touch. When the person is relaxing more and more and you feel...and I am saying *feel* – not that you think. If you feel an urge arises to touch the person – for example he has a stomach ache or a headache or something and you feel that just touching the head will be helpful – then touch, but first let him get in tune with you. First just give an energy massage, not touching the body.

181

Keep about two inches' distance, because the person's body aura is about six inches away from his body. Keep about two, three inches away, so in a way you are touching his energy aura. You are not touching his or her physical body, but you are touching his subtle body – and that's enough. For the energy to penetrate, that's enough. You have really touched him, but he will not be afraid about that. When you feel that the person is participating tremendously, when his trust is immense and you can see that he is flowing with you, and you can feel that your energy is being absorbed – it is not rejected; he has become like a sponge and is soaking it up – then it becomes a pinpoint. On that point the whole energy showers and enters deepest.

After each healing it is better that if you can take a shower, do so. If it is not possible, then at least wash your hands immediately and shake them. It always happens that when you are passing your energy into the other person, his or her energy also sometimes passes into you; they overlap. Sometimes the person can be very strong, even stronger than you. Sometimes the person may not be strong, but his illness may be very strong, so those vibrations of illness can enter you and can be destructive. They can make you ill, tense. Healing is good but not at your own cost, because then it is foolish and you cannot heal much. Sooner or later you will become ill, badly ill, and your body will be confused very much.[66]

Massage is not simply massage. You are sharing energy; and unless you have energy flowing in you, soon you will become tired. Then it is very risky. It is not physical tiredness that comes – that is not important; you will sleep, you will eat, and it will go. But massage is a deeper sharing of energy. When you are massaging somebody's body, not only are your bodies involved – your subtle bodies, two energy bodies, two bio-plasmas. The person who is taking massage can take too much of your bio-plasma, and unless you are a constant inner supply, unless you are joined to the source, you will become very much dissipated by it. It may not immediately affect you because you are young. Even for months and years you may not feel it, but one day suddenly you will feel you are collapsed.

So my understanding is that first one should work upon oneself, and one should become very, very centred. When you are centred, *you* are not. When you are centred, the source starts functioning. Then you are just a passage. The cosmos starts flowing through you – then there is no problem. You can share as much energy as you want, and you will be constantly getting new energy. Then you are not like a reservoir of water which has no springs to it. You are like a well which has many springs to it; you go on taking the water out and new water is flowing in – you cannot exhaust it. In fact you take the old, rotten, stale water out, and the fresh and alive water comes in. So the well is very happy – you are unburdening it from the past and the old and the stagnant. So if you are in a flow and your energy is flowering then there is no problem.

So massage and healing and these phenomena are very subtle. And it is not only a question of knowing the technique, the bigger question is how to be at the source – then there is no problem. Then I don't bother even about the technique and whether you know it or not. You can simply start playing with somebody's body and energy will be flowing, and there will be great benefits. But there is only real benefit when the person who is massaging is also benefited through it – then there is a real benefit. Then the healer is benefited, and the healee too – both are benefited. Nobody is at loss.[67]

 Do you think Rolfing is a helpful technique which can relieve body / mind tensions?

Body and mind move together, but sometimes it happens that the mind gets ahead, is better than the body. Or sometimes it is otherwise – the mind is in a worse state than the body. When alignment breaks between the body and the mind, there is pain.

When people come to me, their body and mind are functioning together – whatsoever their state. If they are miserable, then the body is adjusted to that misery. If they are happy, then the body is adjusted to that happiness. When they start meditating, that adjustment becomes loose because the mind starts growing, but the body is adjusted to the old mind, and that mind is going, almost gone, so the body is at a loss. And the body has not much intelligence – it is a mechanism and it is very slow. But by and by it follows. Rolfing will be helpful at this moment.

Rolfing is nothing but making the tissues loose. At a few points on the body the musculature takes a certain shape. If somebody has been worrying continuously, then the body takes a certain musculature which is adjusted to worrying. Then worries may disappear but the musculature remains and it will feel heavy, painful. Its function is no more there, and the body does not know how to dissolve it. If you don't do anything about it, it will dissolve by and by but it will take a long time. But why wait?

Through Rolfing it can be dissolved by pressure. The musculature disappears, and you will feel almost as new in the body as you are feeling in the mind. Then a new adjustment arises again – at a higher stage.

It is going to be painful, that's certain. It will be really painful because the whole of the past is accumulated in the body, and the musculature has to be melted, reabsorbed in the body. That reabsorption is painful, but it pays.[68]

? *Do you think that bioenergetics is the right start for me to work upon myself?*

Bioenergetics is one of the right directions to work in. It is not complete, it is not yet a whole philosophy of life, but is moving on the right lines. The body is the base, and much work is needed on the body before you can start any work on the mind. Then much work is needed on the mind before you can start any work on the soul. So it is the right grounding; to start with bioenergetics is the right beginning. And if the beginning is right, half of the work is done. It is very essential and significant, but remember only that it is not the whole thing. You will begin with it but you should not end with it. That has to be remembered, otherwise you are moving in a circle.

The body is not all. The human mind tends to be extremist. Christianity was anti-body; it created all anti-life attitudes. Then the pendulum went to the other extreme, full circle, and Freud and Wilhelm Reich and others started to move too much towards the denied part. So the body is the denied part in the West. Christianity never accepted the body; that has been the curse. But now, just to be in reaction, one can become so obsessed with the body that one can forget something which is higher than the body and which is residing in you. The house has not to be forgotten, has not to be neglected – every care has to be taken of it but the house is simply the house; don't forget the master of the house. So bioenergetics is a good beginning, but it cannot be the end.

? *My body has become more alive through meditation. How can I use this new energy?*

If meditation goes rightly, it always makes you more alive, more loving. It gives you energy, passion, life, so don't obstruct it. Once you start obstructing some energy, blocks are created. Now the energy is streaming, so allow it, move with it; wherever it leads, trust it. That's what trusting means: trust your energy. If the thirst for love has arisen, then move into love and don't be afraid. Fear will come, because love needs much courage. It will lead you into involvement, commitment, and into unknown paths. It is always the beginning of a dangerous life.

So fear will be there, naturally, but don't listen to the fear. Go into love in spite of it – whatsoever the cost. When love starts arising in you, uncoils its energy, that is the moment to be courageous, to be daring. Take the risk, and only then more and more life will happen to you. If you recoil, if you obstruct your energy, the same energy will start becoming frozen.

That's what bioenergetics people go on destroying – that rocklike armour around you. You wanted to love but somehow you obstructed it. The energy that was going out cannot go back to the source. There is no way for it to go back. If you are going to be angry and the energy has to come to the hand to hit the person, to slap the person, and you don't slap but go on smiling, the energy will be retained in the hand. It cannot go back – there is no way. That energy will become a heavy load on the hand. It will destroy the beauty and the grace of the hand. It will make your hand dead.

So whenever an energy arises, go with it. If it is something which can be dangerous to somebody – for example, if it is anger – then go into your room, beat a pillow. But do something. There is no need to be destructive to anybody, don't be violent to anybody, but you can be violent with a pillow. Your energy will be released and you will feel fresh energy flowing. Never hold in any energy.

When you are giving energy to life, life goes on giving energy to you. This is the ecology, the inner ecology. Energy moves in a circle. Life gives to you, you give it back; life gives you more, you give it more. And the circle continues. It is like the river which flows into the ocean, then moves to the clouds, and then again rains on the mountains, and flows again in the river to the ocean. And the circle continues – there is no obstruction anywhere.[69]

What is your understanding of the value of the newly-devised therapy called colourpuncture?

This colourpuncture is perfectly right. Colour affects the body, and to have figured it out is great. Peter Mandel (*the innovator*) has done a great work. With this work you can change not the being, but the mind, the emotions and the body. It is good if one is cleansed in this way; then meditation is very simple. These problems are preventing meditation.[70]

? *How does T'ai Chi work?*

Chi means energy. The whole concept is that solidity is false – just as in modern physics. These walls are not real – it is just pure energy, but the electrons are moving so fast, with such terrific speed that you cannot see the blades separately. So it gives a sense of solidarity. The same is true with your body. What modern physics has come to know right now, Taoists have known for thousands of years – that man is energy.

It is said about a T'ai Chi master that he would tell his disciples to attack him, and he would just sit in the middle. Five or ten disciples would rush from every corner of the room to attack him, but when they came near him, they would feel as if he were a cloud; there was nothing solid...as if you could pass through him and you would not be obstructed by anything.

If you continue this idea that you are energy, it is possible to become just like a cloud with no boundaries, melting and merging with existence. This anecdote is not just an anecdote. With a man who has gone deep into T'ai Chi, it is very easily possible that when you come across him, you will not find any obstruction; you can simply go through him. You cannot hurt him because he is not there to be hurt.[71]

? *I found in the encounter group I did, that certain emotions brought out anger, and I could see how to use T'ai Chi for love, but things like pain and fear I cannot come in contact with.*

T'ai Chi can be used for many, many things, and for this also, because each movement of the body can have some relevance to the emotions. That's why they are called emotions, because they are connected with body motions: each emotion has a particular body gesture related to it, corresponding to it.

When you become angry your eyes have a certain gesture, your hands have a certain gesture, your teeth have a certain energy, your jaw is more aggressive; you are ready to destroy, to be aggressive. The energy accumulates in the hands and in the teeth, because when man was an animal that was the only way to be angry. Still animals are angry with their teeth and with their nails; we still carry that mechanism.

If you try to be angry without using your hands and your teeth and your eyes, you will be in an almost impossible situation – you cannot be angry. That particular gesture in the body is a must. And what precedes what cannot be said? In fact it is just like saying: "Which comes first – the hen or the egg?" Does fear come first and then the gesture of being frightened, or does the gesture come and then fear? They both come together, they are simultaneous.

You can work it out…but T'ai Chi masters will not be of much help because they have not used T'ai Chi in that way. T'ai Chi has many potentialities which have not been used in the past. In fact, T'ai Chi has been used to repress, not to express.

All the Eastern techniques are in a way repressive. Rather than expressing your anger, your sadness or your negativity, the techniques have been made in such a way that you can very, very politely persuade them to go into the unconscious, to the basement. So T'ai Chi masters won't be much help…but you can work it out on your own. Learn T'ai Chi from them but then you can work it out in a very cathartic way and you can throw negative emotions through T'ai Chi movements; they can be thrown out. You can develop that thing and it can be helpful for others too. It can become a new dimension in T'ai Chi. I have always been thinking that some time or other, that dimension has to be developed in T'ai Chi. As it is, it doesn't exist right now.

So don't talk about it, otherwise they will say no…because the East is very orthodox. They have a certain use and they have used it down the ages and they have become very fixed; they are not even exploring new possibilities. The same is the case with Yoga in India – it has become a frozen science; for three thousand years, not a single development. So is the case with T'ai Chi: for three thousand years not a single improvement. It remains exactly where it was three thousand years ago…as if three thousand years have not passed.

The East is very orthodox: once it finds that a certain thing works it uses it only in that way. The West is very, very exploring, hence the West could reach from the bullock cart to the space jet. The East could not, the East still carries the bullock cart; it is the same bullock cart! In the same bullock cart Buddha was moving, in the same bullock cart Patanjali was moving, in the same bullock cart Lao Tzu was moving, and in the same bullock cart the East is still moving.

 How to use the movements to cathart?

Just stand, hold your energy in the hara, concentrate at the hara, and then just whatsoever you feel like…. For example if it is anger, then just feel the energy rising from the hara taking the form of anger like flames, spreading all over the body.

Then relax and let the body move with those flames. You will find that gestures start – they may be more like latihan, Subud, they will be more like Subud movements.

So just like flames – if you are thinking about anger, then think of flames.

? *Then you watch the movements and you trace them back?*

Yes, trace them back.

? *You trace the energy back?*

Trace the energy, yes, and just go with the energy and allow the energy to take its own shape and start moving.

By and by experiment and you will be able to fix the movements – that these are the movements that always come whenever you think of anger, and whenever you think of flames arising in you and taking shape, then this happens. But you try with anger for a few days so you come to an exact formulation. Then try with some other things – sadness, hatred, jealousy – but remember not to get confused. If you try with anger then try anger only for three weeks, so it settles. It settles so much that you can tell somebody else to do the movement and if he does the movement, he will suddenly say that anger is arising in him and anger is being thrown out. You follow me?

Then you try something else when you have come to a fixed pattern about anger. And whatsoever your negativities, you can search....

? *In T'ai Chi some of the forms take an hour – there are many, many more movements. When you can separate the parts, when you link it together, you just let each one go out as it goes out.*

Simply let it go out, let it be dissolved into the cosmos. Don't make a circle, don't take it in; simply let it out. It moves into the existence and disappears...you have poured it into existence.

And this can also be done silently?

Yes, you can do it quietly…you can find your own ways.

These sciences – T'ai Chi, Yoga or things like that – are arts, not really sciences, and everybody can play around and find out their own ways. One should be very, very free about them. They are not very fixed things – they have great freedom in them.

So learn the art and then use it in your own individual way – give it your own flavour. And never become an orthodox follower of these things; otherwise, rather than helping, they constrict you. They help in a certain limited way, but if you can improve upon them, innovate, then you can be benefited tremendously.[72]

CHAPTER 12

PAIN

? *Can you please talk about pain and our identification with it?*

The witnessing self is never felt. We always feel some identity; we always feel some identification. And the witnessing consciousness is the reality. So why does this happen? And how does this happen?

You are in pain – what is really happening inside? Analyze the whole phenomenon: the pain is there, and there is this consciousness that pain is there. These are the two points: the pain is there, and there is this *consciousness* that the pain is there. But there is no gap, and somehow, "I am in pain" – this feeling happens – "I am in pain." And not only this – sooner or later, "I am the pain" begins, happens, starts to be the feeling.

"I *am* pain; I am *in* pain; I am *aware of* the pain" – these are three different, very different states. The rishi says, "I am *aware* of the pain." This much can be allowed, because then you transcend pain. The awareness transcends – you are different from the pain, and there is a deep separation. Really, there has never been any relation; the relation begins to appear only because of the nearness, because of the intimate nearness of your consciousness and all that happens around.

Consciousness is so near when you are in pain – it is just there by the side, very near. It has to be; otherwise, the pain cannot be cured. It has to be just near to feel it, to know it, to be aware about it. But because of this nearness, you become identified, and one. This is a safety measure again; this is a security measure, a

190

natural security. When there is pain you must be near; when there is pain your consciousness *must* go in a rush towards the pain – to feel it, to do something about it.

You are on the street and suddenly you feel a snake there – then your whole consciousness just becomes a jump. No moment can be lost, not even in thinking what to do. There is no gap between being aware and the action. You must be very near; only then this can happen. When your body is suffering pain, disease, illness, you must be near; otherwise, life cannot survive. If you are far off and the pain is not felt, then you will die. The pain must be felt immediately – there should be no gap. The message must be received immediately, and your consciousness must go to the spot to do something. That's why nearness is a necessity. But because of this necessity, the other phenomenon happens: so near, you become one; so near, you begin to feel, "This is me – this pain, this pleasure." Because of nearness there is identification: you become anger, you become love, you become pain, you become happiness.

The rishi says that there are two ways to disassociate yourself from these false identities. You are not what you have been thinking, feeling, imagining, projecting; what you are is simply the fact of being aware. Whatsoever happens, you remain just the awareness. You are awareness – that identity cannot be broken, that identity cannot be negated. All else can be negated and thrown; awareness remains the ultimate substratum, the ultimate base. You cannot deny it, you cannot negate it, you cannot disassociate yourself from it.

So this is the process: That which cannot be thrown, that which cannot be made separate from you, is you; that which can be separated, you are not. The pain is there; a moment later it may not be there – but you will be. Happiness has come, and it will go; it has been, and it will not be – but you will be. The body is young, then the body becomes old. All else comes and goes – guests come and go – but the host remains the same. So the Zen mystics say: Do not be lost in the crowd of the guests. Remember your host-ness. That host-ness is awareness. That host-ness is the witnessing consciousness. What is the basic element that remains always the same in you? Only be that, and disidentify yourself from all that comes and goes. But we become identified with the guest. Really the host is so occupied with the guest, he forgets.

Mulla Nasruddin has given a party for some friends and some strangers. The party is very boring, and half the night is just lost and it goes on. So one stranger, not knowing that Mulla is the host, says to him, "I have never seen such a party, such nonsense. It seems never-ending, and I am so bored that I would like to leave."

191

Mulla says, "You have said what I was going to say to you. I myself have never seen such a boring and nonsense party before, but I was not so courageous as you are. I was also thinking to leave it and just run away." So they both run.

Then, in the street Mulla remembers and says, "Something has gone wrong, because now I remember: I am the host! So please excuse me, I have to go back."

This is happening to us all. The host is lost, the host is forgotten every moment. The host is your witnessing self. Pain comes and pleasure follows; there is happiness, and there is misery. And each moment, whatsoever comes you are identified with it, you become the guest.

Remember the host. When the guest is there, remember the host. And there are so many types of guests: pleasurable, painful; guests you would like, guests you would not like to be your guests; guests you would like to live with, guests you would like to avoid – but all guests. Remember the host. Constantly remember the host. Be centred in the host. Remain in your host-ness; then there is a separation. Then there is a gap, an interval – the bridge is broken. The moment this bridge is broken, the phenomenon of renunciation happens. Then you are in it, and not of it. Then you are there in the guest, and still a host. You need not escape from the guest – there is no need.[73]

? *How can I deal with physical pain as well as the pain I feel in spiritual growth?*

Growth is painful because you have been avoiding a thousand and one pains in your life. By avoiding you cannot destroy them – they go on accumulating. You go on swallowing your pains; they remain in your system. That's why growth is painful – when you start growing, when you decide to grow, you have to face all the pains that you have repressed. You cannot just bypass them.

You have been brought up in a wrong way. Unfortunately, until now, not a single society has existed on the earth which has not been repressive of pain. All societies depend on repression. Two things they repress: one is pain, another is pleasure. And they repress pleasure also because of pain. Their reasoning is that if you are not too happy you will never become too unhappy; if joy is destroyed you will never be deep in pain. To avoid pain they avoid pleasure. To avoid death they avoid life.

And the logic has something in it. Both grow together – if you want to have a life of ecstasy you will have to accept many agonies. If you want the peaks of the Himalayas then you will also have the valleys. But nothing is wrong with the valleys; your approach just has to be different. You can enjoy both – the peak is beautiful, so is the valley. And there are moments when one should enjoy the peak and there are moments when one should relax in the valley.

The peak is sunlit, it is in a dialogue with the sky. The valley is dark, but whenever you want to relax you have to move into the darkness of the valley. If you want to have peaks you will need to grow roots into the valley – the deeper your roots go, the higher your tree will grow. The tree cannot grow without roots and the roots have to move deep into the soil.

Pain and pleasure are intrinsic parts of life. People are so much afraid of pain that they repress pain, they avoid any situation that brings pain, they go on dodging pain. And finally they stumble upon the fact that if you really want to avoid pain you will have to avoid pleasure. That's why your monks avoid pleasure – they are afraid of pleasure. In fact they are simply avoiding all possibilities of pain. They know that if you avoid pleasure then naturally great pain is not possible; it comes only as a shadow of pleasure. Then you walk on the plain ground – you never move on the peaks and you never fall into the valleys. But then you are living dead, then you are not alive.

Life exists between this polarity. This tension between pain and pleasure makes you capable of creating great music; music exists only in this tension. Destroy the polarity and you will be dull, you will be stale, you will be dusty – you won't have any meaning and you will never know what splendour is. You will have missed life.

The man who wants to know life and live life has to accept and embrace death. They come together, they are two aspects of a single phenomenon. That's why growth is painful. You have to go into all those pains that you have been avoiding. It hurts. You have to go through all those wounds that somehow you have managed not to look at. But the deeper you go into pain, the deeper is your capacity to go into pleasure. If you can go into pain to the uttermost limit, you will be able to touch heaven.

I have heard: A man came to a Zen master and asked, "How shall we avoid heat and cold?"

Metaphorically, he is asking, "How should we avoid pleasure and pain?" That is the Zen way of talking about pleasure and pain: heat and cold. "How shall we avoid heat and cold?"

The master answered, "Be hot, be cold."

To be free of pain the pain has to be accepted, inevitably and naturally. Pain is pain – a simple painful fact – but suffering is only and always the refusal of pain, the claim that life should not be painful. It is the rejection of a fact, the denial of life and of the nature of things. Death is the mind and mind's dying. Where there is no fear of death, who is there to die?

Man is unique among creatures in his knowledge of death and in his laughter. Wonderfully then, he can even make of death a new thing: he can die laughing. It is only man who knows laughter; no other animal laughs. It is only man who knows death; no other animal knows death – animals simply die, they are not conscious of the phenomenon of death.

Man is aware of two things which no animal is: one is laughter, another is death. Then a new synthesis is possible. It is only man who can die laughing – he can join the consciousness of death and the capacity to laugh. And if you can die laughing, only then will you give a valid proof that you must have lived laughing. Death is the final statement of your whole life – the conclusion, the concluding remark. How you have lived will be shown by your death, how you die. Can you die laughing? Then you were a grown-up person. If you die crying, weeping, clinging, then you were a child. You were not grown-up, you were immature. If you die crying, weeping, clinging to life, that simply shows you have been avoiding death and you have been avoiding all pains, all kinds of pains.

Growth is facing the reality, encountering the fact, whatsoever it is. And let me repeat: Pain is simply pain; there is no suffering in it. Suffering comes from your desire that the pain should not be there, that there is something wrong in pain. Watch, witness, and you will be surprised. You have a headache: the pain is there but suffering is not there. Suffering is a secondary phenomenon, pain is primary. The headache is there, the pain is there; it is simply a fact. There is no judgment about it. You don't call it good or bad, you don't give it any value; it is just a fact. The rose is a fact, so is the thorn. The day is a fact, so is the night. The head is a fact, so is the headache. You simply take note of it.

Buddha taught his disciples that when you have a headache simply say twice "Headache, headache." Take note. But don't evaluate, don't say "Why? Why has this headache happened to me? It should not happen to me." The moment you say, "It should not," you bring suffering in. Now suffering is created by you, not by the headache. Suffering is your antagonistic interpretation, suffering is your denial of the fact.

And the moment you say, "It should not be," you have started avoiding it, you have started turning yourself away from it. You would like to be occupied in something so that you can forget it. You turn the radio or the telly on or you go to the club or you start reading or you go and start working in the garden – you divert yourself, you distract yourself. Now that pain has not been witnessed; you have simply distracted yourself. That pain will be absorbed by the system.

Let this key be very deeply understood. If you can witness your headache without taking any antagonistic attitude, without avoiding it, without escaping from it; if you can just be there, meditatively there – "Headache, headache" – if you can just simply see it, the headache will go in its time. I am not saying that it will go miraculously, that just by your seeing it will go. It will go in its time. But it will not be absorbed by your system, it will not poison your system. It will be there, you will take note of it, and it will be gone. It will be released.

When you witness a certain thing in yourself it cannot enter into your system. It always enters when you avoid it, when you escape from it. When you become absent then it enters into your system. Only when you are absent can pain become part of your being – if you are present your very presence prevents it from becoming part of your being.

And if you can go on seeing your pains you will not be accumulating them. You have not been taught the right clue, so you go on avoiding. Then you accumulate so much pain, you are afraid to face it, you are afraid to accept it. Growth becomes painful – it is because of wrong conditioning. Otherwise growth is not painful, growth is utterly pleasant.

When the tree grows and becomes bigger do you think there is pain? There is no pain. Even when a child is born, if the mother accepts it there will be no pain. But the mother rejects it; the mother is afraid. She becomes tense, she tries to hold the child inside – which is not possible. The child is ready to go out into the world, the child is ready to leave the mother. He is ripe, the womb cannot contain him any more. If the womb contains him any more the mother will die and the child will die. But the mother is afraid. She has heard that it is very painful to give birth to a child – birth pangs, birth pain. She is afraid, and out of fear she becomes tense and closed.

Otherwise – in primitive societies those tribes still exist – childbirth is so simple, with no pain at all. On the contrary, you will be surprised, the greatest ecstasy happens to the woman in childbirth – not pain, not agony at all, but the greatest ecstasy. No sexual orgasm is so satisfying and so tremendous as the orgasm that happens to the woman when she gives birth to the child naturally. The whole sexual mechanism of the woman pulsates as it cannot pulsate in any lovemaking. The child is coming from the deepest core of the woman. No man can ever penetrate a woman to that core. And the pulsation arises from the inside. The pulsation is a must – that pulsation will come like waves, great tidal waves of joy. Only that will help the child to come out, only that will help the passage to open for the child. So there will be great pulsation and the whole sexual being of the woman will have tremendous joy. But what actually has happened to humanity is just the opposite: the woman comes to feel the greatest agony of her life. And this is a mind creation, this is wrong upbringing. The birth can be natural if you accept it.

And so it is with your birth. Growth means you are being born every day. Birth does not end the day you were born – on that day it simply starts, it is only a beginning. The day you left the womb of your mother you were not born, you *started* being born; that was just the beginning. And a man goes on being born till he dies. It is not that you are born in a single moment. Your birth process continues for seventy, eighty, ninety years, however long you live. It is a continuum. And every day you will feel joy – growing new leaves, new foliage, new flowers, new branches, rising higher and higher and touching new altitudes. You will be getting deeper, higher, you will be reaching to peaks. Growth will not be painful. But growth is painful – it is because of you, your wrong conditioning. You have been taught not to grow; you have been taught to remain static, you have been taught to cling to the familiar and the known. That's why each time the known disappears from your hands you start crying. A toy has been broken, a pacifier has been taken away....

Remember, only one thing is going to help you: awareness – nothing else. Growth will remain painful if you don't accept life in all its ups and downs. The summer has to be accepted and the winter too. This is what I call meditation. Meditation is when you are emptied of all that is old and told and done to death. Then you see. Or rather, then there is seeing: the birth of the new.[74]

? *I have had a hard, horrible illness from my early age and this mistake of nature makes me suffer constantly. Could you please talk about suffering?*

The suffering is your interpretation. You have become too much identified with it. That is your decision. You can disidentify, and the suffering disappears. Your suffering is like a nightmare: in the dream you think a great rock has fallen on your chest, it is crushing you to death. Out of fear you awake...and all that you find is nothing – your own hands resting on your chest. But the weight of your hands triggered imagination in you: it became a rock, and you started feeling very, very frightened. And because of the fear, you are awakened...and now you laugh. Ask the buddhas, ask the awakened ones, and they say there is no suffering in the world – people are fast asleep and dreaming all kinds of sufferings.

And I know your difficulty: if you have a physical problem, if you are blind, how can you believe that this is only a dream? If you are crippled, how can you believe that this is only a dream? But have you not watched? – every night you dream, and every morning you know that it was a dream and all nonsense – and again you will dream, and in dream again you will believe that this is truth. How many dreams have you dreamed in your life? Millions of dreams! Each night you are dreaming almost without break; just for a few minutes the dreaming stops, and then again another cycle of dreaming starts.

Millions of dreams you have dreamed. And every morning you have laughed and you have said it was unreal, but you have not learnt much. Tonight again when you dream, the same fallacy will persist: you will know that this is truth – in dream you will know this is true. The day you can remember in your dream that this is a dream, immediately the dream disappears…because you have brought awareness into your life.

It looks very difficult to trust that all that you are suffering is just a dream created by yourself – but it is so, because all those who have become awakened say so. Not a single awakened person has said otherwise. And in lucid moments of awareness you will also feel the same. This is my suggestion for you: your problem cannot be solved only by an intellectual discussion – your problem can be only dissolved, not solved. Your problem can only be dissolved by becoming more aware.

One of my friends, an old friend, fell from a staircase and broke both his legs. I went to see him; he was in tremendous pain. And he was a very active person although he was very old, seventy-five – but very active, almost young, and running so much after this and that, and doing this and that, that it was impossible for him to rest on the bed. And the doctors had said that for three months at least he had to be only in bed. This was more of a calamity than the two broken legs.

When I saw him, he started crying. I had never seen that man cry – he is a strong man, a very strong man, almost a man of steel, and has seen all kinds of things in his life, is a very seasoned man. I asked him, "You, and crying – what is the matter with you?"

He said, "Just bless me so that I can die. I don't want to live anymore – three months just in bed! Can you imagine? This is torture. Just three days have passed and it feels almost as if for three years I have been in bed. You know me," he said, "I cannot rest. Just bless me so that I can die soon! I don't want to live anymore. These three months and then the doctors say I will remain crippled my whole life – so what is the point?"

I said to him, "You please do a meditation. I will sit by your side, you just do a simple meditation: that you are not the body."

He was dubious. He said, "What is that going to do to me? I have heard all that you say about meditation, but I cannot meditate because I cannot sit silently."

I said, "Now there is no question of sitting silently – you are already in the bed.

This is a blessing! Just close your eyes and I will teach you a meditation. And I bless you to die, because if you want to die then perfectly good. But my blessing may work, may not work, so meanwhile you meditate."

He understood the point: "There is nothing to do...so why not meditate?" A simple meditation I told him: "You simply go in, look at the body from the inside, say 'It is not me – the body is far away, far away, going distant and more distant and more distant. I am a watcher on the hills, and the body is down there in the dark valley, and the distance is immense.'"

Half an hour passed. I had to leave, and he was in such a meditation that I didn't want to disturb him, but I didn't want to leave him either because I wanted to know what was happening, what he would say. So I had to shake him. He said, "Don't disturb me!"

I said, "But I have to leave."

He said, "You can leave, but don't disturb me – it is so beautiful. The body is really lying so far away, miles and miles away; I have left it in the valley and I am sitting on the top of the hill, a sunlit hill. It is so beautiful, and I don't feel any pain either." And those three months proved the most valuable time of his life. Those three months made him a totally different man. He is still crippled, cannot walk, has to remain mostly in the bed – but you cannot find a more blissful person. He radiates bliss. Now he says it was not a curse – it was a blessing.

Suffering can be transformed into a blessing. Who knows? – you are transforming your blessings into sufferings.[75]

Chapter 13

Bodily Functions

? *It seems man has fallen to such a level that he cannot even breathe properly anymore. Could you speak on the significance of this?*

Breathing is one of the things to be looked after because it is one of the most important things. If you are not breathing fully, you cannot live fully. Then almost everywhere you will be withholding something, even in love. In talking, even, you will be withholding. You will not communicate completely; something will always remain incomplete.

Once breathing is perfect everything else falls into line. Breathing is life. But people ignore it, they don't worry about it at all, they don't pay it any attention. And every change that is going to happen is going to happen through the change in your breathing. If for many years you have been breathing wrongly, shallow breathing, then your musculature becomes fixed – then it is not just a question of your will. It is as if somebody has not moved for years: legs have gone dead, the muscles have shrunk, blood flows no more. Suddenly the person decides one day to go for a long walk – it is beautiful, a sunset. But he cannot move; just by thinking it is not going to happen. Now much effort will be needed to bring those dead legs to life again.

The breathing passage has a certain musculature around it, and if you have been breathing wrongly – and almost everybody has – then the musculature has become fixed. Now it will take many years to change it by your own effort, and it will be an unnecessary waste of time. Through deep massage, particularly through Rolfing, those muscles relax and then you can start again. But after Rolfing, once you start breathing well, don't fall into the old habit again.

Everybody breathes wrongly because the whole society is based on very wrong conditions, notions, attitudes. For example, a small child is weeping and the mother says not to cry. What will the child do? – because crying is coming, and the mother says not to cry. He will start holding his breath because that is the only way to stop it. If you hold your breath everything stops – crying, tears, everything. Then by and by that becomes a fixed thing – don't be angry, don't cry, don't do this, don't do that.

The child learns that if he breathes shallowly then he remains in control. If he breathes perfectly and totally as every child is born breathing, then he becomes wild. So he cripples himself. Every child, boy or girl, starts playing with the genital organs because the feeling is pleasant. The child is completely unaware of the social taboos and nonsense, but if the mother or father or somebody sees you playing with your genitals they tell you to stop it immediately. And such condemnation is in their eyes you become shocked, and you become afraid of breathing deeply, because if you breathe deeply it massages your genital organs from within. That becomes troublesome, so you don't breath deeply; just shallow breathing so you are cut off from the genital organs.

All societies that are sex-repressive are bound to be shallow-breathing societies. Only primitive people who don't have any repressive attitude about sex breathe perfectly. Their breathing is beautiful, it is complete and whole. They breathe like animals, they breathe like children.[76]

The breathing continuously changes with your emotions. When you are angry, your breathing is unrhythmic, asymmetrical. When you are in sexual lust, your breathing is almost insane. When you are calm and quiet, joyful, your breathing has a musical quality to it; your breathing is almost a song. When you are feeling at home in existence, when you have no desires and are feeling contented, suddenly breathing almost stops. When you are in a state of awe, wonder, breathing stops for a moment. And those are the greatest moments of life, because only in those moments when breathing almost stops are you in utter tune with existence: you are in God and God is in you.

Your experience of breathing has to be more and more profound, scrutinized, observed, watched, analyzed. See how your breathing changes with your emotions, and vice versa, how your emotions change your breathing. For example, when you are afraid, watch the change in your breath. And then, one day, try to change the breath to the same pattern as when you were afraid. And you will be surprised that if you change your breath to exactly what it was when you were afraid, fear will arise in you – immediately. Watch your breathing when you are deeply in love with somebody; holding his hand, hugging your beloved, watch your breathing. And then, one day, just sitting silently under a tree, watch yourself again breathing in the same way. Make the pattern, fall into the same gestalt again. Breathe in the same way as if you were hugging your beloved and you will be surprised; the whole existence becomes your beloved. Again there is great love arising in you. They go together. Hence in Yoga, in Tantra, in Tao – in all these three great systems and sciences of human consciousness and the expansion of human consciousness – breathing is one of the key phenomena. They have all worked on breathing.

Buddha's whole meditation system depends on a certain quality of breath. He says, "Simply watch your breath, without changing it. Without in any way changing it, simply watch." But you will be surprised: the moment you watch, it changes, because watchfulness has its own rhythm. That's why Buddha says, "You need not change it; simply watch." Watchfulness will bring its own kind of breathing – it comes by itself. And slowly, slowly you will be surprised: the more watchful you become, the less you breathe. The breath becomes longer, deeper.

For example, if in one minute you were breathing sixteen breaths, now you may breath six, or four, or three. As you become watchful, the breath goes deeper, becomes longer and you are taking less and less breaths in the same time period. Then you can do it from the other side too. Breathe slowly, quietly, deep, long breaths, and suddenly you will see watchfulness arising in you. It is as if each emotion has a polarity in your breathing system: it can be triggered by your breathing.

But the best way is to watch when you are in love, when you are sitting by the side of your friend. Watch your breath, because that loving rhythm of breath is most important: it will transform your whole being. Love is where you feel most sharply the absurdity, the falsity, of your position as a separated being. Yet by this very separation, this absurdity, you are able to express what you could not express in any other way. By your very otherness you are able to celebrate identity. Hence, the paradox of love; you are two and yet you feel one. You are one, yet you know you are two. Oneness in twoness: that is the paradox of love. And that has to be the paradox of prayer too, and meditation too. Ultimately you have to feel as one with existence as you feel with your beloved, with your lover, with your friend, with your mother, with your child, in some rare valuable moments. By your very otherness you are able to celebrate identity.

Watch your loving moments more and more. Be alert. See how your breathing changes. See how your body vibrates…just hugging your woman or your man, make it an experiment, and you will be surprised. One day, just hugging, melting into each other, sit at least for one hour, and you will be surprised: it will be one of the most psychedelic experiences. For one hour, doing nothing, just hugging each other, falling into each other, merging, melting into each other, slowly, slowly the breathing will become one. You will breathe as if you are two bodies but one heart. You will breathe together. And when you breathe together – not by any effort of your own, but just because you are feeling so much love that the breathing follows – those will be the greatest moments, the most precious; not of this world, but of the beyond, the far out. And in those moments you will have the first glimpse of meditative energy....

You should learn to breathe very silently, as if there were no hurry to breathe, as if you were indifferent to it, aloof, far away, distant. If you can be aloof, far away and distant to your breathing, you will be able to attain to the middle. In that moment you will be neither masculine nor feminine. You will be both and neither, you will be transcendental....

When you are distracted, watch: your breathing will be distracted too. When you are not distracted, when you are sitting silently with no distraction, your breathing will be cool, silent, rhythmic; it will have the quality of subtle music. And that quality is the exact middle, because you are not doing anything, yet you are not fast asleep. You are neither active nor inactive, you are balanced. And in that moment of balance you are closest to reality, to God, to heaven.

Remember, your each breath is not just a breath, it is a thought too, an emotion too, a fantasy too. But this will be understood only if you watch your breathing for a few days. When you are making love, watch your breathing. You will be surprised, your breathing is chaotic; because sexual energy is very rough, raw energy. Sexual fantasies are rough and raw, animalistic. There is nothing special about sexuality – every animal has it. When you are sexually aroused, you are just behaving like any other animal in the world. And I am not saying that there is anything wrong in being an animal, all that I am saying is just a fact. I am stating a fact. So whenever you are in sexual love, watch your breath: it loses all balance.

Hence, in Tantra, love-making is allowed only when you have learnt how to make love and yet keep your breath cool, rhythmic. Then a totally different quality comes to your love-making: it becomes prayerful; then it is sacred. Now for the outsider there will be no difference because he will see you are making love to a woman or making love to a man, and it will be the same for the outsider. But for the insider, for those who know, there will be a great difference. In the old Tantra schools where all those secrets were developed, experimented upon, observed, this was one of the central focuses of their experimentation: if a man can make love without his breath being at all affected by it, then it is no longer sex, then it is sacred. And then it will take you to great depths of your own being; it will open doors and mysteries of life.

Your breath is not just breath, because breath is your life; it contains all that life contains. [77]

> **?** *In Western countries there is a growing need for tranquilizers because people suffer from sleeplessness. Can meditation help people to regain the capacity of falling asleep, and what is the relationship between sleep and meditation?*

In sleep we reach the same place we do in meditation. The only difference is that in sleep we are unconscious, while in meditation we are fully conscious. If someone were to become fully aware, even in his sleep, he would have the same experience as in meditation.

For example, if we were to put a person under anaesthetic, and in his unconscious state bring him on a stretcher to a garden where flowers are in full bloom, where fragrance is in the air, where the sun is shining and the birds are singing, the man would be completely unaware of all this. After we brought him back and he was out of the anaesthesia, if we asked him how he liked the garden, he would not be able to tell us anything. Then, if you were to take him to the same garden when he was fully conscious, he would experience everything present there when he had been brought in before. In both cases, although the man was brought to the same place...he was unaware of the beautiful surroundings in the first instance, while in the second instance he would be fully aware of the flowers, the fragrance, the song of the birds, the rising sun. So, although you will undoubtedly reach as far in an unconscious state, to reach some place in an unconscious state is as good as not reaching there at all.

In sleep, we reach the same paradise we reach in meditation, but we are unaware of it. Each night we travel to this paradise, and then we come back – unaware. Although the fresh breeze and the lovely fragrance of the place touch us, and the songs of the birds ring in our ears, we are never aware of it. And yet, in spite of returning from this paradise totally unaware of it, one might say, "I feel very good this morning. I feel very peaceful – I slept well last night."

What do you feel so good about? Having slept well, what good happened? It cannot be only because you slept, surely you must have been somewhere; something must have happened to you. But in the morning you have no knowledge of it, except for a vague idea of feeling good. One who has had a deep sleep at night gets up refreshed in the morning. This shows the person has reached a rejuvenating source in sleep – but in an unconscious state. One who is unable to sleep well at night finds himself more tired in the morning than he was the previous evening. And if a person does not sleep well for a few days it becomes difficult for him to survive, because his connection with the source of life is broken. He is unable to reach the place it is essential he should....

In New York, at least thirty percent of the people cannot sleep without tranquilizers. Psychologists believe that if this condition prevails for the next hundred years, not a single person will be able to sleep without medication. People have completely lost sleep. If a man who has lost sleep were to ask you how you go to sleep, and your answer were, "All I do is put my head on the pillow and fall asleep," he will not believe you. He will find this impossible and suspect there must be some trick he doesn't know to it – because he lays his head on the pillow too, and nothing happens.

God forbid, but a time may come, after a thousand or two thousand years, when everyone will have lost natural sleep, and people will refuse to believe that, a thousand or two thousand years before their time, people simply rested their heads on their pillows and fell asleep. They will take this as fiction, a mythical story from the *Puranas*. They will not believe it to be true. They will say, "This is not possible, because if that isn't true about us, how can it be true about anyone else?"

I am drawing your attention to all of this because three or four thousand years ago people would close their eyes and go into meditation as easily as you go to sleep today. Two thousand years from now it will be difficult to sleep in New York – it is difficult even today. It is becoming difficult to sleep in Bombay – it is just a matter of time. Today it is hard to believe there was a time when a man could close his eyes and go into meditation – because now, when you sit with your eyes closed, you reach nowhere; inside, thoughts keep hovering around and you remain where you are.

In the past, meditation was as easy for those who were close to nature as sleep is for those who live close to nature. First meditation disappeared; now sleep is on its way out. Those things are first lost which are conscious; after that, those things are lost which are unconscious. With the disappearance of meditation the world has almost become irreligious, and when sleep disappears the world will become totally irreligious. There is no hope for religion in a sleepless world.

You will not believe how closely, how deeply, we are connected to sleep. How a person will live his life depends totally on how he sleeps. If he does not sleep well, his entire life will be a chaos: all his relationships will become entangled, everything will become poisonous, filled with rage. If, on the contrary, a person sleeps deeply, there will be freshness in his life – peace and joy will continuously flow in his life. Underlying his relationships, his love, everything else, there will be serenity. But if he loses sleep, all his relationships will go haywire. He will have messed up life with his family, his wife, his son, his mother, his father, his teacher, his students – all of them. Sleep brings us to a point in our unconscious where we are immersed in God

- although not for too long. Even the healthiest person only reaches to his deeper level for ten minutes of his nightly eight hours' sleep. For these ten minutes he is so completely lost, drowned in sleep, that not even a dream exists.

Sleep is not total as long as one is dreaming – one keeps moving between the states of sleep and wakefulness. Dreaming is a state in which one is half asleep and half awake. To be in a dream means, even though your eyes are closed, you are not asleep; external influences are still affecting you. The people you met during the day, you are still with them at night in your dreams. Dreams occupy the middle state between sleep and wakefulness. And that you don't remember in the morning that you dreamed all night is beside the point. Much research on sleep is being carried out in America. Some ten big laboratories have been experimenting on thousands of people for about eight to ten years.

Americans are showing interest in meditation because they have lost sleep. They think that perhaps meditation may bring their sleep back, that it may bring some peace into their lives. That's why they look upon meditation as nothing more than a tranquilizer. When Vivekananda first introduced meditation in America, a physician came to him and said, "I enjoyed your meditation immensely. It is absolutely a non-medicinal tranquilizer. It's not a medicine and yet it puts one to sleep – it's great." Yogis are not the reason their influence is growing so much in America – the lack of sleep is the real cause. People's sleep is in a mess, and consequently life in America is filled with heaviness, depression, tension. And so in America we see the growing need for tranquilizers – somehow, to bring sleep to people.

Each year, millions of dollars are being spent on tranquilizers in America. Ten big laboratories are conducting research on thousands of people who are being paid to undergo nights of rather uncomfortable, painful sleep. All kinds of electrodes and thousands of wires are attached to people's bodies, and they are examined from all angles to find out what is happening inside them. One incredible discovery these experiments have revealed is that man dreams almost the whole night. Waking up, some people said they didn't dream, while some said they did. But in fact, all of them dreamed. The only difference was that those with better memories remembered dreaming, while those with weaker memories could not recall dreaming. But it was found that a completely healthy person was able to slip into a deep, dreamless sleep for ten minutes.

Dreams can be scanned through machines. Nerves in the brain remain active during our dreaming state, but as the dream stops, the nerves cease to be active as well, and the machine indicates a gap has occurred. The gap shows that, at that time, the man was neither dreaming nor thinking – he was lost somewhere.

It is interesting that the machines keep recording movement inside the man while he is in the dreaming state, but as soon as he falls into dreamless sleep, the machine shows a gap. They don't know where the man disappeared in that gap. So, dreamless sleep means the man has reached a place beyond the machine's range. It is in this gap that man enters the divine. The machine is unable to detect this space in between, this gap. The machine records the internal activity as long as the man is dreaming – then comes the gap and the man disappears somewhere. And then, after ten minutes, the machine starts recording again. It is difficult to say where the man was during that ten-minute interval. American psychologists are very intrigued by this gap; hence they consider sleep the biggest mystery.

You sleep every day, yet you have no idea what sleep is. A man sleeps all through his life, and yet nothing changes – he knows nothing about sleep. The reason you don't know anything about sleep is that when sleep is there, *you* are not. Remember, you *are* only as long as sleep is not, and so you come to know only as much as the machine knows. Just as in the face of the gap the machine stops and is unable to reach where the man has been transported, you cannot reach there either – because you are no more than a machine as well.

Since you do not come across the gap either, sleep remains a mystery; it remains beyond your reach. This is so because a man falls into wakeless sleep only when he ceases to exist in his 'I-am-ness'. And therefore, as the ego keeps growing, sleep becomes less and less. An egoistic person loses his capacity to sleep because his ego, the 'I', keeps asserting itself twenty-four hours a day. It is the 'I' that wakes up, the same 'I' that walks on the street. The 'I' remains so present the entire twenty-four hours that at the moment of falling asleep, when the time approaches to drop the 'I', one is unable to get rid of it. Obviously, it becomes difficult to fall asleep. As long as the 'I' exists, sleep is impossible. And as long as the 'I' exists, entering into existence is impossible.

Entering into sleep and entering into existence are exactly one and the same thing; the only difference is that through sleep one enters into existence in an unconscious state, while through meditation one enters into existence in a conscious state. But this is a very big difference. You may enter existence through sleep for thousands of lives, yet you will never come to know existence. But if, even for a moment, you enter meditation you will have reached the same place you have reached in deep sleep for thousands and millions of lives – although always in an unconscious state – and it will transform your life totally.

The interesting thing is, once a person enters meditation, enters the emptiness where deep sleep takes him, he never remains unconscious – even when he is asleep.

Ananda lived with Buddha for many years, for years he slept near Buddha. One morning he asked Buddha, "For years I have been watching you sleep. Not once do

206

you ever change sides; you sleep the whole night in the same position. Your limbs stay where they were when you laid down at night; there is not the slightest movement. Many times I have got up at night to check whether you have moved. I have stayed up nights watching you – your hands, your feet, rest in the same position; you never ever change sides. Do you keep some kind of a record of your sleep the whole night?"

"I don't need to keep any record," Buddha replied. "I sleep in a conscious state, so I find no need to change sides. I can if I want to. Turning from one side to another is not a requirement of sleep, it's a requirement of your restless mind." A restless mind cannot even rest in one place for a single night, let along during the day. Even sleeping at night, the whole time the body shows its restlessness.

If you watch a person asleep at night you will see he is continuously restless the whole time. You will find him moving his hands in much the same way he does when he is awake during the day. In his dream at night, you will find him running and panting in much the same way it happens with someone during the day – he feels out of breath, tired. At night, in dreams, he fights in much the same way he fights during the day. He is filled with passion during the day, at night as well. There is no fundamental difference between the day and the night of such a person, except that at night he lies down exhausted, unconscious; everything else continues to function as usual. So Buddha said, "I can change sides if I want to, but there is no need."

But we don't realize…. A man sitting in a chair keeps jiggling his legs. Ask him, "Why are your legs jiggling like that? It's understandable if they move when you walk, but why are they moving when you are sitting in a chair?" No sooner do you say this than the man will stop immediately. Then he won't even move for a second, but he will have no explanation as to why he was doing it. It shows how restlessness within causes agitation in the entire body. Inside is the restless mind; it cannot be still, in one position, even for a moment. It will keep the whole body fidgeting: the legs will move, the head will shake; even sitting the body will change sides.

That's why, even for ten minutes, you find it so difficult to sit still in meditation. And from a thousand different spots the body urges you to twitch and turn. We do not notice this until we sit with awareness in meditation. We realize then what sort of a body this is; it doesn't want to remain still in one position even for a second. The confusion, the tension, and the excitement of the mind stir up the entire body.

For about ten minutes everything disappears in wakeless sleep – although these ten minutes are available only to one who is completely healthy and peaceful, not to everyone. Others get this kind of sleep anywhere from one to five minutes; most people get only two, or one minute of deep sleep. The little juice we receive in that one minute of reaching to the source of life we apply to making our next twenty-four hours work. Whatever little amount of oil the lamp receives in that short period, we utilize it to carry on our lives for a full twenty-four hours. The lamp of one's life burns on whatsoever amount of oil it receives then. This is the reason the lamp burns so slow – not enough oil is collected to make the lamp of life burn brightly, so it can become a flaming torch.

Meditation brings you slowly to the source of life. Then it is not that you keep taking a handful of nourishment out of it, you are simply *in* the source itself. Then it is not that you refill your lamp with more oil – then the entire ocean of oil becomes available to you. Then you begin to live in that very ocean. With that kind of living, sleep disappears – not in the sense that one doesn't sleep anymore, but in the sense that, even when one is asleep, someone within remains wide awake. Then dreams no longer exist. A yogi stays awake, he sleeps, but he never dreams – his dreams disappear totally. And when dreams disappear, thoughts disappear. What we know as thoughts in the wakeful state are called dreams in the sleeping state. There is only a slight difference between thoughts and dreams: thoughts are slightly more civilized dreams, while dreams are a little primitive in nature. Of the two, one is the original thought.

In fact, children, or the aboriginal tribes, can think only in pictures, not in words. Man's first thoughts are always in pictures. For example, when a child is hungry he does not think in words, "I am hungry." A child can visualize the mother's breast; he can imagine himself sucking the breast. He can be filled with the desire to go to the breast, but he cannot form the words. The word formation starts much later; pictures appear first....

The language of words is handy during the day, but it is not useful at night. We again become primitive at night. We disappear in sleep as we are. We lose our degrees, university educations, everything. We are transported to a point where the original man once stood. That's why pictures emerge at night in sleep, and words appear during the day. If we want to make love during the day, we can think in terms of words, but at night there is no way to express love except through images.

Thoughts do not seem as alive as dreams. In dreams the whole image appears before you. That's why we enjoy watching a movie based on a novel more than reading the novel itself. The only reason for this is that the novel is in the language of words, while the movie is in the language of images. In the same manner, you feel greater joy being here and listening to me live. You would not feel the same joy listening to this talk on a tape, because here the image is present, on tape there are only words. The language of images is nearer to us, more natural. At night words turn into pictures; that's the difference there is.

The day dreams disappear, thoughts disappear too; the day thoughts disappear, dreams disappear as well. If the day is empty of thoughts, the night will be empty of dreams. And remember, dreams don't allow you to sleep, and thoughts don't allow you to sleep, and thoughts don't allow you to awaken. Make sure you understand both things: dreams do not let you sleep, and thoughts do not let you awaken. If dreams disappear, sleep will be total; if thoughts disappear, awakening will be total. If the awakening is total and the sleep is total, then not much difference exists between the two. The only difference is in keeping the eyes open or closed, and in the body being at work or at rest. One who is totally awakened sleeps totally, but in both states his consciousness remains exactly the same. Consciousness is one, unchangeable; only the body changes. Awake, the body is at work; asleep, the body is at rest.

A friend has asked why God is not attained in sleep. My answer is: he can be attained if you can remain awake even in your sleep. And so my method of meditation is a sleeping method – sleeping in awareness, entering into sleep with awareness. That's why I ask you to relax your body, to relax your breathing, to calm down your thoughts. All this is a preparation for sleep. Therefore, it so often happens that some friends go to sleep during meditation – obviously; this is a preparation for sleep. And, while preparing for it, they don't know when they go to sleep. That's why I repeat the third suggestion: stay awake inside, remain conscious within; let the body be totally relaxed, let the breathing be totally relaxed, more relaxed that it normally is while sleeping. But stay awake within. Within, let your awareness burn like a lamp so you don't fall asleep.

The initial conditions of meditation and sleep are the same, but there is a difference in the final condition. The first condition is that the body should be relaxed. If you suffer from insomnia, the first thing a doctor will teach you is relaxation. He will ask you to do the same thing I am asking: relax your body, don't let any tension remain in your body; let your body be totally loose, just like cotton fluff. Have you ever noticed how a dog or a cat sleeps? They sleep as if they are not. Have you ever noticed a baby sleeping? There is no tension anywhere – its arms and legs remain unbelievably loose. Watch a youth and an old man – you will find everything tense in them. So the doctor would ask them to relax.

The same condition applies to sleep: the breathing should be relaxed, deep and slow. You must have noticed that jogging, the breathing becomes faster. Similarly, when the body exerts itself at work, the breathing becomes faster and the blood circulation increases. For sleeping, the blood circulation should slow down – the situation should be just the opposite to jogging – and then the breathing will relax. So the second condition is: relax your breathing....

So the conditions for meditation are primarily the same as those applicable to sleep: relax your body, relax your breathing, let go of thoughts. And so, for sleep as well as for meditation, the initial conditions are equally true. The difference is in the final condition. In the former you remain in deep sleep; in meditation you remain fully awake – that's all.

So you are right in asking the question. There *is* a deep relationship between sleep and meditation. However, there is one very significant difference between the two: the difference between a conscious and an unconscious state. Sleep is unawareness, meditation is awakening.[78]

? *Any suggestions for a sufferer of insomnia?*

When you are just falling into sleep at night, just ready to fall into sleep, go backwards through the memories of the whole day – *backwards*. Do not start from the morning. Start right from where you are, just on the bed – the last item, and then go back. Then go back by and by, step by step, just to the first experience in the morning when you first became awake. Go back, and remember continuously that you are not getting involved.

For example, in the afternoon someone insulted you. See yourself, the form of yourself, being insulted by someone – but you remain just an observer. Do not get involved; do not get angry again. If you get angry again, then you are identified. Then you have missed the point of meditation. Do not get angry. He is not insulting *you*, he is insulting the form that was in the afternoon. That form has gone now.

You are just like a river flowing: the forms are flowing. In the childhood you had one form, now you do not have that form. That form has gone. River-like, you are changing continuously. So when in the night you are meditating backwards on the happenings of the day, just remember that you are a witness: do not get angry. Someone was praising you: do not get elated. Just look at the whole thing as if you are looking indifferently at a film. And backwards is very helpful – particularly for those who have any trouble with sleep.

If you have any trouble with sleep, insomnia, sleeplessness, if you find it difficult to fall into sleep, this will help deeply. Why? Because this is an unwinding of the mind. When you go back you are unwinding the mind. In the morning you start winding, and the mind becomes tangled in many things, in many places. Unfinished and incomplete, many things will remain on the mind, and there is no time to let them settle at the very moment that they happen.

So in the night go back. This is an unwinding process. And when you will be getting back to the morning when you were just on your bed, to the first thing in the morning, you will again have the same fresh mind that you had in the morning. And then you can fall asleep like a very small child....

So many persons suffer a particular disease, and nothing physiological, nothing medical helps; the disease continues. The disease seems to be psychological. What to do about it? To say to someone that his disease is psychological is no help. Rather, it may prove harmful because no one feels good when you say his disease is psychological. What can he do then? He feels he is helpless.

This going backwards is a miraculous method. If you go back slowly – slowly unwinding the mind to the first moment when this disease happened, if by and by you go back to when for the first time you were attacked by the disease, if you can unwind to that moment, you will come to know that this disease is basically a complex of certain other things, certain psychological things. By going back those things will bubble up.

If you pass through that moment when the disease first attacked you, suddenly you will become aware of what psychological factors contributed to it. And you are not to do anything: you are just to be aware of those psychological factors and go on backwards. Many diseases simply disappear from you because the complex is broken. When you have become aware of the complex, then there is no need of it. You are cleaned of it – purged.

This is a deep catharsis. And if you can do it daily, you will feel a new health, a new freshness coming to you. And if we can teach children to do it daily, they will never be burdened by their past. They will not need ever to go to the past. They will be always here and now. There won't be any hang up; nothing will be hovering over them from the past.[79]

Would you talk on the part that the two hemispheres of the brain play in the personality?

Modern research has come to a very significant fact, one of the most significant achieved in this century, and that is that you don't have one mind, you have two minds. Your brain is divided into two hemispheres: the right hemisphere and the left hemisphere. The right hemisphere is joined to the left hand, and the left hemisphere is joined with the right hand – crosswise. The right hemisphere is intuitive, illogical, irrational, poetic, platonic, imaginative, romantic, mythical, religious; and the left hemisphere is logical, rational, mathematical, Aristotelian, scientific, calculative.

These two hemispheres are constantly in conflict – the basic politics of the world are within you, the greatest politics of the world are within you. You may not be aware of it, but once you become aware, the real thing to be done is somewhere between these two minds.

The left hand is concerned with the right hemisphere – intuition, imagination, myth, poetry, religion – and the left hand is very much condemned. The society is of those who are right-handed – right-handed means left hemisphere. Ten percent of children are born left-handed but they are forced to be right-handed. Children who are born left-handed are basically irrational, intuitive, non-mathematical, non-Euclidian. They are dangerous for society so it forces them in every way to become right-handed. It is not just a question of hands, it is a question of inner politics: the left-handed child functions through the right hemisphere. That, society cannot allow, it is dangerous, so he has to be stopped before things go too far.

It is suspected that in the beginning the proportion must have been fifty-fifty – left-handed children fifty percent and right-handed children fifty percent – but the right-handed party has ruled so long that by and by the proportion has fallen to ten percent and ninety percent. Even amongst you here many will be left-handed but you may not be aware of it. You may write with the right hand and do your work with the right hand but in your childhood you may have been forced to be right-handed.... This is a trick because once you become right-handed your left hemisphere starts functioning....

The left-handed minority is the most oppressed minority in the world, even more than negroes, even more that the poor people. If you understand this division, you will understand many things. With the bourgeoisie and the proletariat, the proletariat is always functioning through the right hemisphere of the brain: the poor people are more intuitive. Go to the primitive people, they are more intuitive. The poorer the person, the less intellectual – and that may be the cause of his being poor. Because he is less intellectual he cannot compete in the world of reason. He is less articulate as far as language is concerned, reason is concerned, calculation is concerned – he is almost a fool. That may be the cause of his being poor. The rich person is functioning through the left hemisphere; he is more calculative, arithmetical in everything, cunning, clever, logical – and he plans. That may be the reason why he is rich....

The same applies to men and women. Women are right-hemisphere people, men are left-hemisphered. Men have ruled women for centuries. Now a few women are in revolt, but the amazing thing is that these are the same type of women. In fact they are just like men – rational, argumentative, Aristotelian. It is possible that one day, just as the communist revolution has succeeded in Russia and China, somewhere, maybe in America, women can succeed and overthrow men. But by the time the women succeed, the women will no longer be women, they will have become left-hemisphered.

Just superficial things change, deep down the same conflict remains. The conflict is in man. Unless it is resolved there, it cannot be resolved anywhere else. The politics is within you; it is between the two parts of the mind. A very small bridge exists. If that bridge is broken through some accident, through some physiological defect or something else, the person becomes split, the person becomes two persons – and the phenomenon of schizophrenia or split personality happens. If the bridge is broken – and the bridge is very fragile – then you become two, you behave like two persons. In the morning you are very loving, very beautiful; in the evening you are very angry, absolutely different. You don't remember your morning – how can you remember? Another mind was functioning – and the person becomes two persons. If this bridge is strengthened so much that the two minds disappear as two and become one, then integration, then crystallization, arises. What George Gurdjieff used to call the crystallization of being is nothing but these two minds becoming one, the meeting of the male and the female within, the meeting of yin and yang, the meeting of the left and right, the meeting of logic and illogic, the meeting of Plato and Aristotle. If you can understand this basic bifurcation in your tree of life then you can understand all the conflict that goes on around and inside you....

The female mind has a grace, the male mind has efficiency, and of course, in the long run, if there is a constant fight, grace is bound to be defeated – the efficient mind will win, because the world understands the language of mathematics, not of love. But the moment your efficiency wins over your grace, you have lost something tremendously valuable: you have lost contact with your own being. You may become very efficient, but you will be no more a real person. You will become a machine, a robot-like thing.

Because of this there is constant conflict between man and woman. They cannot remain separate, they have to get into a relationship again and again – but they cannot remain together either. The fight is not outside, the fight is within you. And this is my understanding: unless you have resolved your inner fight between the right and the left hemispheres, you will never be able to be peacefully in love – never, because the inner fight will be reflected outside. If you are fighting inside and you are identified with the left hemisphere, the reason hemisphere, and you are continuously trying to overpower the right hemisphere, you will try to do the same with the woman you fall in love with. If the woman is continuously fighting her own reason inside, she will continuously fight the man she loves.

All relationships – almost all, the exceptions are negligible, can be left out of account – are ugly. In the beginning they are beautiful; in the beginning you don't show the reality; in the beginning you pretend. Once the relationship settles and you relax, your inner conflict bubbles up and starts being mirrored in your relationship. Then come fights, then come a thousand and one ways of nagging each other, destroying each other. Hence the attraction for homosexuality. Whenever a society becomes too divided between man and woman, homosexuality erupts immediately, because at least a man in love with a man is not that much in conflict. The love relationship may not be very satisfying, may not lead to tremendous bliss and orgasmic moments, but at least it is not so ugly as the relationship between a man and a woman. Women become lesbians whenever the conflict becomes too much, because at least the love relationship between two women is not so deep in conflict. The same meets the same; they can understand each other.

Yes, understanding is possible, but the attraction is lost, the polarity is lost. It is a very great cost. Understanding is possible, but the whole tension, the challenge, is lost. If you choose challenge, then comes conflict, because the real problem is somewhere within you. Unless you have settled, come to a deep harmony between your female and male mind, you will not be able to love.

People come to me and they ask how to go deep in a relationship, I tell them, "First you go deep in meditation. Unless you are resolved within yourself you will create more problems than you already have. If you move in relationship, all your problems will be multiplied. Just watch: the greatest and the most beautiful thing in the world is love, but can you find anything more ugly, more hell-creating?"

Mulla Nasruddin once told me, "Well, I have been putting off the evil day for months but I have got to go this time."

"Dentist or doctor?" I inquired.

"Neither," he said, "I am getting married."

…If you are outside of it, it may look like a beautiful oasis in the desert, but as you come close the oasis starts drying and disappearing. Once you are caught in it, it is an imprisonment. But remember, the imprisonment doesn't come from the other, it comes from within you.

If the left-hemisphere brain goes on dominating you, you will live a very successful life – so successful that by the time you are forty you will have ulcers; by the time you are forty-five you will have had at least one or two heart attacks; by the time you are fifty you will be almost dead – but successfully dead. You may become a great scientist, but you will never become a great being. You may accumulate enough wealth, but you will lose all that is of worth. You may conquer the whole world like an Alexander, but your own inner territory will remain unconquered.

There are many attractions to follow the left-hemisphere brain – that is the world brain. It is more concerned with things; cars, money, houses, power, prestige.

The right-hemisphere brain is the orientation of the sannyasin, one who is more interested in his own inner being, his inner peace, his blissfulness, and is less concerned about things. If they come easily, good; if they don't come that is also good. He is more concerned with the moment, less concerned with the future; more concerned with the poetry of life, less concerned with the arithmetic of it.

I have heard an anecdote.

Finkelstein had made a huge killing at the races and Muscovitz, quite understandably, was envious. "How did you do it, Finkelstein?" he demanded.

"Easy," said Finkelstein. "It was a dream."

"A dream?"

"Yes; I had figured out a three-horse parley, but I was not sure about the third horse. Then the night before, I dreamed that an angel was standing over the head of my bed and kept saying, 'Blessings on you, Finkelstein, seven times seven blessings on you.' When I woke up I realized that seven times seven is forty-eight, and that horse number forty-eight was Heavenly Dream. I made Heavenly Dream the third horse in my parley and I just cleaned up, simply cleaned up."

Muscovitz said, "But Finkelstein, seven times seven is forty-nine! "

And Finkelstein said, "So, you be the mathematician."

There is a way to follow life through arithmetic and there is another way to follow life through dream – through dreams and visions. They are totally different.

Just the other day somebody asked, "Are there ghosts, fairies, and things like that?" Yes there are – if you move through the right-hemisphere brain there are. If you move through the left-hemisphere brain, there are not. All children are right-hemisphered – they see ghosts and fairies all around, but you go on talking to them and putting them in their places and saying to them, "Nonsense! You are stupid! Where is the fairy? There is nothing, just a shadow." By the time you convince the child, the helpless child… by and by you convince him and he moves from the right-hemisphered orientation to the left-hemisphered orientation – he has to. He has to live in your world: her has to forget his dreams, he has to forget all myth, he has to forget all poetry, he has to learn mathematics. Of course he becomes efficient in mathematics – and becomes almost crippled and paralyzed in life. Existence goes on getting farther and farther away and he becomes just a commodity in the market, his whole life becomes just rubbish... although, of course, valuable in the eyes of the world.

A sannyasin is one who lives through the imagination, who lives through the dreaming quality of his mind, who lives through poetry, who poeticizes about life, who looks through visions. Then trees are greener than they look to you, then birds are more beautiful, then everything takes on a luminous quality. Ordinary pebbles become diamonds; ordinary rocks are no longer ordinary – nothing is ordinary. If you look from the right hemisphere, everything becomes divine, sacred. Religion is from the right hemisphere.[80]

? *Please speak about the physical senses.*

Never for a single moment think that your physical senses are as they should be – they are not. They have been trained. You see things if your society allows to to see them. You hear things if your society allows you to hear them. You touch things if your society allows you to touch things.

Man has lost many of his senses – for example, smell. Man has almost lost smell. Just see a dog and his capacity to smell – how sensitive is his nose! Man seems to be very poor. What has happened to man's nose? Why can't he smell as deeply as a dog or a horse? The horse can smell for miles. The dog has an immense memory of smells. Man has no memory. Something is blocking his nose.

Those who have been working deep into these layers say that it is because of the repression of sex that smell is lost. Physically man is as sensitive as any other animal, but psychologically his nose has been corrupted. Smell is one of the most sexual doors into your body. It is though smell that animals start feeling whether a male is in tune with the female or not. The smell is a subtle hint. When the female is ready to make love to the male she releases a certain kind of smell. Only through that smell does the male understand that he is acceptable. If that smell is not released by the feminine sexual organism, the male moves away; he is not accepted.

Man has destroyed smell because it will be difficult to create a so-called cultured society if your sense of smell remains natural. You are going along the road and a woman starts smelling and gives you a hint of acceptance. She is somebody else's wife; her husband is with her. The signal is there that you are acceptable. What will you do? It will be awkward, embarrassing!...

You don't see people eye to eye; or, if you do see them, it is only for a few seconds. You don't see people really; you go on avoiding. If you look, it is thought to be offensive. Just remember, do you really see people? Or do you go on avoiding their eyes? – because if you don't avoid them then you may be able to see a few things which the person is not willing to show. It is not good manners to see something that he is not willing to show, so it is better to avoid. We listen to the words, we don't see the face – because many times the words and the face are contradictory. A man is saying one thing and he is showing another. Gradually we have completely lost the sense of seeing the face, the eyes, the gestures. We only listen to the words. Just watch this and you will be surprised how people go on saying one thing and showing another. And nobody detects it because you have been trained not to look directly into the face. Or, even if you look, the look is not that of awareness, not that of attention. It is empty; it is almost as if you are not looking.

We hear sounds by choice. We don't hear all kinds of sounds – we choose. Whatsoever is useful we hear. And to different societies and different countries, different things are valuable. A man who lives in a primitive world, in a forest, in a jungle, has a different kind of receptivity for sounds. He has to be continuously alert and aware of the animals. His life is in danger. You need not be alert. You live in a cultured world where animals don't exist anymore and there is no fear. Your survival is not at stake. Your ears don't function perfectly because there is no need....

People don't touch each other, they don't hold hands, they don't hug each other. And when you hold somebody's hand, you feel embarrassed, he feels embarrassed. Even if you hug somebody, it feels as if something wrong is happening. And you are in a hurry to get away from the other's body, because the other's body can open you. Even children are not allowed to hug their parents. There is great fear, and all fear is basically, deep down, rooted in the fear of sex. There is a taboo against sex. A mother cannot hug her son because the son may get sexually aroused – that is the fear. A father cannot hug his daughter – he is afraid he may get physically aroused. Warmth has its own way of working. Nothing is wrong in being physically aroused or sexually aroused. It is simply a sign that one is alive, that one is immensely alive. But the fear, the sex taboo, says keep away, keep a distance....

That is the whole effort of Yoga: to make your body alive, sensitive, young again, to give your senses their maximum functioning. Then one functions with no taboos around; then lucidity, grace, beauty flow. Warmth arises again, openness – and growth happens. One is constantly new, young, and is always on an adventure. The body becomes orgasmic. Joy surrounds you. Through joy the first corruption disappears; hence my insistence to be joyous, to be celebrating, to enjoy life, to accept the body. Not only to accept it, but to feel grateful that God has given you such a beautiful body, such a sensitive body, with so many doors to relate to reality: eyes and ears and nose and touch. Open all these windows and let life's breezes flow in, let life's sun shine in. Learn to be more sensitive. Use every opportunity to be sensitive so that the first filter is dropped....

When you are sitting on the grass, close your eyes, become the grass – be grassy. Feel that you are the grass, feel the greenness of the grass, feel the wetness of the grass. Feel the subtle smell that goes on being released by the grass. Feel the dewdrops on the grass – that they are on you. Feel the sunrays playing on the grass. For a moment be lost in it, and you will have new sense of your body. And do it in all kinds of situations: in a river, in a swimming pool, lying on the beach in the sunrays, looking at the moon in the night, lying down with closed eyes on the sand and feeling the sand. Millions of opportunities are there to make your body alive again. And only you can do it. Society has done its work of corruption, you will have to undo it. And once you start hearing, seeing, touching, smelling through joy, then you hear the reality, then you see the reality, then you smell the reality.[81]

? *I have been experiencing times of feeling negative. What is happening to us when we come into this state?*

There are three cycles in human existence. The first cycle is the physical. It takes twenty-three days to complete, and it affects a broad range of physical factors, including resistance to disease, strength, coordination, and the other basic body functions, and the sensation of physical well-being.

The second cycle is emotional. It takes twenty-eight days to complete, just as it takes twenty-eight days in the feminine body for the menstruation to come. Just now science is becoming alert that even man has a kind of monthly period and that after each twenty-eight days it happens. The feminine period is visible and physical. Man's period is not visible and not physical; more psychological, more emotional, but it happens. The emotional cycle governs creativity, sensitivity, mental health, mood, perception of the world and ourselves.

When a woman has her period, for three, four or five days she is in misery, sad, negative, dull, dead, feeling very low, jumpy, shaken. But women become accustomed to it because it is so visible. By and by they learn that it has to be so, so by and by they are not so miserable. It is an every month thing and so visible, so things settle. But man's problem is more difficult. The period is there – the male period – but it is not visible and you don't know where it comes from and when it goes.... This is a twenty-eight day cycle in the body; it follows the moon. So whenever there is a moon you will be more happy, and when there is no moon you will be less happy.

And then, finally, the third cycle. The third cycle is the intellectual cycle. It takes place over a thirty-three day period. It regulates memory, alertness, receptivity to knowledge and the logical and analytical functions. The first half of each period is positive and the second half, negative. Sometimes you have a time in the negative phase, others in the positive, and vice versa. When all the three cycles are in the positive, peaks of joy and ecstasy happen. And when all the three are in the negative, one lives in hell. Heaven means all the three are in the positive and hell is the other end. And to be free of both is nirvana, *moksha,* absolute freedom....

You have just to understand your phases, and you have to be a little more watchful. Start keeping a diary about these negative phases. Within three, four months, you will be able to make your chart, and then you can predict that the next Monday you are going to be in a bad mood,

In ancient days yogis used to make such charts. The science of bio-rhythm was well-known and practiced in the Yoga and Sufi schools. And these charts were very helpful because if you know that for the first week of every month you become very, very negative, then a few things can be avoided. In the first week don't do anything for which you can repent later on; don't fight, don't get angry. The people who are really following these charts will not move out of their rooms. They will not do anything for those seven or four or three days, because whatsoever they do will be wrong.

And then you know when your positive mood comes. That is the time to relate, to go to people, to meet, and nothing will go wrong. You will be in a different state altogether. Watching this way, within six, eight months you will be able to become a witness, and then nothing disturbs. Then you know it is just part of nature – nothing to do with you. Seeing it, you start transcending.[82]

 Why do I always feel destructive when I have my period?

For many women the days of the period are a little destructive, and the reason is very biological. You have to understand and become a little alert and aware so that you can rise a little higher than your biology; otherwise you are in the grip of it.

If you are pregnant, the period stops because the same energy that has been released in the period starts being creative: it creates the child. When you are not pregnant, every month the energy accumulates and if it cannot be creative then it becomes destructive. So when a woman is having her period, for these four or five days she has a very destructive attitude, because she does not know what to do with the energy. And the energy vibrates, it haunts the innermost core of your being, and you cannot give any creativity.

All creative energy can become destructive, and all destructive energy could have become creative. For example, Hitler: he wanted to be a painter in the very beginning, but he was not allowed. He could not manage to pass the examination and enter an art school. The man who could have been a painter became one of the most destructive men in the world. With the same energy he may have become a Picasso. And one thing is certain – he had energy. The same energy could have been infinitely creative.

Ordinarily, women are not destructive. In the past they were never destructive because they were continuously pregnant. One child is born, then again they were pregnant. For their whole life they used their energy. Now, for the first time in the world a new danger is arising, and that is the destructiveness of women, because now there is no need for them to be pregnant continuously – in fact pregnancy is almost out of date – but the energy is there.

I see a deep connection between birth control methods and the Women's Liberation Movement. Women are becoming destructive and they are destroying family life, their relationships. They may be trying to rationalize it in many ways, but they are trying to be liberated from the slavery. In fact it is a destructive phase. They have the energy and they don't know what to do with it. The birth control methods have stopped their creative channelization. Now if some channels are not opened to them they will become very destructive.

In the West the family life is almost gone. There is continual conflict, continual fighting, quarreling and being nasty to each other. And the reason is – and nobody understands what the reason is – a biological problem.

So whenever you feel the period is coming, be more alert; and before it starts, do wild dancing. You can go beyond nature because you have a higher nature also. One can go beyond biology, and one has to, otherwise one is a slave to hormones! So whenever you feel destructive, start dancing. What I am saying is that dancing will absorb your energy. You are doing the opposite. You say you like to rest and not do anything during these days, but do something – anything, go for a long walk – because the energy needs release. Once you catch the point, once you know that the dance relaxes you completely, those four days of your period will become the most beautiful because you will never have so much energy as then.[83]

?

Living with myself when I have my period is one thing. Now I have to stay centred with my husband's period too!

It is very good to know which days you will be suffering from your monthly period – whether you are a man or a woman – because when somebody is suffering from their menstrual period, you have to be more compassionate and more loving towards the person. He is not his usual self…. The only thing to be remembered is that if you both have menstrual crises on the same date, then one of you has to go for a honeymoon – just one. Each month you can alternate – next month the other one can go for the honeymoon. But don't remain together, because that will be a very explosive situation….

Unless you become a watcher, unless you become a witness to your own mental states – this is what I call meditation. And these are great opportunities: when you are feeling sad, just watch it. It is chemistry – you are consciousness. Don't get mixed up with chemistry; don't get identified with chemistry. It is physiology, it is chemistry, it is biology – you are consciousness, a watcher.

Slowly, slowly, even when your whole chemistry is going berserk, you will remain centred, grounded, unaffected – and this is true for both, man or woman.[84]

?

I have heard you mention the seven-year cycles in the life of a human being. What is the significance of these cycles?

In fact there is a seven-year cycle in each life. We change each seven years – one cycle is complete. And all great changes happen between the end of one cycle and the beginning of the second cycle.

First, at the age of seven the child is no longer a child; a totally different world starts. Up to then he was innocent. Now he starts learning the cunningness of the world, the cleverness, all the deceptions, games; he starts learning to be pseudo, he starts wearing masks. The first layer of falsity starts surrounding him.

At the age of fourteen, sex, which was never a problem up to now suddenly arises in his being…and his world changes, utterly changes! For the first time he becomes interested in the other sex…. A totally new vision of life arises and he starts dreaming and fantasizing. And this way it goes on….

At the age of twenty-one, again: now a power trip, an ego trip, ambition – now he is ready to go into some power trip, to attain more money, to become more famous, this and that. That is the age of twenty-one; again a cycle is complete.

At the age of twenty-eight, again – he becomes settled, starts thinking of security, comfort, the bank balance. So hippies are right if they say, "Don't trust anybody beyond thirty." In fact they should say twenty-eight, because that is the time when a person becomes straight.

By the age of thirty-five again a change starts happening, because thirty-five is almost the peak of life. If a man is going to die at seventy, which is normal, then thirty-five seems to be the peak. The bigger cycle has come halfway and a man starts thinking of death, starts being afraid. Fear arises. This is the age, between thirty-five and forty-two, where ulcers and blood pressure, heart attacks and all sorts of things happen – because of the fear. Fear creates all these things – cancer, TB.... A man becomes prone to all sorts of accidents because the fear has entered into his being. Now death seems to be coming close: he has taken the first step towards death the day he passes thirty-five.

At the age of forty-two a person starts becoming religious. Now death is not an intellectual thing; he becomes more and more alert about it and wants to do something, *really* do something – because if he waits anymore it will be too late.... At the age of forty-two a person needs some religion, just as at the age of fourteen he needed a woman or she needed a man to relate to. Sexual relationship was needed; exactly the same happens at forty-two – now a religious relationship is needed. One needs a God, a master, somewhere to surrender, somewhere to go and unburden oneself.

At the age of forty-nine a person becomes settled about religion. The search is over, he settles.

At the age of fifty-six, if things go naturally and a person follows his rhythm, a person will start attaining a few glimpses of the divine.

At the age of sixty-three, if everything goes naturally, he will have his first *satori*. And if this happens at the age of sixty-three, that he has had his first satori, he will die a beautiful death at the age of seventy. Then death will not be death – it will be a door to the divine, it will be a meeting with the beloved.[85]

?   *Can you talk about sex and health?*

Everything that the religions have called bad can be used in a tremendously beneficial way.

For example, sex they have condemned as bad and the doing of the devil, but if you condemn sex, then you become unable to transform its energy....

And it is simply energy. It can move in any direction, downwards, upwards. If you accept it, in the very acceptance it starts moving upwards because you are befriending it. The moment you reject it you are creating an enmity, a division in yourself.

This division between God and devil is not just there in the holy books. It has penetrated you, it has made you schizophrenic. One part thinks, "This is me – the good part – and the bad part must belong to the devil." You are split. Now, how are you going to change that part you have rejected from your being as not yours? It is there, and it is intensely powerful. Your rejection makes it more intense because you don't use it, you go on collecting it, you go on repressing it.

Ninety percent of the mind diseases in the world are nothing but repressed sexuality, and fifty percent of body diseases are repressed sexuality. If we can accept sexuality naturally, ninety percent of your mental diseases will simply disappear, and fifty percent of physical diseases will simply disappear, leaving no trace behind. And you will find human beings, for the first time, in a totally new age of health, well-being, wholeness.

To me only that wholeness is holy, when your schizophrenia is no longer there; when you are one, integratedly one – and courageous enough to accept everything, that, "This is me. Whatsoever it is, it is me, and I am going to make use of it the best I can."[86]

? *Would you talk about sexual energy?*

Sexual energy is another name for your life-force. The word 'sex' has become condemned by the religions; otherwise there is nothing wrong in it. It is your very life. Sexual energy is a natural energy: you are born out of it. It is your creative energy. When the painter paints or the poet composes or the musician plays or the dancer dances, these are all expressions of your life-force.

Not only are children born out of your sexual energy, but everything that man has created on the earth has come out of sexual energy. Sexual energy can have many transformations: at the lowest it is biological; at the highest it is spiritual. It has to be understood that all creative people are highly sexual. You can see the poets, you can see the painters, you can see the dancers: all creative people are highly sexual, and the same is true about the people whom I call the mystics. Perhaps they are the most sexual people on the earth, because they are so full of life energy, abundant, overflowing....

Sexual energy is your potentiality for spiritual growth. You can become enlightened only because of your sexual energy.

I have been searching for almost thirty-five years, in all kinds of books, strange scriptures from Tibet and Ladakh and China and Japan – India has the greatest number of scriptures in the world – and I have been looking for one thing: Has there ever been an enlightened, impotent person? There is no incidence recorded anywhere. An impotent person has never been a great poet either, or a great singer, or a great sculptor, or a great scientist. What is the problem with the impotent person? He has no life-force; he is hollow. He cannot create anything – and to create oneself as an enlightened being needs tremendous energy....

Sex has become a thing of the marketplace. On the one hand, religions have been repressing sexual energy and creating perversions which have culminated in the dangerous disease AIDS, which has no cure. The whole credit goes to religions, and if they have any sense of being human, then all the churches and all the monasteries and the Vatican itself should be turned into hospitals for the people suffering from AIDS, because these are the people who have created them. Theirs is the responsibility. They have forced men to live separately from women; they have insisted that celibacy is the very foundation of a religious life. But celibacy is unnatural, and anything unnatural cannot be the foundation of a religious life.

Because celibacy is unnatural, and religions have divided men and women into different monasteries, they have created the situation for homosexuality. They are the pioneers of homosexuality, and homosexuality has led to AIDS, which cannot be called simply a disease because it does not come into the category of diseases. It is death itself. So on the one hand religions have created perversions; on the other hand they insisted on monogamy, which in fact means monotony. That has created the profession of the prostitute. The priest is responsible for the prostitute. It is so ugly and sick that we have created objects, commodities, things to be exploited out of so many beautiful women.

Even today, it is not understood exactly what sex is. It need not be repressed, because it is your very energy. It has to be transformed, certainly; it has to be raised to its highest purity. And as you start moving upwards – the name of the ladder is meditation – sex becomes love, sex becomes compassion, and ultimately sex becomes the explosion of your inner being, the illumination, the awakening, the enlightenment. But it is sexual energy: it can rot, it can go into perversions. But if it is to be understood naturally and helped through meditation to move upwards towards silent spaces, to pass through your heart and reach to the seventh centre at the highest point in your body, you will feel grateful towards the energy. Right now you feel only ashamed.

This shame and guilt is created by the religious organizations, founders of religion. Naturally the question arises: Why did they make sex a mess? And through making a mess of sex they have messed up the whole world and its mind and its growth. Why? – because this was the simplest way to keep humanity in slavery. This was the simplest way to keep people guilty, and anybody who feels guilty can never raise his head in revolt. So all the vested interests wanted man to lose his dignity, self-respect, to feel guilty, ashamed. They have been condemning sex continuously, and their condemnation has led the whole world into a very miserable, psychologically abnormal state....

All these crimes are perpetuated by your so-called virtuous leaders, religious saints. But they have been doing this harm for thousands of years. Rather than helping man to sublimate his energies, to make them creative, they have only been able to force man to repress his energies. And repressed energies become a cancer, repressed energies create all kinds of perversions.

The teacher asked her childrens' art class to draw on the blackboard their impressions of the most exciting thing they could think of.

Little Hymie got up and drew a long jagged line.

"What is that?" asked the teacher.

"Lightning," said Hymie. "Every time I see lightning I get so excited, I scream."

"Very good," said the teacher.

Next, little Sally drew a long wavy line. She explained that it was the sea which always excited her. The teacher thought that was excellent too.

Then little Ernie came up to the blackboard, made a single dot and sat down.

"What is that?" asked the puzzled teacher.

"It is a period," said Ernie.

"Well," said the teacher, "what is so exciting about a period?"

"I don't know," said Ernie to the teacher, "but my sister has missed two of them and my whole family is excited."

This excitement has made the whole world a mad asylum, and it goes on growing so fast that it always defeats all scientific calculations.

Just forty years ago, when India became free, it had four hundred million people. Now, after only forty years, it has nine hundred million people. Five hundred million people have been produced in forty years; and by the end of this century, the calculations of the scientists are that it will be the biggest nation in the world for the first time – up to now China has been the first – it will go beyond one billion people. And Jayendra Saraswati is talking about no family planning, no birth control....

When one thousand people were dying per day in Ethiopia, even then the pope was continuously talking about no birth control, Mother Teresa was talking about no birth control. You have to see the implications: Mother Teresa needs orphans; without orphans she does not have any qualifications to have a Nobel prize. But from where can you get orphans if birth control methods are applied? And strangely enough, they condemn birth control methods because they are not God's creation, but they don't condemn medicine, which is also not God's creation. At least there is no mention of medicine in those six days when he made the world.

Medicine has given man longer life. There are people in the Soviet Union who have passed their one hundred and eightieth year, and they are still young; there is every possibility that they will pass their second century. There are thousands who have passed beyond one hundred and fifty, and no religious leader condemns it, saying that medicine should be stopped from giving people health and longevity. No religious leader goes on saying that diseases should be allowed because they are God-created.

Medicine can be used; people can be made more healthy...and naturally when they are more healthy they are more sexually powerful. But birth control methods cannot be used because they will reduce the numbers of their congregations. It is a competition of numbers. Catholics are six hundred million in number. It is the greatest religion in the world – only because of the numbers; otherwise it is the most third-rate religion in the world, there is nothing much in it which can be called religious. But it is the biggest religion, the greatest religion, only on the strength of numbers. It cannot allow numbers to decline – even if these numbers are going to kill the whole of humanity.

I am in absolute favour of birth control methods for two reasons: birth control methods will keep the world healthy, nourished; secondly, once birth control methods are used, sex loses its profanity – or its sacredness. It becomes simple fun, it becomes just a joyful exchange of energies. According to me, birth control is the greatest invention that man has made. It is the greatest revolution because it can make man and woman equal, liberated. Otherwise the woman is constantly pregnant, and because of her pregnancy she cannot be independent financially, she cannot be independent educationally, she cannot be independent from man's domination.

Once she is free from being pregnant compulsorily she will have as much time, as much energy to be creative. Until now half of humanity has remained uncreative:

o great poets, no great saints, no great musicians, no great artists. Women have had
o time. I was surprised to know that even the books on cookery are written by
nen, not by women. And the best cooks are men, not women: in all the great five-
tar hotels you will find great cooks, always men. Strange...that has been the domain
f the woman forever, but she has no energy left. Because of these religious people
he will never be liberated.

Sex energy has to be welcomed and transformed through the alchemy of
neditation into higher states of being, into creativity in different dimensions, not
nly creating more and more children. Life has to be planned – it should not be
ccidental.[87]

? *I feel so imprisoned by the fear of being intimate and totally losing control with a*
man. This outrageous woman is locked up inside. When she comes out once in a
while, men usually freak out, so she goes back into hibernation, plays safe, and is
totally frustrated. Could you please speak about this fear of intimacy?

Mankind, especially womankind, suffers from many sicknesses. Up to now all
the so-called civilizations and cultures have been psychologically sick. They
ave never dared even to recognize their sickness; and the first step of treatment is
o recognize that you are sick. The relationship between man and woman has been
specially unnatural.

A few facts have to be remembered. Firstly, man has the capacity for only one
rgasm; woman has the capacity for multiple orgasms. This has created a tremendous
roblem. There would not have been any problem if marriage and monogamy had
ot been imposed on them; it seems it was not the intention of nature. The man
ecomes afraid of the woman for the simple reason that if he triggers one orgasm in
er, then she is ready for at least half a dozen more orgasms – and he is incapable of
atisfying her. The way that man has found is: don't give the woman even one orgasm.
ven take away from her the conception that she can have an orgasm.

Secondly, man's sex is local, genital. The same is not the case with woman. Her
exuality, her sensuality is spread all over her body. It takes a longer time for her to
varm up, and before she even gets warmed up, the man is finished. He turns his back
owards her and starts snoring. For thousands of years, millions of women around
ne world have lived and died without knowing the greatest natural gift – of
rgasmic joy. It was a protection for man's ego. The woman needs a long foreplay so
nat her whole body starts tingling with sensuality, but then there is the danger – what
o do with her capacity for multiple orgasm?

Looked at scientifically, either sex should not be taken so seriously and friend should be invited to give the woman her whole range of orgasms, or some scientifi vibrator should be used. But with both there are problems. If you use scientifi vibrators, they can give as many orgasms as the woman is capable of; but once a woman has known...then the man's organ looks so poor that she may choose a scientific instrument, a vibrator, rather than a boyfriend. If you allow a few friend to join you, then it becomes a social scandal – that you are indulging in orgies. So the simplest way man has found is that the woman should not even move while he i making love to her; she should remain almost like a corpse. And man's ejaculation i quick – two minutes, three minutes at the most; by that time the woman is not at al aware of what she has missed.

As far as biological reproduction is concerned, orgasm is not a necessity. But a far as spiritual growth is concerned, orgasm is a necessity. According to me, it is the orgasmic experience of bliss that has given humanity in the early days the idea o meditation, of looking for something better, more intense, more vital. Orgasm i nature's indication that you contain within yourself a tremendous amount o blissfulness. It simply gives you a taste of it – then you can go on the search.

The orgasmic state, even the recognition of it, is a very recent thing. Just in thi century, psychologists became aware of what problems women are facing. Throug psychoanalysis and other psychological schools the conclusion was the same, that sh is being prevented from spiritual growth; she remains just a domestic servant.

As far as reproducing children is concerned, man's ejaculation is enough – s biology has no problem; but psychology has. Women are more irritable, nagging bitchy, and the reason is that they have been deprived of something that is thei birthright; and they don't even know what it is. Only in Western societies has th younger generation become aware of the orgasm. And it is not coincidental that th younger generation has gone into the search for truth, for ecstasy – because orgasn is momentary, but it gives you a glimpse of the beyond.

Two things happen in orgasm: one is, mind stops the constant yakkety yak – i becomes for a moment no-mind; and second, time stops. That single moment c orgasmic joy is so immense and so fulfilling that it is equal to eternity. In the ver early days man became aware that these are the two things which give you th greatest pleasure possible, as far as nature is concerned. And it was a simple an logical conclusion that if you can stop your chattering mind and become so silent tha everything stops – time included – then you are free from sexuality. You nee not depend on the other person, man or woman; you are capable of attainin this state of meditation alone. And orgasm cannot be more than momentary, bu meditation can be spread over the whole twenty-four hours. A man like Gautan

Buddha is living every moment of his life in orgasmic joy – it has nothing to do with sex.

I have been asked again and again why very few women became enlightened. Amongst other reasons, the most important reason is: they never had any taste of orgasm. The window to the vast sky never opened. They lived, they produced children, and they died. They were used by biology and man, just like factories, producing children. In the East, even now, it is very difficult to find a woman who knows what orgasm is. I have asked very intelligent, educated, cultured women – they don't have any idea of it. In fact, in the Eastern languages there is no word which can be used as a translation for 'orgasm.' It was not needed; it was simply never touched on.

And man has taught woman that it is only prostitutes who enjoy sex: they moan and they groan and they scream, and they go almost crazy. To be a respectable lady you should not do such things. So the woman remains tense, and feels humiliated deep down – that she has been used. And many women have reported to me that after making love, when their husband goes on snoring, they have wept. A woman is almost like a musical instrument; her whole body has immense sensitivity, and that sensitivity should be aroused. So there is a need for foreplay. And after making love, the man should not go to sleep; that is ugly, uncivilized, uncultured. A woman who has given you such joy needs some afterplay too – just out of gratitude.

Your question is very important – and is going to become more and more important in the future. This problem has to be solved; but marriage is a barrier, religion is a barrier, your rotten old ideas are barriers. They are preventing half of humanity from being joyous, and their whole energy – that should have blossomed in flowers of joy – turns sour, poisonous, in nagging, in being bitchy. Otherwise all this nagging and this bitchiness would disappear.

Men and women should not be in a contract, like marriage. They should be in love – but they should retain their freedom. They don't owe anything to each other. And life should be more mobile. A woman coming into contact with many friends, a man coming into contact with many women should be simply the rule. But it is possible only if sex is taken as playfulness, as fun. It is not sin, it is fun. And since the introduction of the Pill, of birth control, now there is no fear about having children.

Birth control, in my opinion, is the greatest revolution that has happened in history. All its implications have not yet been made available to man. In the past it was difficult because making love meant more and more children. That was destroying the woman, she was always pregnant; and to remain pregnant and give birth to twelve or twenty children is a torturous experience. Women were used like cattle. But the future can be totally different – and the difference will come not from man.

Just as Marx said about the proletariat, "Proletariat of the world unite, you have nothing to lose ..." and everything to gain.... He had seen society divided into two classes, the rich and the poor. I see society divided into two classes, man and woman.

Man has remained the master for centuries, and woman the slave. She has been auctioned, she has been sold, she has been burnt alive. Everything inhuman that can be done has been done to women – and they constitute half of humanity.

The whole future can be a totally different phenomenon. All the women of the world just need to fight for a separate voting system, so that a woman will vote only for a woman, and a man should vote only for a man. Then in every parliament there will be half women and half men. And men are divided into small parties. Women have to be aware not to create divisions, but to agree on fundamentals – because it is a question of thousands of years of slavery: you cannot afford parties. There should be only one international party of women, and they could take over all the governments of the world.

That seems to be the only way to change the status of women: to allow science full freedom to transform the relationship between man and woman and to drop the idea of marriage, which is absolutely ugly because it is simply a kind of private ownership. Human beings cannot be owned, they are not property. And love should be just a joyful play. And if you want children, then children should belong to the society, so the woman is not labelled as mother, as wife, or as prostitute. These labels should be removed.

You are asking, "I feel so imprisoned by the fear of being intimate and totally losing control." Every woman is afraid, because if she loses control with a man, the man freaks out. He cannot handle it; his sexuality is very small. Because he is a donor, he loses energy while making love. The woman does not lose energy while making love – on the contrary, she feels nourished. Now these are facts which have to be taken into account. Man has for centuries forced the woman to control herself and has kept her at a distance, never allowing her to be too intimate. All his talk about love is bullshit.

You say: "This outrageous woman is locked up inside. When she comes out once in a while, men usually freak out, so she goes back into hibernation, plays safe, and is totally frustrated." This is not only your story; it is the story of all women. They are all living in deep frustration. Finding no way out, knowing nothing about what has been taken away from them, they have only one opening: they will be found in churches, in temples, in synagogues, praying to God. But that God is also a male chauvinist. In the Christian trinity there is no place for a woman. All are men: the Father, the Son, the Holy Ghost. It is a gay men's club.

I am reminded that when God first created the world he created man and woman from the mud, and then breathed life into them. He created them equal. But looking at the world, you can understand – whoever has created it is a little stupid. He created man and woman, and made a small bed for them to sleep in. The bed was so small that only one person could sleep on it. They were equal, but the woman insisted: she would be on the bed – he should sleep on the floor. And the problem was the same with the man – he was not willing to sleep on the floor. You will be surprised to know that the first night in existence was the beginning of pillow fights.

They had to go to God. And the solution was very simple – just make a king-size bed; any carpenter could have done it. But God is a man, and is as prejudiced as any other man: he demolished the woman, destroyed her. And then he created Eve, but now woman was no longer equal to man – she was created from one of Adam's ribs; so she was just to serve man, to take care of man, to be used by man.

Christians don't tell you the whole story. They start their story from Adam and Eve – but Eve is already reduced to a state of slavery. And since that day woman has lived in slavery in thousands of ways. Financially she has not been allowed to be independent. Educationally she has not been allowed to be equal to man – because then she could be financially independent. Religiously she has not been allowed even to read the scriptures or listen to somebody else reading the scriptures.

Woman's wings have been cut in many ways. And the greatest harm that has been done to her is marriage, because neither man nor woman is monogamous; psychologically they are polygamous. So their whole psychology has been forced against its own nature. And because woman was dependent on man she had to suffer all kinds of insults – because man was the master, he was the owner, he had all the money.

To satisfy his polygamous nature, man created prostitutes. Prostitutes are a by-product of marriage. And this ugly institution of prostitution will not disappear from the world unless marriage disappears. It is its shadow – because man does not want to be tied to a monogamous relationship, and he has the freedom of movement, he has the money, he has the education, he has all the power. He invented prostitutes; and to destroy a woman by making her a prostitute is the ugliest murder you can do. The strange fact is, all religions are against prostitution – and they are the cause of it. They are all for marriage, and they cannot see a simple fact – that prostitution came into existence with marriage.

Now the women's liberation movement is trying to imitate all the stupidities that men have done to women. In London, in New York, in San Francisco, you can find male prostitutes. That is a new phenomenon. This is not a revolutionary step, this is a reactionary step.

The problem is that unless you lose control while making love, you will not have an orgasmic experience. So at least my people should be more understanding, that

231

the woman will moan and groan and scream. It is because her whole body is involved – total involvement. You need not be afraid of that. It is tremendously healing: she will not be bitchy towards you, and she will not nag you, because all the energy that becomes bitchiness has been transformed into an immense joy. And don't be afraid about the neighbours – it is their problem if they are worried about your groaning and moaning, it is not your problem. You are not preventing them....

Make your love a really festive affair, don't make it a hit and run affair. Dance, sing, play music – and don't let sex be cerebral. Cerebral sex is not authentic; sex should be spontaneous. Create the situation. Your bedroom should be a place as holy as a temple. In your bedroom don't do anything else; sing and dance and play, and if love happens on its own, as a spontaneous thing, you will be immensely surprised that biology has given you a glimpse of meditation. And don't be worried about the woman who is going crazy. She *has* to go crazy – her whole body is in a totally different space. She cannot remain in control; if she controls it she will remain like a corpse. Millions of people are making love to corpses.

I have heard a story about Cleopatra, the most beautiful woman. When she died, according to the old Egyptian rituals her body was not buried for three days. She was raped in those three days – a dead body. When I first came to know about it, I was surprised – what kind of man would have raped her? But then I felt, perhaps it is not so strange a fact. All men have reduced women to corpses, at least while they are making love.

The most ancient treatise on love and sex is Vatsyayana's *Kamasutras,* aphorisms about sex. It describes eighty-four postures for making love. And when the Christian missionaries came to the East, they were surprised to realize that they knew only one posture: man on top – because then man has more mobility, and the woman is lying like a corpse underneath him.

Vatsyayana's suggestion is very accurate, that the woman should be on top. The man on top is very uncultured; the woman is more fragile. But why men have chosen to be on the top is so that they can keep the woman under control. Crushed under the beast, beauty is bound to be under control. The woman is not even to open her eyes, because that is like a prostitute. She has to behave like a lady. This posture, man on top, is known in the East as the missionary posture.

A great revolution is ahead in the relationship between man and woman. There are institutes evolving around the world, in the advanced countries, where they teach you how to love. It is unfortunate that even animals know how to love, and man has to be taught. And in their teaching, the basic thing is foreplay and afterplay. Then love becomes such a sacred experience.

You should drop the fear of being intimate and totally losing control with a man.

Let the idiot be afraid; if he wants to be afraid, that is his business. You should be authentic and true to yourself. You are lying to yourself, you are deceiving yourself, you are destroying yourself. What is the harm if the man freaks out and runs out of the room naked? Close the door! Let the whole neighbourhood know that this man is mad. But you need not control your possibility of having an orgasmic experience. The orgasmic experience is the experience of merging and melting, egolessness, mindlessness, timelessness. This may trigger your search for finding a way that, without any man, without any partner, you can drop the mind, you can drop time, and you can enter into orgasmic joy on your own. I call this authentic meditation.

So you have to stop going into hibernation, stop playing safe, and all your frustration will disappear. Why should you be worried about the man? Let him ask the question, "What am I supposed to do? This woman goes crazy, jumps on top of me, starts scratching my face…!" But here in my place, among my people, he cannot make much fuss about it. He has to accept it as a natural phenomenon. Otherwise simply meditate – who is telling him to make love to a woman? Women have not discovered meditation. Perhaps it was these freak-outs who discovered meditation to avoid the woman and all the problems, and just sit silently, doing nothing – and the spring comes, and the grass grows by itself. He can do that.

I have heard: a fat American walking down the street saw a sign: "Amazing Slimming Treatment! Twenty-four-hour cure – one thousand dollars. Six-hour cure – five thousand dollars."

Curious, he went inside and asked the receptionist about the twenty-four-hour cure. He was shown inside a large room, and there stood a beautiful naked girl with a sign around her neck, "You catch me, you make love to me; but first you have to catch me."

That was the process of slimming! He was very impressed, and thought, "If this is the one-thousand-dollar cure, the five-thousand-dollar one must be five times as good." So he immediately signed up for the five-thousand-dollar, six-hour cure.

He was undressed and taken into another large room, and the door was locked behind him. Alone in the room with him was an enormous gorilla, with a sign around his neck saying, "I catch you, I make love to you."

Don't be worried, enjoy the whole game – be playful about it. If one man freaks out…there are millions of men: one day you will find some mad guy who does not freak out. And anyway, freaking out and running all around the bed will give him a slimming treatment – and without paying a single dollar![88]

? *At what point did the human mind become perverted?*

The human mind became perverted when it started following priests and politicians against its own nature. Perversion happens the moment you go against your nature. You cannot throw your nature out of the window; it is within you. But if you go against it, its natural expression is closed. And when the natural expression is closed, the unnatural energy starts finding some other way, it has to come out.

For example, celibacy creates millions of people who are perverted. Their perversion is rooted in their idea of celibacy; then homosexuality arises, lesbianism arises, sodomy arises, pornography arises. And now all that perversion has brought a new disease in the world, AIDS, which knows no cure. Still, no man of any importance is saying that it is because of celibacy – because that means irritating and annoying all the religions.

I have never thought that humanity is so poor that there are not even a dozen people who will say the truth – that when the time comes they will not hesitate to risk all their respectability. But I am utterly disappointed in the intelligentsia of the world: nobody is saying that it is celibacy that should be made a crime. On the contrary, governments are making laws saying that homosexuality is a crime. You are making the symptoms a crime, and nobody is even asking why people turn out to be homosexuals.

And who are the people who turn to homosexuality in the first place? – the monks, the soldiers, the prisoners, the boys living separately in university hostels. They become sexually mature at the age of fourteen and they have to wait at least ten more years for their marriage. And the biologists have found that men's sexuality, their sexual energy, is at its peak when they are nearabout eighteen years of age. By the time they get married they are already going down. And when they were at the peak of their energy, you prevented them from meeting girls; and the same is the situation of the girls. You don't allow mixed hostels, otherwise there would be no homosexuality. You don't allow nuns and monks to live in the same monastery, otherwise there would be no need for homosexuality. Destroy the basis and the perversion disappears.

Shepherds living far away in the forest or in the mountains, alone with their sheep, start making love to the sheep. That is sodomy; they can't even find a man, they are so alone there, and their sexual energy wants some way to be relieved.

Perversion has been around man since religions began dominating him. They started giving disciplines to people without any understanding of human nature, without any knowledge of human psychology. They are still doing that, and they are forcing governments to make homosexuality a crime punishable by at least five years in jail. And the strangest thing is, in the jail, homosexuality is the most prevalent thing. So by sending homosexuals into jails, you are giving them new pastures, new possibilities. But nobody will say that celibacy is the cause, because all the religions preach celibacy.

Perhaps I am the only person who is saying that celibacy should be completely banned, and that all monks and all nuns should be made to live together. This unnaturalness should be prevented.

Perversions arise because religions are against nature. And God is the most important cause of all perversions. Those who want perversions to disappear have to declare the death of God, because only with the death of God can those religions disappear and leave man in freedom to live according to his nature.

Elsie the Cow was on one side of the fence, and Ferdinand the Bull was on the other side. Elsie gave Ferdinand a wink, and he leaped over the fence to her side, "Aren't you Ferdinand the Bull?" she asked.

"Just call me Ferdinand," he said. "The fence was higher than I thought."

That's how things become perverted.

Religion has proved to be the greatest man-made calamity, a disaster, a suicidal attempt by man himself. It has created institutions which are all unnatural: celibacy on one hand, marriage on the other hand. And they have praised marriage as highly as possible. Marriages, they say, are made in heaven. But ask the married people – they live in hell. It is strange, marriages happen in heaven, and married people live in hell. But to say anything against marriage annoys even those people who are living in hell, and they will not raise their hands in support.

I have heard about Leo Tolstoy, Chekhov, and Gorky – three great novelists of Russia: before the revolution they were sitting in the garden of Leo Tolstoy just talking about things and, by the way, they started talking about women. Chekov said something, Gorky said something, but Tolstoy remained silent. They both turned to him and said, "Why aren't you saying anything about it?"

He said, "I will, but I will say something only when one of my feet is in the grave. I will say it and jump into the grave, because if I say anything and my wife hears it.... I am already living in hell – why make it even worse? I will just keep quiet."

Hymie Goldberg knocked on the door of the psychiatric hospital. A nurse answered the door, and he asked whether any of their patients had escaped recently.

"Why do you want to know?" asked the nurse.

"Well," said Goldberg, "someone has run off with my wife."[89]

? *What, in your opinion, is the most beneficial way to bring a child into the world?*

The child in the mother's womb has no fear, there is no reason for it. But once he comes out of the mother's womb, a great fear runs through his whole being. He is being taken...as if you take a tree out of the earth, uproot it. The whole tree is shaking and trembling; you are taking out its roots, you are destroying its very base. It know no other nourishment, it knows no other way to exist. The earth has taken care of it, and you are uprooting it....

When the child comes out of the womb, it is the greatest shock of his life. Even death will not be this big a shock, because death will come without warning. Death will come most probably when he is unconscious. But while he is coming out of the mother's womb, he is conscious. In fact, for the first time he is becoming conscious. His nine months' long sleep, peaceful sleep, is disturbed – and then you cut the thread which joins him with the mother.

The moment you cut that thread that joins him with the mother, you have created a fearful individual. This is not the right way; but this is how it has been done up to now. Unknowingly, this has helped the priest and the so-called religions to exploit man.

The child should be taken away from the mother more slowly, more gradually. There should not be that shock – and it can be arranged. A scientific arrangement is possible. There should not be glaring lights in the room, because the child has lived for nine months in absolute darkness, and he has very fragile eyes which have never seen light. And in all your hospitals there are glaring lights, tube lights, and the child suddenly faces the light.... Most people are suffering from weak eyes because of this; later on they have to use glasses. No animal needs them. Have you seen animals with glasses reading the newspaper? Their eyes are perfectly healthy their whole life, to the point of death. It is only man...and the beginning is at the very beginning. No, the child should be given birth to in darkness, or in a very soft light, candles perhaps. Darkness would be the best, but if a little light is needed, then candles will do.

And what have the doctors been doing up to now? They don't even give a little time for the child to be acquainted with the new reality. The way they welcome the child is so ugly. They hang the child by his feet in their hands and they slap his bottom. The idea behind this stupid ritual is that this will help the child to breathe — because in the mother's womb he was not breathing on his own; the mother was breathing for him, eating for him, doing everything for him. But to be welcomed into the world hanging upside down, with a slap on your bottom, is not a very good beginning. But the doctor is in a hurry; otherwise the child would start breathing on his own.

He has to be left on the mother's belly, on top of the mother's belly; before the joining thread is cut, he should be left on the mother's belly. He was inside the belly, beneath — now he is outside. That is not a great change. The mother is there, he can touch her, he can feel her. He knows the vibe. He is perfectly aware that this is his home. He has come out, but this is his home. Let him be with the mother a little longer, so he becomes acquainted with the mother from the outside; from the inside he knows her. And don't cut the thread that joins him till he starts breathing on his own. Right now, what is done? We cut the thread and slap the child so he has to breathe. But this is forcing him, this is violent, and absolutely unscientific and unnatural.

Let him first breathe on his own. It will take a few minutes. Don't be in such a hurry. It is a question of a man's whole life. You can smoke your cigarette two or three minutes longer; you can whisper sweet nothings to your girlfriend a few minutes longer. It is not going to harm anybody. What is the rush? You can't give him three minutes? A child needs no more than that. Just left on his own, within three minutes he starts breathing. When he starts breathing, he becomes confident that he can live on his own. Then you can cut the thread. It is useless now; it will not give a shock to the child.

Then the most significant thing is, don't put him in blankets and in a bed. No, for nine months he was without blankets, naked, without pillows, without bed sheets, without a bed — don't make such a change so quickly. He needs a small tub with the same solution of water that was in his mother's womb — it is exactly ocean water: the same amount of salt, the same amount of chemicals, exactly the same. That is again proof that life must have happened first in the ocean. It still happens in the oceanic water.

That's why when a woman is pregnant she starts eating salty things, because the womb goes on absorbing the salt — the child needs exactly the same salty water that exists in the ocean. So just make up the same water in a small tub, and let the child lie down in the tub, and he will feel perfectly welcomed. This is the situation he is acquainted with.

In Japan, one Zen monk has tried a tremendous experiment showing that a three-month-old child can swim. Slowly he has been coming down. First he tried with nine-month-old children, then with six-month-old children, now with three-month-old children. And I say to him that you are still far away. Even the child just born is capable of swimming, because he has been swimming in his mother's womb.

So give the child a chance, similar to the mother's womb. He will be more confident; and no priest can exploit him so easily, telling him about hellfire, and all that nonsense.[90]

CHAPTER 14

AGEING

In Western society, at least, youth is considered to be everything — and to a certain extent it seems this is as it should be if we are to continue growing in every dimension of life. But the natural corollary of that is that as one moves away from youth, birthdays are no longer a cause for congratulations, but are an embarrassing and unavoidable fact of life. It becomes impolite to ask someone their age; grey hair is dyed, teeth capped or replaced entirely, demoralized breasts and faces have to be lifted, tummies made taut, and varicose veins supported — but under cover. You certainly don't take it as a compliment if someone tells you that you look your age. But my experience is that as I am becoming older, each year is only better and better; yet nobody told me this would be so, and one never hears people singing the praises of growing older. Would you speak of the joys of growing older?

The question you have asked implies many things. First, the Western mind is conditioned by the idea that you have only one life — seventy years — and youth will never come again. In the West, the spring comes only once; naturally, there is a deep desire to cling as long as possible, to pretend in every possible way that you are still young.

In the East the older person was always valued, respected. He was more experienced, he had seen many, many seasons coming and going; he had lived through all kinds of experiences, good and bad. He had become seasoned; he was no longer immature. He had a certain integrity that comes only with age. He was not childish, carrying his teddy bears; he was not young, still fooling around thinking that this was love.

He had passed through all these experiences, had seen that beauty fades; he had seen that everything comes to an end, that everything is moving towards the grave. From the very moment he left the cradle, there was only one way – and it was from cradle to the grave. You cannot go anywhere else; you cannot go astray even if you try. You will reach to the grave whatever you do.

The old man was respected, loved; he had attained a certain purity of the heart because he had lived through desires, and seen that every desire leads to frustration. Those desires are past memories. He had lived in all kinds of relationships, and had seen that every kind of relationship turns into hell. He had passed through all the dark nights of the soul. He had attained a certain aloofness – the purity of an observer. He was no longer interested in participating in any football game. Just living his life, he had come to a transcendence; hence, he was respected, his wisdom was respected.

But in the East, the idea has been that life is not just a small piece of seventy years in which youth comes only once. The idea has been that, just as in existence everything moves eternally – the summer comes, the rains come, the winter comes, and the summer again; everything moves like a wheel – life is not an exception. Death is the end of one wheel and the beginning of another. Again you will be a child, and again you will be young, and again you will be old. It has been so since the beginning, and it is going to be so to the very end – until you become so enlightened that you can jump out of the vicious circle and can enter into a totally different law. From individuality, you can jump into the universal. So there was no hurry, and there was no clinging.

The West is based on the Judaic tradition which believes in only one life. Christianity is only a branch of the Judaism. Jesus was a Jew, born a Jew, lived a Jew, died a Jew; he never knew that he was a Christian. If you meet him somewhere and greet him with, "Hello, Jesus Christ," he will not recognize who you are addressing because he never knew that his name is Jesus and he never knew that he is Christ. His name was Joshua, a Hebrew name, and he was a messiah of God, not a Christ. Jesus Christ is a translation in Greek from Hebrew. Mohammedanism is also a by-product of the same tradition – the Jewish. These three religions believe in one life. To believe in one life is very dangerous because it does not give you chances to make mistakes, it does not give you chances to have enough experience of anything; you are always in a hurry.

The whole Western mind has become the mind of a tourist who is carrying two, three cameras, and rushing to photograph everything because he only has a three-week visa. And in three weeks, he has to cover the whole country – all the great monuments. There is no time for him to see them directly; he will see them at home, at ease, in his album. Whenever I remember the tourists, I see the old women rushing from one place to another – from Ajanta to Ellora, from Taj Mahal to Kashmir – in a hurry, because life is short.

It is only the Western mind which has created the proverb that time is money. In the East things go slowly; there is no hurry – one has the whole of eternity. We have been here and we will be here again, so what is the hurry? Enjoy everything with intensity and totality.

So, one thing: because of the idea of one single life, the West has become too concerned about being young, and then everything is done to remain young as long as possible, to prolong the process. That creates hypocrisy, and that destroys an authentic growth. It does not allow you to become really wise in your old age, because you *hate* old age; old age reminds you only of death, nothing else. Old age means the full stop is not far away; you have come to the terminus – just one whistle more, and the train will stop.

I had an agreement with my grandfather. He loved his feet to be massaged, and I had told him, "Remember, when I say 'comma,' that means be alert; the semicolon is coming close. When I say 'semicolon,' get ready, because the full stop is coming close. And once I say 'full stop,' I mean it." So he was so much afraid of "comma," that when I would say, "Comma," he would say, "It is okay, but let the semi colon be a little longer. Don't make it short and quick!"

Old age simply reminds you, in the West, that a full stop is coming close – prolong the semicolon-colon. And who are you trying to deceive? If you have recognized that youth is no longer there, you can go on deceiving the whole world but you are not young, you are simply being ridiculous.... People are trying to remain young, but they don't know that the very fear of losing youth does not allow you to live it in its totality.

And secondly, the fear of losing youth does not allow you to accept old age with grace. You miss both youth – its joy, its intensity – and you also miss the grace, and the wisdom, and the peace that old age brings. But the whole thing is based on a false conception of life. Unless the West changes the idea that there is only one life, this hypocrisy, this clinging, and this fear cannot be changed.

In fact, one life is not all; you have lived many times, and you will live many times more. Hence, live each moment as totally as possible; there is no hurry to jump to another moment. Time is not money, time is inexhaustible; it is available to the poor as much as to the rich. The rich are not richer as far as time is concerned, and the poor are not poorer. Life is an eternal incarnation.

What appears on the surface is very deep-rooted in the religions of the West. They are very miserly in giving you only seventy years. If you try to work it out, almost one-third of your life will be lost in sleep, one-third of your life will have to be wasted in earning food, clothes, housing. Whatever little is left has to be given to education, football matches, movies, stupid quarrels, fights. If you can save, in seventy years' time, seven minutes for yourself, I will count you a wise man. But it is difficult to save even seven minutes in your whole life; so how can you find yourself? How can you know the mystery of your being, of your life? How can you understand that death is not an end? Because you have missed experiencing life itself, you are going to miss the great experience of death, too; otherwise, there is nothing to be afraid of in death. It is a beautiful sleep, a dreamless sleep, a sleep that is needed for you to move into another body, silently and peacefully. It is a surgical phenomenon; it is almost like anaesthesia. Death is a friend, not a foe.

Once you understand death as a friend, and start living life without any fear that it is only a very small timespan of seventy years – if your perspective opens to the eternity of your life – then everything will slow down; then there is no need to be speedy. In everything, people are simply rushing. I have seen people taking their office bag, pushing things into it, kissing their wife, not seeing whether she is their wife or somebody else, and saying good-bye to their children. This is not the way of living! And where are you reaching with this speed?

I have heard about a young couple who had purchased a new car, and they were going full speed. The wife was asking the husband again and again, "Where are we going?" – because women are still old-minded: "Where are we going?"

The man said, "Stop bothering me, just enjoy the speed we are going at. The real question is not where we are going; the real question is at what great speed are we going?"

Speed has become more important than the destination, and speed has become more important because life is so short. You have to do so many things, that unless you do everything with speed, you cannot manage. You cannot sit silently even for a few minutes – it seems a wastage. In those few minutes you could have earned a few bucks.

Just wasting time closing your eyes, and what is there inside you? If you really want to know, you can go to any hospital and see a skeleton. That is what is inside you. Why are you unnecessarily getting into trouble by looking in? Looking in, you will find a skeleton. And once you have seen your skeleton, life will become more difficult; kissing your wife, you know perfectly well what is happening – two skeletons. Somebody just needs to invent X-ray glasses, so people can put on X-ray glasses and see all around skeletons laughing. Most probably, he will not be alive to take his glasses off; so many skeletons laughing is enough to stop anybody's heartbeat. "My God, this is the reality! And this is what all these mystics have been telling people, 'Look inwards' – avoid them!"

The West has no tradition of mysticism. It is extrovert: Look outward, there is so much to see. But they are not aware that inside there is not only the skeleton, there is something more within the skeleton. That is your consciousness. By closing your eyes you will not come across the skeleton, you will come across your very life source. The West needs a deep acquaintance with its own life source, then there will be no hurry. One will enjoy when life brings youth, one will enjoy when life brings old age and one will enjoy when life brings death. You simply know one thing – how to enjoy everything that you come across, how to transform it into a celebration. I call the authentic religion the art of transforming everything into a celebration, into a song, into a dance.

An old man walked into a health clinic and told the doctor, "You have got to do something to lower my sex drive."

The doctor took one look at the feeble old man and said, "Now, now sir, I have got the feeling that your sex drive is all in your head."

"That's what I mean, sonny," the old man said. "I have got to lower it a little."

Even the old man is wanting to be a playboy. It shows one thing with certainty – that he has not lived his youth with totality. He has missed his youth, and he is still thinking about it. Now he cannot do anything about it, but his whole mind is continuously thinking about the days he had in youth which have not been lived; at that time he was in a hurry.

If he had lived his youth he would be free in his old age of all repressions, sexuality; there would be no need for him to drop his sexual instinct. It disappears, it evaporates in living. One just has to live uninhibited, without any interference from your religions, from your priests, and it disappears; otherwise, when you are young you are in church, and when you are old, you are reading the *Playboy* by hiding it in your *Holy Bible*. Every *Holy Bible* is used only for one purpose, hiding magazines like *Playboy*, so you are not caught by children – it is embarrassing.

I have heard of three men, old men. One was seventy, the other was eighty and the third was ninety. They were all old friends, retired, who used to go for a walk and sit on a bench in the park, and have all kinds of gossips. One day the youngest of the three, the seventy-year-old man, looked a little sad. The second one, the eighty-year-old, asked, "What is the matter? You are looking very sad."

He said, "I am feeling very guilty. It will help me to unburden myself if I tell you. It is an incident: A beautiful lady was taking a bath – she was a guest in our house – and I was looking through the keyhole and my mother caught hold of me."

Both the old friends laughed; they said, "You are an idiot. Everybody does such things in childhood."

He said, "It is not a question of childhood, it happened today."

The second man said, "Then it is really serious. But I will tell you something which has been happening to me for three days, and I am keeping it like a stone, a rock on my heart. Continuously for three days my wife has refused to love me."

The first man said, "That is really very bad."

But the third, the oldest laughed and he said, "First you ask him what he means by love."

So he asked, and the second old man said, "Nothing much. Don't make me feel more embarrassed. It is a simple process. I hold my wife's hand and press it three times, then she goes to sleep and I go to sleep. But for three days, whenever I try to hold her hand, she says, 'Not today, not today! Feel ashamed; you are old enough – not today!' So for three days I have not loved."

The third old man said, "This is nothing. What has been happening to me I must confess, because you are young and it will help you in your future. Last night, as the night was passing and the morning was coming closer, I started to make preparations to make love to my wife and she said to me, 'What are you trying to do, you idiot?' I said, 'What am I trying to do? I am simply trying to make love to you,' and she said, 'This is the third time in the night; neither you sleep nor you allow me to sleep. Love, love, love!' So I think it seems I am losing my memory. Your problems are nothing; I have lost my memory."

If you listen to old people, you will be surprised; they are talking only of things which they should have lived, but the time has passed when it was possible to live them. At that time they were reading the *Holy Bible* and listening to the priest. Those priests and those holy scriptures have corrupted people, because they have given them ideas against nature and they cannot allow them to live naturally. If we need a new humanity, we will have to erase the whole past and start everything anew. And the first basic principle will be: allow everybody, help everybody, teach everybody to live according to his nature, not according to any ideals, and live totally and intensely without any fear. Then children will enjoy their childhood, the young people will enjoy their youth and the old people will have the grace that comes naturally, out of a whole life lived naturally.

Unless your old age is graceful and wise and full of light and joy, contentment, fulfillment, a blissfulness...in your very presence, unless flowers blossom and there is a fragrance of eternity, then it is certain that you have not lived. If it is not happening that way, that means somewhere you have gone astray, somewhere you have listened to the priests, who are the corrupters, the criminals, somewhere you have gone against nature – and nature takes revenge. And its revenge is to destroy your old age and make it ugly, ugly to others and ugly in your own eyes; otherwise old age has a beauty which even youth cannot have.

Youth has a maturity, but it is unwise. It has too much foolishness in it; it is amateurish. Old age has given the last touches to the paintings of one's own life. And when one has given the last touches, one is ready to die joyously, dancingly. One is ready to welcome death.[91]

CHAPTER 15

DEATH, EUTHANASIA, SUICIDE

? *What is a natural death?*

It is a significant question, but there are many possible implications in it. The simplest and the most obvious is that a man dies without any cause; he simply becomes old, older, and the change from old age to death is not through any disease. Death is simply the ultimate old age – everything in your body, in your brain, has stopped functioning. This will be the ordinary and obvious meaning of a natural death.

But to me natural death has a far deeper meaning: one has to live a natural life to attain a natural death. Natural death is the culmination of a life lived naturally, without any inhibition, without any repression – just the way the animals live, the birds live, the trees live, without any split...a life of let-go, allowing nature to flow through you without any obstructions from your side, as if you are absent and life is moving on its own. Rather than you living life, life lives you, you are secondary; then the culmination will be a natural death. According to my definition only an awakened man can die a natural death; otherwise all deaths are unnatural because all lives are unnatural.

How can you arrive at a natural death, living an unnatural life? Death will reflect the ultimate culmination, the crescendo of your whole life. In a condensed form, it is all that you have lived. So only very few people in the world have died naturally because only very few people have lived naturally. Our conditionings don't allow us to be natural. Our conditionings, from the very beginning, teach us that we have to be something more than nature, that just to be natural is to be animal; we have to be supernatural. And it seems very logical. All the religions have been teaching this – that to be man means going above nature – and they have convinced centuries of humanity to go above nature. Nobody has succeeded in going above nature. All that they have succeeded in is destroying their natural, spontaneous beauty, their innocence. Man need not transcend nature. I say unto you, man has to fulfill nature – which no animal can do. That is the difference.

The religions were cunning, cheating and deceiving people. They made the distinction that animals are natural and you have to be supernatural. No animal can do fasting; you cannot convince any animal that fasting is something divine. The animal only knows that it is hungry, and there is no difference between fasting and being hungry. You cannot convince any animal to go against nature.

This gave an opportunity to the so-called religious people, because man has the capacity at least to fight against nature. He will never be victorious, but he can fight. And in fighting he will not be destroying nature; he will be destroying only himself. That's how man has destroyed himself – all his joy, all his love, all his grandeur – and has become not something higher than animals, but something lower, in every possible way. Perhaps you have never thought about it: no animal in the wild is homosexual. The very idea, and the whole world of animals will burst into laughter. It is simply stupid! But in a zoo, where females are not available, animals turn into homosexuals out of sheer necessity.

But man has turned the whole world into a zoo: millions and millions of people are homosexuals, lesbians, sodomists, and what-not – all kinds of perversions. And who is responsible? The people who were teaching you to go beyond nature, to attain supernatural divineness....

Whenever you enforce something, the result is not going to bring a betterment. In many spheres, by different religions, it has been tried to make man something above nature. The result has been, without any exception, failure. You are born as a natural being. You cannot go above yourself. It is just like trying to lift yourself off the ground by pulling your legs. You may hop a little, but sooner or later you are going to fall to the ground, and you may have a few fractures. You cannot fly.

And that's what has been done. People have been trying to raise themselves above nature, which means above themselves. They are not separate from nature, but the idea suited their egos: you are not animals so you have to be above nature; you cannot behave like animals. People have even tried to make animals not behave like animals; they have tried to make them go a little above nature.

In the Victorian age in England dogs were clothed when people used to take them for a walk. The dogs had coats to prevent them being natural, to prevent them being naked and nude – which is suitable to animals. These kind of people are trying to raise their dogs a little higher than animals.

You will be surprised to know that in the Victorian age in England, even the legs of chairs were covered – for the simple reason that they were called legs, and legs should be covered. Bertrand Russell, who lived almost one century – a long life – remembers in his childhood that seeing the feet of a woman was enough to get sexually excited. The dresses were made in such a way that they covered the feet; you could not see the feet.

It was believed, even just one hundred years ago, that the women of the royal family don't have two legs. Royalty has to be somehow different than ordinary, common humanity, and nobody had seen – and there was no possibility to see – whether their legs were separate from each other. But the ego...neither did those royal people make it clear: "This is nonsense, we are as human as you are." The ego prevented them. If the people are putting them on a higher pedestal, then why bother? – just remain royal. That was one of the reasons why royal families would not allow anybody, a commoner, to be married into the royal family, because he may expose the whole thing: "These people are just as human as everybody else; there is nothing royal about them." But for centuries they maintained the idea.

I would also like you to be different from the animals, but not in the sense that you can go above nature – no. You can go deeper into nature, you can be more natural than animals. They are not free, they are in a deep coma; they cannot do anything other than what their ancestors have been doing for millennia.

You can be more natural than any animal. You can go to the abysmal depths of nature, and you can go to the very heights of nature, but you will not be going beyond in any way. You will be becoming more natural, you will be becoming more multi-dimensionally natural. To me the religious man is not one who is above nature, but is the man who is totally natural, fully natural, who has explored nature in all its dimensions, who has not left anything unexplored.

Animals are prisoners; they have a certain limited area of being. Man has the capacity, the intelligence, the freedom to explore. And if you have explored nature totally, you have come home – nature is your home. And then death is a joy, is a celebration. Then you die without any complaint; you die with deep gratitude, because life gave you so much, and death is simply the ultimate height of all that you have lived.

It is just like before the flame of a candle goes out it burns brightest. The natural man, before he dies, lives brightest for a moment; he is all light, all truth. To me this is natural death. But it has to be earned, it is not given to you. The opportunity is given to you, but you have to explore, you have to earn, you have to deserve.

Even to see the death of an authentic man, just to be near him while he is dying, you will be filled suddenly with a strange joy. Your tears will not be of sadness, sorrow; they will be of gratitude and blissfulness — because when a man dies naturally, living his life fully, he spreads his being into the whole of nature. Those who are present and close to him are bathed…a sudden freshness, a breeze, a new fragrance and a new feeling that death is not something bad, that death is not something to be afraid of, that death is something to be earned, to be deserved.

I teach you the art of life. But it can be called also the art of death. They are both the same.[92]

? *I am trained as a physician, and I have always felt deeply that it is a good thing. But intrinsic in my work, in my activity, is a refusal to accept illness and death, disease and human suffering. Could you please say something about this?*

Now, a distinction has to be made. Illness, disease and suffering are one thing, death is totally different. In the Western mind, illness, disease, suffering and death are all together — packed in one package. From there problems arise.

Death is beautiful; illness is not, suffering is not, disease is not. Death is beautiful. Death is not a sword that cuts your life, it is like a flower — an ultimate flower — that blooms at the last moment. It is the peak. Death is the flower on the tree of life. It is not the end of life but the crescendo. It is the ultimate orgasm. There is nothing wrong in death; it is beautiful — but one needs to know how to live and how to die. There is an art of living and there is an art of dying, and the second art is of more value than the first art. But the second can be known only when you have known the first. Only those who know how to live rightly know how to die rightly. And then death is a door to the divine.

So, the first thing: please keep death apart. Only think of illness, disease and suffering. You need not fight against death. That is creating trouble in the Western mind, in the Western hospitals, in Western medicine. People are fighting against death. People are almost vegetating in the hospitals, just alive on drugs. They are forced to live unnecessarily when they would have died naturally. Through medical support their death is being postponed. They are of no use, life is of no use to them; the game is over, they are finished. Now to keep them alive is just to make them suffer more. Sometimes they may be in a coma, and a person can be in a coma for months and years. But because there is an antagonism towards death it has become a great problem in the Western mind: what to do when a person is in a coma and will never recover, but can be kept alive for years? He will be a corpse, just a breathing corpse, that's all. He will simply vegetate, there will be no life. What is the point? Why not allow him to die? There is the fear of death. Death is the enemy – how to surrender to the enemy, to death?

So there is great controversy in the Western medical mind. What to do? Should a person be allowed to die? Should a person be allowed to decide whether he wants to die? Should the family be allowed to decide whether they would like him to die? – because sometimes the person may be unconscious and cannot decide. But is it right to help somebody to die? Great fear arises in the Western mind. To die? That means you are murdering the person! The whole of science exists to keep him alive. Now this is stupid! Life in itself has no value unless there is joy, unless there is dance, unless there is some creativity, unless there is love – life in itself is meaningless. Just to live is meaningless. A point comes when one has lived, a point comes when it is natural to die, when it is beautiful to die. Just as when you have been doing work the whole day, a point comes when you fall asleep; death is a kind of sleep – a deeper sleep. You will be born again in a newer body with a newer mechanism, with new facilities, with new opportunities, new challenges. This body is old and one has to leave it; it is just a dwelling....

In the East we have a different outlook: death is not the enemy but the friend. Death gives you rest. You have become tired, you have lived your life, you have known all the joys that can be known in life, you have burned your candle totally. Now go into darkness, rest for a while and then you can be born again. Death will revive you again in a fresher way.

So the first thing: Death is not the enemy.

The second thing: Death is the greatest experience in life if you can die consciously. And you can die consciously only if you are not afraid of it. If you are against it you become very panicky, very afraid. When you are so afraid that you cannot tolerate that fear, there is a natural mechanism in the body which releases drugs into the body and you become unconscious. There is a point beyond which endurance will not be possible; you become unconscious. So millions of people die unconsciously and miss a great moment, the greatest of all. It is *samadhi*, it is *satori*, it is meditation happening to you. It is a natural gift.

If you can be alert and you can see that you are not the body... You will have to see, because the body will disappear. Soon you will be able to see that you are not the body, you are separate. Then you will see you are separating from the mind too; then the mind will disappear. And then you will be just a flame of awareness, and that is the greatest benediction there is. So don't think of death as illness, disease and human suffering.[93]

?

A few months ago my friend and I were visiting his dying father. Lots of people were around. His body was about finished. To most people he was indifferent, but when everyone left he suddenly opened his eyes and told us, "I feel like I have two bodies; one body is sick and the other is completely healthy." We told him, "That's right! The healthy body is the real you, so stay with that one." He said, "Okay," and closed his eyes, and as we sat with him, the sick energy around the hospital bed changed. We couldn't believe this new energy; it was as if we were sitting in your presence...such beautiful silence. After we left he improved for a while, went home and died peacefully in his bed. Even though I've been with you for ten years, I felt so ignorant in front of this man who was so ready to let go of everything with such trust and clarity and peace.

The experience that you went through is always possible when someone is dying. All that is required is a little alertness. The man who was dying was aware – not much awareness is needed for this experience.

At the moment of death your physical body and your spiritual body start separating. Ordinarily, they are so much involved with each other that you don't feel their separation. But at the moment of death, just before death happens, both the bodies start getting unidentified with each other. Now their ways are going to be different; the physical body is going to the physical elements, and the spiritual body is on its pilgrimage onwards to a new birth, in a new form, in a new womb.

If the person is a little alert he can see it himself, and because you said to him that the healthier body is you, and the body that is sick and dying is not you.... In those moments, to trust is very easy because it is happening just before the eyes of the person himself; he cannot identify with the body that is falling apart, and he can immediately recognize the fact that he is the healthier one, the deeper one.

But you could have helped the man even a little more – this was good, but not good enough. Even this experience of the man, of getting unidentified with the physical body, immediately changed the energy in the room; it became silent, peaceful. But if you had learned the art of how to help a dying man, you would not have stopped where you stopped. A second thing was absolutely necessary to tell him because he was in a trusting state – everybody is, at the moment of death.

It is life which creates problems and doubts and postponements, but death has no time to postpone. The man cannot say, "I will try to see," or, "I will see tomorrow." He has to do it right now, this very moment, because even the next moment is not certain. Most probably he is not going to survive. And what is he going to lose by trusting? Death, anyway, is going to take away everything. So the fear of trust is not there; time to think about it is not there. And a clarity is there that the physical body is getting farther and farther away.

It was a good step to tell him, "You are the healthier body." The second step would have been to tell him, "You are the witness of both the bodies; the body that is dying is physical, and the body that you are feeling is healthy is psychological. But who are *you?* You can see both the bodies...certainly you must be the third; you cannot be one of these two." This is the whole process of the *Bardo.* Only in Tibet have they developed the art of dying. While the whole world has been trying to develop the art of living, Tibet is the only country in the world which has developed the whole science and art of dying. They call it the *Bardo.*

If you had told the person, "This is good that you have taken one step, you are out of the physical body; but now you have got identified with the psychological body. You are not even that, you are only awareness, a pure consciousness, a perceptivity...." If you could have helped the person to understand that he is neither this body nor that body, but something bodiless, formless, a pure consciousness, then his death would have been a totally different phenomenon.

You saw the change of energy; you would have seen another change of energy. You saw silence descending; you would have seen music also, a certain dancing energy also, a certain fragrance filling the whole space. And the man's face would have shown a new phenomenon – the aura of light. If he had taken the second step also, then his death would have been the last death. In the *Bardo* they call it "the great death," because now he will not be born into another form, into another imprisonment; now he will remain in the eternal, in the oceanic consciousness that fills the whole universe.

So remember it – it may happen to many of you. You may be with a friend or with a relative, your mother, your father. While they are dying, help them to realize two things: first, they are not the physical body – which is very simple for a dying man to recognize. Second – which is a little difficult, but if the man is able to recognize the first, there is a possibility of the second recognition too – that he is not even the second body; he is beyond both the bodies. He is pure freedom and pure consciousness.

If he had taken the second step then you would have seen a miracle happening around him – something, not just silence, but something more alive, something belonging to eternity, to immortality. And all of you who were present there would have been overwhelmed with gratitude that this death has not been a time of mourning but it has become a moment of celebration.

If you can transform a death into a moment of celebration, you have helped your friend, your mother, your father, your brother, your wife, your husband. You have given them the greatest gift that is possible in existence. And close to death it is very easy. The child is not even worried about life or death; he has no concern. The young man is too much involved in biological games, in ambitions, in becoming richer, in becoming powerful, in having more prestige; he has no time to think of eternal questions. But at the moment of death, just before death is going to happen, you don't have any ambition. And whether you are rich or poor makes no difference; whether you are a criminal or a saint makes no difference. Death takes you beyond all discriminations of life and beyond all stupid games of life.

But rather than helping people, people destroy that beautiful moment. It is the most precious in a man's whole life. Even if he has lived one hundred years, this is the most precious moment. But people start crying and weeping and showing their sympathy, saying, "This is very untimely, it should not happen." Or they start consoling the person, saying, "Don't be worried, the doctors are saying that you will be saved."

These are all foolishnesses. Even the doctors play a part in these stupid things. They don't tell you that your death is coming. They avoid the subject; they go on giving you hope. They say, "Don't be worried, you will be saved," knowing perfectly well that the man is going to die. They are giving him a false consolation, not knowing that this is the moment when he should be made fully aware of death – so acutely and so impeccably aware that pure consciousness is experienced. That moment has become a moment of great victory. Now there is no death for him, but only eternal life.[94]

?

The main issue in the coming parliamentary election in Holland is euthanasia. Politicians are fighting about the right formula for legislation of the issue. Please comment.

Euthanasia, or the freedom to choose your death, should be accepted as a birthright of every human being. A limit can be put to it, for example, seventy-five years. After the age of seventy-five the hospitals should be ready to help anybody who wants to get rid of their body. Every hospital should have a place for dying people, and those who have chosen to die should be given special consideration and help. Their death should be beautiful.

Every hospital should have a teacher of meditation.

The person who is going to die should be given one month and will be allowed... if he changes his mind he can go back, because nobody is forcing him. Emotional people who want to commit suicide cannot remain emotional for one month — emotionality can be momentary. Most of the people who commit suicide, if they had waited one moment longer, they would not have committed suicide at all. It is out of anger, out of jealousy, out of hatred or something that they forget the value of life.

The whole problem is that the politicians think accepting euthanasia means suicide is no longer a crime. No, it does not mean that. Suicide is still a crime.

Euthanasia will be with the permission of the medical board. One month's rest in the hospital – every kind of help that can be given to the person to become calm and quiet...all friends coming to meet him, his wife, his children, because he is going on a long journey. There is no question of preventing him – he has lived long, and he does not want to go on living, his work is finished.

And he should be taught meditation in this one month, so that he can do meditation while death comes. And for death, medical help should be given so it comes like a sleep – slowly, slowly, side by side with meditation, sleep going deeper. We can change thousands of people's deaths into enlightenment. And there is no fear of suicide, because he is not going to commit suicide; if somebody tries to commit suicide he will still be committing a crime. He is asking permission. With the permission of the medical board...and he has one month's time in which he can change his mind at any moment. On the last day he can say, "I don't want to die" – then he can go home. There is no problem in it: it is his decision.

Right now there is a very strange situation in many countries. People try to commit suicide: if they succeed, good; if they don't succeed, then the court gives them the death sentence. Strange! – they themselves were doing that. They were caught in the middle. Now for two years a trial will go on; judges and advocates will be arguing, and this and that, and finally the man has to be hanged, again. He was doing that in the very first place, by himself! Why all this nonsense?

Euthanasia is becoming more and more a need, because with medical science progressing people are living longer. Scientists have not come across any skeleton from five thousand years ago of a person who was more than forty years old when he died. Five thousand years ago the longest a person was going to live was forty, and out of ten children born nine were going to die within two years – only one would survive – so life was immensely valuable.

Hippocrates gave the oath to the medical profession that you have to help life in every case. He was not aware – he was not a seer – he had not the insight to see that a day could come when out of ten children, all ten would survive. Now that is happening. On the one hand, nine more children are surviving; and on the other hand, medical science helps people to live longer – ninety years, one hundred years is not rare. In developed countries it is very easy to find a ninety-year-old person or a one-hundred-year-old person.

In the Soviet Union there are people who have reached one hundred and fifty years, and there are a few thousand people who have reached one hundred and eighty years of age – and they are still working. But now life has become boring. One hundred and eighty years, just think of it, doing the same thing – even the bones will be hurting – and yet they still have no possibility of death. Death still seems to be far away – they are still working and healthy.

In America there are thousands of people in the hospitals just lying in their beds with all kinds of instruments connected to them. Many are on artificial breathing machines. What is the point if the person himself cannot breathe? What do you expect him to do? And why are you burdening the whole nation with this person when there are many people dying on the streets, starving?

Thirty million people in America are on the streets without shelter, without food, without clothes, and thousands of people are taking up hospital beds, doctors, nurses – their work, their labour, medicines. Everybody knows they will die sooner or later, but as long as you can you should keep them alive. They *want* to die. They shout that they want to die, but the doctor cannot help in that. These people certainly need some rights; they are being forced to live, and force is in every way undemocratic.

So I want it to be a very rational thing. Make it seventy-five years or eighty years; then life is lived enough. The children are grown up…when you are eighty your children will be fifty, fifty-five; *they* are getting old. Now there is no need for you to be bothered and worried. You are retired; now you are simply a burden, you don't know what to do.

And that is why old people are so irritable – because they don't have any work, they don't have any respect, they don't have any dignity. Nobody bothers about them, nobody takes note of them. They are ready to fight and be angry and shout. These are simply their frustrations that are showing; the real thing is they want to die. But they cannot even say it. It is unchristian, it is irreligious – the very idea of death.

They should be given freedom, but not only to die; they should be given the freedom of one month's training in how to die. In that training meditation should be a basic part; physical care should be a basic part. They should die healthy, whole, silent, peaceful – slowly slipping deep into sleep. And if meditation has been joined with sleep they may die enlightened. They may know that only the body is left behind, and they are part of eternity.

Their death will be better than the ordinary death, because in the ordinary death you don't have the chance of becoming enlightened. In fact more and more people will prefer to die in the hospitals, in the special institutes for death where every arrangement is made. You can leave life in a joyous, ecstatic way, with great thankfulness and gratitude.

I am all for euthanasia but with these conditions.[95]

?

A friend of mine committed suicide some time ago, and I feel so much emotion about it. He was a sannyasin, and I feel you didn't protect him.

A few things have to be understood. First you don't accept death; that is where the problem is. You are clinging too much to life.

And do you think that I have to protect people from dying? I have to help them to live totally, to die totally – that's my work. To me, death is as beautiful as life. You have a certain idea that I have to protect people from their death. Then I will be against them. Death is beautiful, nothing is wrong with it. In fact sometimes life may be wrong, but death is never wrong because death is a relaxation, death is a surrender.

You are creating the problem out of your fear; it has nothing to do with your friend. His death has disturbed you: it has brought the fact into your consciousness that you will also have to die, and that you cannot accept. Now you want some consolation from me. I am not going to give any consolation to anybody. I give only truth, and death is as true as life. But people live with this idea that death is something inimical, it has to be avoided; as long as it is avoided, it is good. One has to live anyhow, one has to go on dragging. Even if life has no meaning, one has to go on living. One may be suffering, one may be paralyzed, one may be mad. One may not be of any use to anybody, one may be burden to oneself and each moment may be of ugly suffering, but still one has to live on as if life has some intrinsic value. This is the idea people carry in their mind: death is a taboo. But to me it is not. To me both life and death are beautiful; they are two aspects of the same energy.

So I have to help you to live and I have to help you to die: that is my way of protecting you. Let it be completely clear, otherwise you will always be confused. Somebody is ill, a sannyasin falls ill and then he starts wondering whether he can trust me because he has fallen ill. I am not here to protect you from illness. I am here to help you to understand illness, to go through it silently, witnessing it, seeing it, undisturbed. Illness is part of life. Now, if somebody thinks that I have to protect him against illness then he will never be able to understand me; he is here for the wrong reasons. If he is dying, I will help him to die.

Death can be a great glory, it can be a great peak. Death always disturbs people because they reject it. You have a rejection, you are against death. You don't want to die, you would like to remain forever and ever; but that is not possible. This is the first thing.

The second thing is: because it was not even a natural death, it was a suicide, you have the idea that I should protect sannyasins. I should prevent suicide, no sannyasin should commit a suicide. Why? It is part of your freedom. If a sannyasin decides that

256

the game is over and he wants to go home, then who am I to prevent him? I will simply say, "Go happily and dancingly. Don't go sadly; make it a happy journey back home."

But that sannyasin never asked me. Even if he had, I would have told him. "This is your freedom, I don't interfere in your freedom. It is your life, it is your death; who am I to interfere? All that I can do is make available to you the skill that makes everything beautiful." And a suicide can also be beautiful.

You will be surprised that in India there exists a religion, Jainism, that allows suicide; allows it as a religious act! It allows its sannyasins to commit suicide if they decide to do it. I think that is one of the greatest acceptances of freedom; no other religion has dared that much. Sooner or later every nation in the world will have to accept suicide as a fundamental right, because if a person wants to die, then who are you — your courts, your police and your law — to prevent him? Who are you? Who has given you the right? Why should he be made to feel guilty? Why should he be made to feel a criminal? Why can't he invite his friends and die dancing and singing? Why should he commit it like a crime?

Suicide is not a crime; your law makes it a crime. In a better world where freedom is respected more, if a person wants to die, he will invite his friends along. For a few days he will live with his friends, he will dance and sing and listen to good music, read poetry and go visiting neighbours to say good-bye. One day all will gather together and he will simply die. And they will have given him a good send-off! In a better world suicide will not be a crime.

You just have to change your attitude. And you have to be very clear about me: I am not an ordinary teacher who consoles people. My commitment is towards truth, not towards consolation. Howsoever uncomfortable the truth is, my commitment is towards truth. This to me is a sacred phenomenon, freedom.

If he decides to commit suicide, that's perfectly okay; you should be able to give that freedom to him. You are resisting it; he has already committed suicide and you are not giving him permission to go through with it. That is your problem, that is not his problem. He has not created the problem, he has simply provoked a problem which has always been in you. Now let him go, say good-bye, relax and understand it.

This moment of sadness can become one of great understanding, because something has been touched deep down in your heart. Now don't waste time! Meditate over it, look at it from every corner, from every angle. Don't just be angry, don't just be sad; let it become a great moment of meditation too. Yes, sadness is there, anger is there, as if he had cheated you. He was your friend and he didn't even say anything to you. How dare he? He deceived you! That's why you are feeling great anger deep down. And you are angry at me too; how could I allow it? He never asked me, but if he had, I would have allowed him. But he never asked me. In fact there is no need to ask; if he wants to go, he wants to go.

All is good. Yes, even suicide is good. It takes guts to accept that. The first taboo in the world was sex, and sex is by and by being accepted. Now suicide needs a Freud in the world, someone like a Freud, who destroys the second taboo. These two are the taboos: sex and death. Now somebody is needed to make death acceptable, rejoice-able; someone to destroy the myth that something is wrong in it, that only cowards commit suicide. That is wrong. In fact just the reverse is the case: cowards go on clinging to life. But sometimes a man comes to a point where he sees there is no sense in living. He gives the ticket back to God. He says, "Keep your world, I am going. I don't want to see this film any more."

I have heard about George Bernard Shaw that he was invited to see a drama. In the middle he suddenly got up. The author asked, "Where are you going?"

He said, "I have seen half of it."

The author said, "But half is still to come!"

Bernard Shaw said, "But it is written by the same man, so I have finished with it!" One has seen half of life, then one sees that it is written by the same man, so what is the point in staying? You go home and rest!

Meditate over it — it is a beautiful moment. You are sad, angry, yes; but meditate on it. And you will be benefited. That sannyasin has done some good service to a few people. Don't waste this moment just in being angry and sad; bring meditation to it, think over it: why are you feeling this? And make it a problem of yours. Don't throw the responsibility on him, because that is pointless. That's what we do: we ask ourselves *why* did he commit suicide? That is not the point. Why it hurts *you* — that is the problem. Why he killed himself is for him to decide. Why didn't he say anything to you? That is also for him to decide. Who knows why he decided not to say anything to anybody? Who knows why he decided to do it on that particular day?

He seems to have died very peacefully. One of the commune's doctors was there to see him when he died: he was lying on the road very peacefully, almost as if he had fallen asleep there, one hand under his head, as if the turmoil is gone, the storm is finished.

That is not the problem — why he did it, why he didn't say anything. This is also not the problem — why Osho didn't prevent him doing it, why he didn't take care. That too is not a problem for you. The problem for you is: Why can't you accept it? Where does it hurt? You have to go into it deeply, find the wound and go into it. And it will be a great revelation to you that you don't accept death, that you are afraid of death, that even your relationship with me is not a relationship of trust but only of onsolation, of greed. You want to use me for some of *your* ideas: that I should rotect you, that I am a kind of security to you. I am not! I am not a guarantee for nything. I am a very irresponsible man. Those who join hands with me have to join ands with me in total awareness that they are coming along with an irresponsible aan who follows no morality, who knows no principles, who has no so-called alues, who is utterly chaotic and who trusts life and its chaos absolutely. So hatsoever life brings is good for me.

Go into these things and see how your relationship to me is affected by his death, hy your trust is shaken, what you were hoping for. There must have been some deep iotive behind it, and that motive is disturbed. If you can meditate, you will come ut of it very fresh and new, and you will be thankful to him. And don't be worried bout him: he is already born, he has found a mother. There are so many foolish omen around the world – you cannot avoid being born again! So don't be worried. here is every possibility that within two, three years, he will be back here as a child. he day he comes I will declare, "This is him!" Just wait![96]

? *I have attempted suicide a number of times, and I feel really attracted to death. This disturbs me, but at the same time gives me joy. Will you say something about it?*

This is great! One can commit suicide only once, and you have attempted many times – and you are still alive. Those attempts were not true, they were all bogus, id you knew it even then.

I have heard: Mulla Nasruddin wanted to commit suicide. Being a man of great everness he made all the arrangements, left no loopholes. Perhaps nobody else had tempted suicide in that way. He went on top of a hill taking a pistol with him. Just nderneath the hill, deep down, was a river, very dangerous, deep, and surrounded y all kinds of rocks. On the hill there was a tree – he had also brought a rope. Not take any chances he figured out all the possible things so that suicide was absolutely ertain. He also carried with him a big container full of kerosene oil.

He hanged himself from the tree, but because he was going to do many more iings, he could not take his feet from the earth – because then how was he going to o other things? So he was hanging from the tree and standing on the earth. Then he oured kerosene oil over himself; he had brought a lighter too. He created a fire, the erosene oil was burning all around him. But he was not a man to take any chances, he also shot a bullet into his head. But the bullet cut the rope, he fell down into te river, and the river water destroyed the fire!

Desperately, he was coming back home when I met him. I asked, "You are still alive after all that arrangement?"

He said, "What to do? I know how to swim!" Everything failed!

You say you have attempted suicide many times. One thing is certain: you don't want to commit suicide, you want to play with the idea. And you feel also that there is fear about death and there is also a certain joy. This is not only your situation. It is a very common human phenomenon. Life is a torture, a burden; it is anguish. One wants to get rid of it. To get rid of it means getting rid of all the anguish, the despair, the hopelessness, the meaninglessness, this wife, this husband, these kids, this job; hence there is an attraction towards death, because death will put an end to all your misery. But it will also put an end to you – that creates fear.

You really want to live, and live forever, but you want to live in paradise. And you are living in a hell! You want to get rid of the hell, you don't want to get rid of yourself. And I want to emphasize that you are your own hell. So suicide is attractive from one side in that it will put an end to all your miseries, but on the other hand there is a great fear: it will finish you too.

Isn't there some way that the miseries can be finished and you can live more intensely? I also teach you that a certain suicide can help you – the suicide of the ego, not of you. Let the ego die, and then see that with it all problems disappear. You are left full of joy, blessedness, and each moment goes on opening new doors to new mysteries. Each moment becomes a moment of discovery – and it is an unending process.

You have attempted so many times to commit suicide. This time you commit suicide *my* style! And anyway, you have failed so much that you must have become very much of an expert in failing. And deep down you don't want to die because you are afraid of death – which is natural. Why should one put an end to one's life when life has not even been lived? You have not even tasted it, you have not explored the multi dimensional beauties, joys and blessings of life. Naturally you are afraid. But still you go on attempting it because you don't know how to get rid of all the miseries. Suicide seems to be the simplest way. You are in a split: half of your mind says, "Commit suicide and be finished with all this nonsense – enough is enough." The other part tries to sabotage your effort, because the other part wants to live; you have not lived yet.

Suicide is not going to help. Only more life, more abundant life, is going to help. So this time kill the ego, and see the miracle happen. With the ego gone there is no misery, no anguish, and no need to commit suicide. With the ego gone all the doors that were closed by the ego suddenly open and you are available to the sun, to the moon, to the stars. And it is easier, because to kill the ego you don't need a pistol, kerosene oil, a rope to hang the ego, fire to burn the ego, and if everything fails, the

260

deep mountainous river underneath to finish the ego. You don't need any of these things, because the ego is only a creation of the society, of the religions, of the culture. It does not exist in fact. You have only to look deeply into it; it is a shadow. You have to look into it, and it is not there. Meditation is simply a method of looking into what this ego is. And whoever has ever looked in has not found it. Without any exception, throughout the history of man, whoever has looked inwards has not come across any ego.

This is the suicide of the ego. Nothing has to be done, just a little turning in. And once you know it is not there, then all the sufferings that you were carrying because of a non-existential ego disappear. They cannot have any nourishment anymore. All these things have been created in your mind by conditioning, by programming; that's what the society has done to you. We have lived the whole of history in an ugly way....

You think you are a Christian? It is just an idea implanted in you. Do you think there is a God? An idea implanted in you. Do you think there is a heaven and hell? It is nothing but programming. You are all programmed.

My work with you is to deprogram you. And I am showing you all the notes — day after day, continuously — that these are the things that have made you almost dull, stupid, even attracted towards suicide, towards death. My religion is unique in this way: all the religions of the past have programmed people; I deprogram you, and then I leave you alone, to yourself.

People have been asking me, "What is your religion? What is your philosophy? Can't you give us something like a Christian catechism so we can understand that these are your principles?"

I have none, because that will be programming you again. When a Hindu becomes a Christian, what happens? The Christians deprogram him as a Hindu, and re-program him as a Christian. There is no difference. From one ditch he has fallen into another ditch. Perhaps the newness of it may keep him happy for a few days, but soon he will start looking for another ditch. Now he is addicted to ditches! And in this way he is simply digging his own grave. That is the final ditch into which he will fall.

I deprogram you, and I don't give you any other program. I leave you alone, empty, just a zero. In that zero, the ego disappears and all the blessings start showering on you.[97]

Is there anything you can say about what is happening to Vimalkirti, who has been in a coma for the past week?

Nothing is happening to Vimalkirti – exactly nothing, because nothing i
nirvana. The West has no idea of the beauty of nothingness. The whol
Western attitude is extrovert, oriented towards things, oriented towards action:
'Nothing' sounds like emptiness – it is not so. This is one of the greatest discoverie
of the East, that nothing is not empty, on the contrary it is just the opposite c
emptiness. It is fullness, it is overflowingness. Break the word 'nothing' in two
make it 'no-thingness', and then suddenly its meaning changes, the gesta
changes.

Nothing is the goal of sannyas. One has to come to a space where nothing i
happening; all happening has disappeared. The doing is gone, the doer is gone, th
desire is gone, the goal is gone. One simply is – not even a ripple in the lake c
consciousness, no sound.

The Zen people call it "the sound of one hand clapping." Now, one hand clappin
cannot create sound; it is soundless sound, the *omkar,* just silence. But silence is nc
empty, it is very full. The moment you are absolutely silent, absolutely attuned wit
nothingness, the whole descends in you, the beyond penetrates you.

But the Western mind has overpowered the whole world: we have becom
workaholics. And my whole approach is to help you to become zeros. The zero is th
most perfect experience in life; it is the experience of ecstasy.

Vimalkirti is blessed. He was one of those few of my chosen sannyasins who neve
wavered for a single moment, whose trust has been total the whole time he was here
He never asked a question, he never wrote a letter, he never brought any problem
His trust was such that he became by and by absolutely merged with me. He has on
of the rarest hearts; that quality of the heart has disappeared from the world. He i
really a prince, really royal, really aristocratic! Aristocracy has nothing to do wit
birth, it has something to do with the quality of the heart. And I experienced him a
one of the rarest, most beautiful souls on the earth. It is not a question at all c
asking about him: What is happening?

Of course, one tends to think in the old ways in which one was brought up, an
more particularly so about a German!

I have heard: One German reached heaven and knocked on the doors. St. Pete
opened a small window and looked out. He asked, "How old are you?" Then he looke
in the records and was very puzzled because the German said, "Seventy."

He said, "This can't be right. According to your record of working hours yo
must be at least one hundred and forty-three years old!"

The German continuously works. The German represents the ultimate in th
Western mind, just as the Indian represents the ultimate in the Eastern mind. Th

Indian is always sitting silently, doing nothing, waiting for the spring to come so that the grass can grow by itself. And it really grows!

Little Joey was sitting outside under a tree when he heard his mother cry out from the house, "Joey, what are you doing?"

"Nothing, Mum," he answered.

"No, really, Joey, what are you doing?"

"I said I ain't doing anything."

"Don't lie to me! Tell me what you are doing!"

At this point Joey gave a deep sigh, picked up a stone and tossed it a few feet. "I'm throwing rocks!" he said.

"That's what I thought you were doing! Now stop it immediately!"

"Golly," Joey said to himself. "No one will let ya do just nothin' anymore!"

Something has to be done.... Nobody believes — *you* will not believe me when I say Vimalkirti is doing nothing, is just being.

The day he had the haemorrhage I was a little worried about him, hence I told my doctor sannyasins to help him remain in the body at least for seven days. He was doing so beautifully and so fine, and then just to end suddenly when the work was incomplete....He was just on the edge — a little push and he would become part of the beyond. In fact, that's the reason why I want one of the most modern medical centres to be in the commune. If somebody is just on the verge and can be helped medically to remain in the body for a few more days, then he need not come back to life again.

Many questions have come to me about what I think of living through artificial methods. Now, he is breathing artificially. He would have died the same day — he almost did die. Without these artificial methods he would have already been in another body, he would have entered another womb. But then I will not be available here by the time he comes. Who knows whether he will be able to find a master or not? — and a crazy master like me! And once somebody has been so deeply connected with me, no other master will do. They will look so flat, so dull, so dead! Hence I wanted him to hang around a little more. Last night he managed: he crossed the boundary from doing to non-doing. That 'something' that was still in him dropped. Now he is ready, now we can say good-bye to him, now we can celebrate, now we can give him a send-off. Give him an ecstatic *bon voyage!* Let him go with your dance, with your song!

When I went to see him, this is what transpired between me and him. I waited by his side with closed eyes — he was immensely happy. The body is not at all usable anymore…. The surgeons, the neurosurgeons and the other doctors were worried; they were asking again and again, inquiring about what I was up to, why I wanted him to be in the body, because there seemed to be no point in it – even if he somehow managed to survive, his brain would never be able to function rightly. And I would not like him to be in that state – it is better that he goes. They were worried about why I wanted him to go on breathing artificially. Even his heart stopped once in a while and then, artificially, his heart had to be stimulated again. His kidneys began to fail yesterday, his skull has been drilled – there was such a great swelling inside. This was something congenital; it was bound to happen – it was a program in his body.

But he managed beautifully: before *it* could happen he used this life for the ultimate flowering. Just a little bit had remained; last night even that disappeared. So last night when I told him, "Vimalkirti, now you can go into the beyond with all my blessings," he almost shouted in joy, "F-a-a-r out!" I told him, "Not that long!"

And I told him a story….

The crow came up to the frog and said, "There is going to be a big party in heaven!"

The frog opened his big mouth and said, "F-a-a-r out!"

The crow went on, "There will be great food and drinks!"

And the frog replied, "F-a-a-r out!"

"And there will be beautiful women, and the Rolling Stones will be playing!"

The frog opened his mouth even wider and cried, "F-a-a-r out!"

Then the crow added, "But anyone who has a big mouth won't be allowed in!"

The frog pursed his lips tightly together and mumbled, "Poor alligator! He will be disappointed!"

Vimalkirti is perfectly beautiful. He will not need to come back again into a body; he is going awakened, he is going in the state of buddhahood.

So you all have to rejoice, dance and sing and celebrate! You have to learn how to celebrate life and how to celebrate death. Life is really not as great as death can be, but death can be great only if one achieved the fourth state, *turiya*.

Ordinarily it is difficult to get disidentified from the body and the brain and the heart, but it happened very easily to Vimalkirti. He had to become disidentified because the body was already dead – it has been dead for five days – the brain was already lost, the heart was far away. This accident is an accident for the people who are on the outside, but for Vimalkirti himself it has proved a blessing in disguise. You cannot get identified with such a body: the kidneys not functioning, the breathing not functioning, the heart not functioning, the brain totally damaged. How can you get identified with such a body? Impossible. Just a little alertness and you will become separate — and that much alertness he had, that much he had grown. So he immediately became aware that "I am not the body, I am not the mind, I am not the heart either." And when you pass beyond these three, the fourth, *turiya,* is attained, and that is your real nature. Once it is attained it is never lost.

He used to love my jokes and this will be the last lecture for him, so two jokes for him:

An Italian couple was rushing to the hospital as the wife was about to have a baby. On the way there was a terrible automobile accident and the husband ended up in the hospital in a coma. When he finally came to he was told he had been in a coma for three months and that his wife was fine and he was the proud father of twins, a boy and a girl.

As soon as he could he left the hospital to be with his family, and after being home for a little while he asked his wife the names she had given the children. The wife replied, "Well-a, in keeping with-a Italian-a tradition, I didn't name them. It's-a the man's-a place to name-a the newborn babies, and since you were unconscious the job-a went-a to your brother."

Hearing this, the husband got very upset, saying, "My brother is an idiot-a! He doesn't know-a anything! So what-a did-a he name them?"

The wife said, "He named the girl-a, Denise."

"Hey," the husband said, "that's-a not-a bad! And-a the bambino?"

"The boy he named Da nephew."

Abe Einstein owned a company which manufactured nails in Ohio. He was doing so well that he could afford to spend the winter vacationing in Miami. The only problem was that he did not believe that his son, Max, had the good sense to run the business in his absence. Abe's friend, Moishe, convinced him to take the winter off, pointing out that Max was going to inherit the business some day anyway, so he ought to give himself a chance to prove himself now.

Abe was having a great time in Miami until he received a copy by post of the magazine, *Nails Quarterly.* In the magazine was a full-page color ad for Einstein's Nails with a picture of Jesus nailed to the cross. The caption read: "They Used Einstein's Nails!"

Abe called Max immediately, "Don't ever say such a thing again!"

Max assured his father that he understood. Abe felt assured until he got the next issue of *Nails Quarterly,* containing an ad showing Jesus lying on the ground below the cross with the caption: "They Didn't Use Einstein's Nails!"

These are the 'three L's' of my *philosia:* life, love, laughter. Life is only a seed, love is a flower, laughter is fragrance. Just to be born is not enough, one has to learn the art of living; that is the A of meditation. Then one has to learn the art of loving; that is the B of meditation. And then one has to learn the art of laughing; that is the C of meditation. And meditation has only three letters: A,B,C.

So today you will have to give a beautiful send-off to Vimalkirti. Give it with great laughter. Of course, I know you will miss him – even I will miss him. He has become such a part of the commune, so deeply involved with everybody. I will miss him more than you because he was the guard in front of my door, and it was always a joy to come out of the room and see Vimalkirti standing there always smiling. Now it will not be possible again. But he will be around here in your smiles, in your laughter. He will be here in the flowers, in the sun, in the wind, in the rain, because nothing is ever lost – nobody really dies, one becomes part of eternity.

So even though you will feel tears, let those tears be tears of joy – joy for what he has attained. Don't think of yourself, that you will be missing him, think of him, that he *is* fulfilled. And this is how you will learn, because sooner or later many more sannyasins will be going on the journey to the farther shore and you will have to learn to give them beautiful send-offs. Sooner or later I will have to go, and this is how you will also learn to give me a send-off – with laughter, dance, song.

My whole approach is of celebration. Religion to me is nothing but the whole spectrum of celebration, the whole rainbow, all the colours of celebration. Make it a great opportunity for yourself, because in celebrating his departure many of you can reach to greater heights, to new dimensions of being; it will be possible. These are the moments which should not be missed; these are the moments which should be used to their fullest capacity.

I am happy with him…and many of you are getting ready in the same way. I am really happy with my people! I don't think there has ever been a master who had so many beautiful disciples. Jesus was very poor in that sense – not a single disciple became enlightened. Buddha was the richest in the past, but I am determined to defeat Gautam Buddha![98]

CHAPTER 16

ESOTERICS

Wilhelm Reich says in his book, Listen, Little Man, *that he found that man reaches out with his life energy when he feels well and loving; that he retracts that energy when he is afraid. Reich says that he found that man's life energy — which he termed 'orgone' — is "found in the atmosphere," outside the body. He says he succeeded in seeing it and devised apparatus which magnified it.*
Is what he observed so?

Wilhelm Reich was one of the unique intelligences born in this century. What he has found has been known to the East as *aura*. You must have seen around the statues of Buddha or Mahavira or Krishna — a round aura around the head. That round aura is a reality. What Wilhelm Reich said was authentically true, but the people to whom he said it were not the right people to understand it. They thought he was mad because he described life as an energy surrounding the body. It is exactly true.

Life is an energy that surrounds your body. Not only your body, but flowers, trees — everything has its own aura. And that aura, that energy surrounding you shrinks and expands in different situations. Any situation where your energy shrinks should be thought bad, sick. And every situation where your energy expands, should be respected and loved. In love your energy reaches out, you become more alive. And when you are in fear, your energy shrinks, you become less alive.

Now, poor Wilhelm Reich was thought by Americans to be mad because he was not only magnifying that energy — he had found a few exercises in which that energy magnifies — he was even catching that energy in boxes, big boxes in which a man could enter. And if the man was sick he would come out whole and healthy. Naturally such a man should be thought mad. He was selling those boxes, empty boxes – but they were not empty. He had found ways to collect the energy which is available in the atmosphere. Around a tree you can find that energy showering, but with your bare eyes you cannot see it.

After he was declared mad and imprisoned, another man in the Soviet Union even managed to photograph it. And now it has become a recognized psychology in the Soviet Union, that life has an aura. And the man, Kirlian, has developed a certain sensitive plate to photograph it. He would photograph the hand, and the hand would come with an aura around it. In a very strange way his photographs even showed if a man would be sick within six months: "Right now he does not show any pattern of sickness, but his aura is shrinking at a certain point...." And if at a certain point the aura is shrinking – maybe the person will become deaf or blind if the aura around the eyes is shrinking. And all his photographs proved to be right. When he said, "This man is in danger of losing his eyesight," there was no visible sign, there was no reason to believe it, but within six months that man became blind. Now in Soviet psychology, Kirlian photography is recognized by the government. It is spreading into other countries also. A man can be cured before he becomes sick. Kirlian photography is very predictive. It shows, at least six months ahead, what is going to happen.

In the East it has been known for centuries that before your death, six months before, you stop being able to see the tip of your nose. Because your eyes start turning upwards, they cannot see the tip of your own nose. The moment you recognize you cannot see the tip of your nose means that within six months your energy will shrink, go back to its source. And the aura, without any photographic technology, has been recognized by yoga for five thousand years. But now, it can be accepted on scientific grounds.

Wilhelm Reich was a unique genius. He could manage to see and feel what is not ordinarily possible. But if you are very meditative, you will start seeing the auras of people, even your own aura. You will see your own hand with the light rays around it, radiating. And when you are healthy you will feel your aura expanding. When you are sick you will feel your aura shrinking – something is shrinking within you.

When you are by the side of a sick person, you will have a strange feeling that he somehow makes you feel sick, because the sick person exploits the auras of the other without his knowing. He needs more life, so whoever has life and comes around him, he takes his life. And you know by experience, without understanding, that there are people you want to avoid, because meeting them you feel sick, meeting them you feel that something has been taken away from you. And there are people you want to meet, because meeting them you feel an expanding, you feel more alive.

Wilhelm Reich was right, but unfortunately the masses never accept their own geniuses; on the contrary, they condemn them, because if Wilhelm Reich is right, then everybody else is almost blind. And in anger he wrote the book, *Listen, Little Man*. But that book is beautiful, and his anger can be forgiven because he was mistreated by 'the little man', by the masses. He was first thought to be mad, then forced into a madhouse, and he died in a madhouse. In the East he would have become a Gautam Buddha. He had the quality, the insight. But a wrong society, a society of very little men, of very small people, small-minded, who cannot conceive the vast, who cannot conceive the mysterious....

The whole atmosphere is full of life. And if you understand your own sources of life you will be suddenly aware that birds are alive, trees are alive, grasses are alive – everywhere there is life! And you can dance with this life, you can start having a dialogue with the atmosphere. Of course, people will think you are mad, because people are still the same. The same people crucified Jesus, the same people forced Wilhelm Reich into a madhouse, the same people poisoned Socrates...but those little people are in the majority.

Wilhelm Reich's anger is right, but still I would say, rather than anger, the little man needs compassion. He was angry because they misbehaved with him, they destroyed his whole life. Rather than understanding him – he would have opened a new door to experiencing, to loving, to living – they destroyed the man completely. Obviously, he became angry.

In the East, the same little men are there, but the Eastern genius has never been angry with them. Rather than being angry it has shown compassion, it has felt compassion for their blindness, and it has tried in every way to bring light to them, a little understanding to their hearts.[99]

? *The other day, you talked about the third eye as a door for connecting with oneself and existence. Whenever I feel open, flowing, connecting with you, other people, nature or myself, I mostly feel it in my heart as silence and expanding spaciousness, and sometimes as radiating light. Is this the same kind of experience you were talking about, or is there a difference between connecting through the third eye or the heart; or are there different stages?*

What you are experiencing is in itself valuable, but it is not the experience of the third eye. The third eye is a little higher than your experience.

The way the mystics in the East have categorized the evolution of consciousness is in seven centres. Your experiences belong to the fourth centre, the heart. It is one of the most important centres, because it is exactly in the middle. Three centres are below it and three centres are above it. That's why love is such a balancing experience.

Your description is, "Whenever I feel open, flowing, connecting with you, other people, nature or myself, I mostly feel it in my heart as silence and expanding spaciousness, and sometimes as radiating light. Is this the same kind of experience you were talking about?"

I was talking about the third eye, which is above the heart. There are three centres above the heart. One is in your throat, which is the centre of creativity; one is between your two eyebrows, exactly in the middle, which is called the third eye. Just as you have two eyes to know the outside world...the third eye is only a metaphor, but the experience is knowing oneself, seeing oneself.

The last centre is *sahasrar,* the seventh; that is at the top of your head. As consciousness goes on moving upwards, first you know yourself, and in the second step you know the whole universe; you know the whole and yourself as part of it.

In the old language, the seventh is 'knowing God', the sixth is 'knowing yourself', the fifth is 'being creative', and the fourth is 'being loving, sharing and knowing others'. With the fourth, your journey becomes certain; it can be guaranteed that you will reach the seventh. Before the fourth, there is a possibility you may go astray.

The first centre is the sex centre, which is for reproduction – so that life continues. Just above it...the sex energy can be moved upwards, and it is a great experience; for the first time you find yourself self-sufficient. Sex always needs the other. The second centre is the centre of contentment, self-sufficiency: you are enough unto yourself. At the third centre you start exploring – who are you? who is this self-sufficient being? These centres are all significant. The moment you find who you are, the fourth centre opens and you find you are love.

Before the fourth the journey has started, but there is a possibility you may not be able to complete it. You can go astray. For example, finding yourself self-sufficient, contented, you can remain there; there is no need to do anything anymore. You may not even ask the question, "Who am I?" The sufficiency is so much that all questions disappear.

A master is needed in these moments, so that you don't settle somewhere in the middle without reaching the goal. And there are beautiful spots to settle – feeling contented, what is the need to go on? But the master goes on nagging you and wants you to know who you are; you may be contented, but at least know who you are. The moment you know who you are, a new door opens, because you become aware of life, of love, of joy. You can stay there; it is so much, there is no need to move anymore. But the master goads you on, "Move to the fourth! Unless you find the purest energy of love, you will not know the splendour of existence."

After the fourth, you cannot go astray. Once you have known the splendour of existence, creativity arises on its own. You have known beauty; you would like to create it also. You want to be a creator. A tremendous longing for creativity arises. Whenever you feel love, you always feel creativity just as a shadow coming with it. The man of creativity cannot simply go on looking outside. There is much beauty outside…but he becomes aware that just as there is an infinite sky outside, to balance it there must be the same infinity inside. If a master is available, it is good; if he is not available, these experiences will lead you onwards.

Once your third eye is opened, and you see yourself, the whole expanse of your consciousness, you have come very close to the temple of God; you are just standing on the steps. You can see the door and you cannot resist the temptation to go inside the temple and see what is there. There you find universal consciousness, there you find enlightenment, there you find ultimate liberation. There you find your eternity.

So these are the seven centres – just arbitrarily created divisions, so the seeker can move from one to another in a systematic way; otherwise, there is every possibility, if you are working by yourself, to get muddled. Particularly before the fourth centre there are dangers, and even after the fourth centre.

There have been many poets who have lived at the fifth centre of creativity and never gone ahead – many painters, many dancers, many singers who created great art, but never moved to the third eye. And there have been mystics who have remained with the third eye, knowing their own inner beauty; it is so fulfilling that they thought they had arrived. Somebody is needed to tell you that there is still something more ahead; otherwise, in your ignorance, what you will do is almost unpredictable.

Mike had decided to join the police force and went along for the entrance examination. The examining sergeant, realizing that the prospective recruit was an Irishman, decided to ask him a simple question. "Who killed Jesus Christ?" he asked.

Mike looked worried and said nothing, so the sergeant told him not to worry and that he could have some time to think about it. Mike was on his way home when he met Paddy.

"Well," said Paddy, "are you a policeman yet?"

"Not only that," says Mike, "but I am on my first case."

Man is such that he needs someone who has known the path and knows the pitfalls, knows the beautiful spots where one can remain stuck, and has compassion enough to go on pushing you – even against you – until you have reached to the final stage of your potentiality.[100]

? *Some years ago I had been very emotionally expressive but felt uncentred. And at that time you told me to keep my energy inside and bring it to my hara. Could you please say something more about the hara and guide me further?*

The *hara* is the centre from where a life leaves the body. It is the centre of death. The word 'hara' is Japanese; that's why, in Japan, suicide is called *hara-kiri*. The centre is just two inches below the navel. It is very important, and almost everybody in the world has felt it. But only in Japan have they gone deeper into its implications.

Even the people in India, who had worked tremendously hard on centres, had not considered the hara. The reason for their missing it was because they had never considered death to be of any significance. Your soul never dies, so why bother about a centre that functions only as a door for energies to get out, and to enter into another body? They worked from sex, which is the life centre. They have worked on seven centres, but the hara is not even mentioned in any Indian scriptures.

The people who worked hardest on the centres for thousands of years have not mentioned the hara, and this cannot be just a coincidence. The reason was that they never took death seriously. These seven centres are life centres, and each centre is of a higher life. The seventh is the highest centre of life, when you are almost a god.

The hara is very close to the sex centre. If you don't rise towards higher centres, towards the seventh centre which is in your head, and if you remain for your whole life at the sex centre, then just by the side of the sex centre is the hara, and then, when then life will end, the hara will be the centre from where your life will move out of the body.

Why have I told you this? You were very energetic, but not aware of any higher centres; your whole energy was at the sex centre, and you were overflowing. Energy overflowing at the sex centre is dangerous, because it can start releasing from the hara. And if it starts releasing from the hara, then to take it upwards becomes more difficult. So I had told you to keep your energy in, and not to be so expressive: Hold it in! I simply wanted the hara centre, which was opening and which could have been very dangerous, to be completely closed.

You followed it, and you have become a totally different person. Now when I see you, I cannot believe the expressiveness that I had seen at first. Now you are more centred, and your energy is moving in the right direction of the higher centres. It is almost at the fourth centre, which is the centre of love and which is a very balancing centre. There are three centres below it, and three centres above it.

Once a person is at the centre of love, there is very rarely a possibility for him to fall back down, because he has tasted something of the heights. Now valleys will be very dark, ugly; he has seen sunlit peaks, not very high, but still high; now his whole desire will be....

And that is the trouble with all lovers: they want more love, because they don't understand that the real desire is not for more love, but for something more than love. Their language ends with love; they don't know any way that is higher than love, and love does not satisfy. On the contrary, the more you love the more thirsty you become.

At the fourth centre, of love, one feels a tremendous satisfaction only when energy starts moving to the fifth centre. The fifth centre is in your throat, and the sixth centre is your third eye. The seventh centre, the *sahasrar,* is on the top of your head. All these centres have different expressions and different experiences.

When love moves to the fifth centre then whatever talents you have, any creative dimension, is possible for you. This is the centre of creativity. It is not only for songs, not only for music; it is for all creativity.

Hindu mythology has a beautiful story. It is a myth, but the story is beautiful, and particularly for explaining to you the fifth centre. Indian mythology says that there is a constant struggle between evil forces and good forces. They both discovered that if they made a certain search in the ocean they could find nectar, and that whoever drank it would become immortal. So they all tried to find it. But as life balances everywhere, there too.... Before they found the nectar they found poison which was hiding the nectar underneath it. Nobody was ready to test it; even the very sight of it created sickness. One of them thought that the first hippie of the world perhaps might be willing – he was the god Shiva. So they asked Shiva, "You test it." He said, "Okay." He not only tested it, he drank it all, and it was pure poison. He kept it just in his neck, at the fifth centre. The fifth centre is the creative center. It became completely poisoned, and Shiva became the god of destruction. So Hindus have three gods: Brahma who creates the world, Vishnu who sustains the world, and Shiva who destroys the world. His destructiveness came from his creative centre being poisoned. And the poison was so great that it cannot be a small destruction; he can only destroy the whole of existence....

Shiva became the destroyer of the world because his fifth centre had accumulated the whole poison of existence in it. It is our creative centre, that's why lovers have a certain tendency to creativity. When you fall in love, you suddenly feel like creating something – it is very close. If you are guided rightly, your love can become your great creative act. It can make you a poet, it can make you a painter, it can make you a dancer, it can make you reach to the stars in any dimension.

The sixth centre which we call the third eye is between the two eyes. This gives you a clarity, a vision of all your past lives, and of all the future possibilities. Once your energy has reached your third eye, then you are so close to enlightenment that something of enlightenment starts showing. It radiates from the man of the third eye, and he starts feeling a pull towards the seventh centre.

Because of these seven centres, India never bothered about the hara. The hara is not in the line; it is just by the side of the sex centre. The sex centre is the life centre, and hara is the death centre. Too much excitement, too much uncentredness, too much throwing your energy all over the place is dangerous, because it takes your energy towards the hara. And once the route is created, it becomes more difficult to move it upwards. The hara is parallel to the sex centre, so the energy can move very easily.

It was a great discovery by the Japanese: they found that there was no need to cut your head off, or shoot your brains out to kill yourself – they are all unnecessarily painful; just a small knife forced in exactly at the hara centre, and without any pain life disappears. Just make the centre open and life disappears, as if the flower opens and the fragrance disappears.

The hara should be kept closed. That's why I had told you to be more centred, to keep your feelings inside, and to bring it to your hara…. If you can keep your hara consciously controlling your energies, it does not allow them to go out. You start feeling a tremendous gravity, a stability, a centredness, which is a basic necessity for the energy to move upwards….

A Pole is walking down the street, and passes a hardware store advertising the sale of a chain saw that is capable of cutting seven hundred trees in seven hours. The Pole thinks that it is a great deal and decides to buy one.

The next day he comes back with the saw, and complains to the salesman, "The thing did not come close to chopping down the seven hundred trees that the ad said it would."

"Well," said the salesman, "let us test it out back." Finding a log, the salesman pulls the starter cord, and the saw makes a great roaring sound.

"What is that noise?" asked the Pole.

So he must have been cutting by hand and it was an electric saw!

Your hara centre has so much energy that, if it is rightly directed, enlightenment is not a faraway place.

So these two are my suggestions: keep yourself as much centred as possible. Don't get moved by small things – somebody is angry, somebody insults you, and you think about it for hours. Your whole night is disturbed because somebody said something. If the hara can hold more energy, then naturally that much more energy starts rising upwards. There is only a certain capacity in the hara, and every energy that moves upwards moves through the hara; but the hara should just be closed.

So one thing is that the hara should be closed. The second thing is that you should always work for higher centres. For example, if you feel angry too often you should meditate more on anger, so that anger disappears and its energy becomes compassion. If you are a man who hates everything, then you should concentrate on hate; meditate on hate, and the same energy becomes love. Go on moving upwards, think always of higher ladders, so that you can reach to the highest point of your being. And there should be no leakage from the hara centre.

India has been too concerned about sex for the same reason: sex can also take your energy outside. It takes…but at least sex is the centre of life. Even if it takes energy out, it will bring energy somewhere else, life will go on flowing. But the hara is a death centre. Energy should not be allowed through the hara. A person whose energy starts through the hara you can very easily detect. For example, there are people with whom you will feel suffocated, with whom you will feel as if they are sucking your energy. You will find that, after they are gone, you feel at ease and relaxed, although they were not doing anything wrong to you.

You will find just the opposite kind of people also, whose meeting you makes you joyful, healthier. If you were sad, your sadness disappears; if you were angry, your anger disappears. These are the people whose energy is moving to higher centres. Their energy affects your energy. We are affecting each other continually. And the man who is conscious chooses friends and company which raises his energy higher.

One point is very clear. There are people who suck you – avoid them! It is better to be clear about it, say good-bye to them. There is no need to suffer, because they are dangerous; they can open your hara too. Their hara is open, that's why they create such a sucking feeling in you.

Psychology has not taken note of it yet, but it is of great importance that psychologically sick people should not be put together. And that is what is being done all over the world. Psychologically sick people are put into psychiatric institutes together. They are already psychologically sick, and you are putting them in a company which will drag their energy even lower. Even the doctors who work with psychologically sick people have given enough indication of it. More psychoanalysts commit suicide than any other profession, more psychoanalysts go mad than any other profession. And every psychoanalyst once in a while needs to be treated by some other psychoanalyst. What happens to these poor people? Surrounded by psychologically sick people, they are continually sucked, and they don't have any idea how to close their haras.

There are methods, techniques to close the hara, just as there are methods for meditation, to move the energy upwards. The best and simplest method is: try to remain as centred in your life as possible. People cannot even sit silently, they will be changing their position. They cannot lie down silently, the whole night they will be turning and tossing. This is just unrest, a deep restlessness in their souls. One should learn restfulness. And in these small things, the hara stays closed. Particularly psychologists should be trained. Also, psychologically sick people should not be put together.

In the East, particularly in Japan in Zen monasteries, where they have become aware of the hara centre, there are no psychologists as such. But in Zen monasteries there are small cottages, far away from the main campus where Zen people live, but in the same forest or in the same mountain area. And if somebody who is psychologically sick is brought to them, he is given a cabin there and he is told to relax, rest, enjoy, move around in the forest – but not to talk. Anyway there is nobody to talk to! Only once a day a man comes to give food; he is not allowed to talk to that man either, and even if he talks, the man will not answer. So his whole energy is completely controlled. He cannot even talk; he cannot meet anybody.

You will be surprised to know that what psychoanalysis cannot do in years, is done in three weeks. In three weeks time the person is as healthy as normal people are. And nothing has been done – no technique, nothing. He has just been left alone so he cannot talk. He has been left alone so he can rest and be himself. He is not expected to fulfill somebody else's expectations.

You have done well. Just continue whatever you are doing, accumulating your energy in yourself. The accumulation of energy automatically makes it go higher. And as it reaches higher you will feel more peaceful, more loving, more joyful, more sharing, more compassionate, more creative. The day is not far away when you will feel full of light, and the feeling of coming back home.[101]

Man has lost contact with the solar plexus because of the fear of sex, because of the repression of sex, because of life-negation.

The solar plexus is the centre of life and death both. That's why Japanese call it *hara*; 'hara' means death. And the Indians call it *manipura*. 'Manipura' means the diamond, the most precious diamond, because life comes from there. In the solar plexus is your seed. It is the first thing that is created in the womb of the mother; then everything else grows around it.

In the solar plexus your father's seed and your mother's seed are both present. The life cell from the father and the life cell from the mother create your solar plexus. That is your first blueprint; from there everything grows and it remains the centre forever and ever. You can forget about it, you can become oblivious to it, you can repress, you can start hanging in the head, but it remains in the centre. You just become less and less alive. The farther away you go, the less and less alive you become and the farther you are from the solar plexus. You live more on the periphery; you lose centreing, you lose grounding. It is very alive. Start living more and more.

That is the primitive mind, the most primal mind. The primal therapists are not yet aware that the primal scream comes from the solar plexus. It is the first mind. Then the second mind arises – the heart, feeling. Then the third mind arises – the head, thinking.

Solar plexus is being, heart is feeling, head is thinking. Thinking is the farthest, feeling is just in the middle; that's why when you feel you are more alive; just a little more alive than when you think. Thoughts are dead things: they are corpses; they don't breathe. Feelings breathe, feelings have a pulsation, but nothing to be compared with the first, primal mind. If you reach the solar plexus and be there and live from there, you will have a totally different kind of life – the real life.

The few moments you feel that you are real are the moments when you are at the solar plexus. That's why sometimes people seek danger, they go mountain climbing, because when danger is very real you simply go into the solar plexus. That's why whenever you are in a shock your solar plexus has the first pulsation. In a shock you cannot think, you cannot feel: you can only be.

If you are driving and suddenly you feel an accident is going to happen, your solar plexus is hit. That's the reason why people like speed in driving, and the speedier your car becomes, the more alive you feel, thrilled. You are coming closer to the solar plexus. That's why there is such attraction in war. People go to the cinema to see a murder story. It is creating a situation in which you can feel your solar plexus again. People read detective novels and when the story really comes to its peak they cannot think, they cannot feel: they *are!*

Try to understand it. All meditations lead to it. It is your *élan vital,* it is the source of your vitality. Go into it, and you can go easily, that's why I am saying to go into it. Whenever you are sitting silently, be there. Forget the head, forget the heart, forget the body: just be a throb behind the navel. If you go deeper into it, it will become possible for you to understand the real concept of trinity – because your father is there, your mother is there. If you are also there, the trinity arises. That is the basic idea of the trinity – not God and the son and the holy ghost. If you are there, then the trinity, a triangle, the father and mother are already there. If you are also there then the Christ is born, the son is born. And when the son is born there is real unity.

Two cannot meet: the third is needed to bridge the two. So your father and mother are there, consummated but not consumed, in a kind of union but not yet a unity. The feminine and the masculine are there but still not bridged, and that is the whole conflict – that you are two, dual. You are bound to be two; something has been given by the father and something has been given by the mother. They are both there, flowing together like two currents but still there is a subtle separation.

If your presence reaches there, if you become more and more aware of it, your very awareness will become the catalytic agent: the two will disappear and there will be oneness. That oneness is called Christ consciousness.[102]

CHAPTER 17
ATTITUDE TO ILLNESS

What is your insight about the cause of cancer?

Cancer is basically a psychological disease; it is basically a disease of the mind, not a physical one. When the mind becomes very tense, so tense that it is intolerable, it starts affecting the body tissues. That's why cancer exists only when civilization becomes very, very sophisticated. In primitive societies you cannot find cancer. People are not so sophisticated. The higher – by 'higher' I mean complicated – the more sophisticated, the more complex a society is, the more cancer will happen....

Cancer has to disappear. Cancer can exist only in a certain neurotic state of mind. If the mind relaxes, sooner or later the body will follow and will relax. It is because of this fact that scientific investigation has not yet been able to find a cure for cancer. It is almost impossible to find a cure for cancer – and the day they find a cure for cancer they will create even more dangerous diseases in the world – because the cure will mean repression. The day they can find strong enough drugs to repress cancer, then some other disease will erupt. That poison will start flowing through some other channel.

That's how it has happened down the ages. Simple diseases were cured and difficult diseases came into being. You cure one disease, another disease comes in and the second one is more complex than the first. The first was a natural reaction of the body, the second is an unnatural, abnormal reaction of the body. You repress the second and the third will come, and the third will be even more difficult to tackle…and so on, so forth. Now cancer is at the top. If cancer is repressed then even more difficult diseases will erupt in the human body and the human mind.[103]

? *For the last week I have known that I have cancer. From that time, except for a few moments of panic and fear, I have felt a deep calmness and relaxation coming into my being. Have I already given up my life, or is this the quietness of acceptance?*

We have given up our lives at the very moment when we were born, because the birth is nothing but a beginning of death. Each moment you will be dying more and more.

It is not that on a certain day, at seventy years old, death comes; it is not an event, it is a process that begins with the birth. It takes seventy years; it is mighty lazy, but it is a process, not an event. And I am emphasizing this fact so that I can make it clear to you that life and death are not two things. They become two if death is an event which ends life. Then they become two; then they become antagonistic, enemies.

When I say that death is a process beginning with birth, I am saying that life is also a process beginning with the same birth – and these are not two processes. It is one process: it begins with birth, it ends with death. But life and death are like two wings of a bird, or two hands, or two legs. Even your brain has two hemispheres, separate – the right hemisphere and the left hemisphere. You cannot exist without this dialectic.

Life is a dialectic – and if you understand this, a tremendous acceptance of death naturally comes to you. It is not against you, it is part of you; without it you cannot be alive.

It is just like the background of a blackboard on which you write with white chalk: the blackboard is not against the white chalk; it simply gives it emphasis, prominence. Without the blackboard your white writing will disappear. It is like day and night – you see it everywhere, but you go on behaving like blind people. Without the night there is no day.

The deeper you enter into the dialectics…it is a miraculous experience. Without inaction there is no action; if you cannot relax, you cannot act. The more you can relax, the more perfection will be in your action. They appear to be opposites; they are not. The better you dissolve into sleep in the night, the sharper, the younger you will wake up in the morning. And everywhere in life you will find the same dialectical process.

The mystics of Zen have a koan: they ask the disciples to meditate on the sound of one hand clapping. It is absurd, there cannot be any sound of one hand clapping. Clapping with what? For clapping two hands are needed, apparently opposed to each other but deep down creating a single clap; united in their efforts, coherent, neither opposed to each other nor contradictory to each other, but complementary.

The meditation is given for the simple reason so that you can become aware that in life you cannot find a single instance supporting the sound of one hand clapping. The whole existence is two hands clapping: man and woman, day and night, life and death, love and hate. The deeper the disciple meditates...slowly, slowly he becomes aware that in existence it is impossible to find anything.

And the master asks everything – "Have you found it? Have you heard the sound of one hand clapping?" Many ideas come to their minds: the sound of running water, and they think perhaps this is it. And they run to the master to tell him, "I have got it: the sound of running water." And they will get a hit from the master's staff: "You idiot! This is not the sound of one hand clapping. There is duality; just go and see. All those rocks in the water, they are creating a sound; it is not the sound of one, it is always the sound of two." In fact, there cannot be a sound of one. Frustrated thousands of times, each answer that the disciple finds is rejected. He comes to the realization that sound is always of the two. Silence is of the one; only silence can be the answer. It is not a clapping. But going through all this process to reach to the silence...and then he comes to the master and the master asks, "Have you heard it?"

The disciple bows down to his feet, tears of joy flowing from his eyes. He cannot even say, "Yes, I have found it." That will not be accurate. He has not found silence; on the contrary, he has disappeared in silence. It is not a finding, it is a disappearing. He is no more, only silence is. Who is there to say now, "I have found the answer?" – hence the tears of joy and a grateful head touching the feet of the master. And the master says, "I do understand, don't be worried. Don't be worried that you cannot say it. Nobody can say it. That's why sometimes when you had come before, rushing with an answer, even before you told me the answer I hit you with my staff and told you, 'You idiot! Go back!' And you were puzzled, that you have not even said the answer and it has been rejected. Now you can understand: it is not a question of this answer or that answer. All answers are wrong. Only silence – which is an existential presence, not an intellectual answer – is right."

You are fortunate to know that within seven days you are going to die, that you have cancer. Everybody has cancer, just a few people are lazy. You are speedy! American! Most people are Indians; even in dying, they will take time. They are always late, always missing the train.

I say you are blessed to know – because everybody is going to die, but because it is unknown when, where, people go on living under the illusion that they are going to live forever. They always see *others* dying. That logically supports their standpoint that, "It is always the other who dies. I never die." You must have seen many people dying, giving you a strong support, a rational background that it is always the other who dies. And when you die, you will not know, you will be unconscious – you will miss the opportunity of knowing death. Those who have known death are unanimous in their opinion that it is the greatest orgasmic experience of life.

But people die unconsciously. It is good that there are diseases which are predictable. Cancer means that you have known seven days before – or seven months, whatever the time may be – that death is coming closer each moment. These seven days are not allowed to everybody. Cancer seems to be something you must have earned in your past life – because J. Krishnamurti died of cancer, Ramana Maharshi died of cancer, Ramakrishna died of cancer. Strange...three enlightened people who are not mythological, who have lived just now, died of cancer. It seems to be something spiritual! It certainly has a spiritual dimension.

I am not saying that all those who die of cancer are enlightened beings, but they can become enlightened beings more easily than anybody else because others go on living under the illusion that they are going to live; there is no hurry. Meditation can be postponed – tomorrow, the day after tomorrow. What is the hurry? – and there are more urgent things which have to be done today. Meditation is never urgent because death is never urgent.

For the man who comes to know that cancer is going to strike within seven days, everything in life becomes meaningless. All urgencies disappear. He was thinking of making a beautiful palace; the very idea disappears. He was thinking to fight the next election; the whole idea disappears. He was worried about the third world war; he is no longer worried. It doesn't matter to him. What happens after him does not matter – he has only seven days to live.

If he is a little alert in those seven days he can live seventy years or seven hundred years or the whole eternity – because now meditation becomes a priority, love becomes a priority...dance, rejoicing, experiencing beauty, which were never priorities before. This week, the full moon night will be a priority because he will never see the full moon again. This is his *last* full moon. He has lived for years: moons have come and gone, and he has never bothered about it; but now he has to take it seriously. This is the *last* moon, this is the *last* chance to love, this is the *last* chance to be, this is the *last* chance to experience all that is beautiful in life. And he has no energy anymore for anger, for fighting. He can postpone; he can say, "After a week I will see you in the court, but this week let me be on a holiday."

Yes, in the beginning you will feel sadness, despair that life is slipping out of your hands. But it is always slipping out of your hands, whether you know it or not. It is slipping out of everybody else's hands whether he knows it or not. You are fortunate that you *know* it.

I am reminded of a great mystic, Eknath. A man used to go to Eknath for years. One day he went early in the morning when nobody was there and he asked Eknath, "Please forgive me. I have come early so that there is nobody else, because I am going to ask a question which I have always wanted to ask but I felt so embarrassed that I suppressed it."

Eknath said, "There was no reason to be embarrassed. You could have asked any question, any time. Sit down here."

So in the temple they sat down. And the man said, "It is difficult for me; how to present it? My question is that for years I have been coming to you and I have never seen you sad, frustrated. I have never seen you in anxiety, in any kind of worry. You are always happy, always fulfilled, contented. I cannot believe this. My doubting mind says, 'This man is pretending.' I have been fighting with my mind, telling it that for years you cannot pretend: 'If he's pretending, *you* try.' And I have tried — for five minutes, seven minutes at the most, and I forget all about it. Worries come, anger comes, sadness comes, and if nobody comes then the wife comes! — and all pretensions are gone. How do you manage day after day, month after month, year after year? I have always seen the same joy, the same grace. Please forgive me, but the doubt persists that somehow you are pretending. Perhaps you don't have a wife; that seems to be the only difference between me and you."

Eknath said, "Just show me your hand."

He took his hand in his own hands, watched it, looked very seriously.

The man said, "Is something wrong? What happened?" He forgot all about his doubt and his pretension and Eknath.

Eknath said, "Before I start answering your question, just by the way, I see that your lifeline is finished...just seven days more. So I wanted to tell it to you first because I may forget. Once I start explaining and answering your question, I may forget."

The man said, "I am no longer interested in the question, and I am no longer interested in the answer. Just help me to stand up." He was a young man. Eknath said, "You cannot stand up?"

He said, "I feel all energy gone. Just seven days, and I had so many plans... everything shattered. Help me! My house is not far away, just take me to my house."

Eknath said, "You can go. You can walk — you have come walking perfectly well just a few seconds ago." The man somehow tried to stand up; he looked as if all his energy had been sucked out. And when he was going down the steps you could see that suddenly he had become old, he was taking the support of the railing. As he was walking on the road you could see — he could fall at any moment, he was walking like a drunkard. Somehow he reached home.

Everybody was getting up – it was early morning – and he went to sleep. They all asked, "What is the matter? Are you sick, not feeling well?"

He said, "Now even sickness does not matter. Feeling well or not well is irrelevant. My lifeline is finished – only seven days. Today is Sunday; the next Sunday, as the sun is setting, I will be gone. I am already gone!"

The whole house was sad. Relatives started gathering, friends – because Eknath had never spoken a lie, he was a man of truth. If he has said it, death is certain. On the seventh day, just before the sun was setting – and the wife was crying, and the children were crying, and the brothers were crying, and the old father and the old mother had become unconscious. Eknath reached the house, and they all said, "You have come right in time. Just bless him; he is going for an unknown journey."

In seven days that man had changed so much; even Eknath had to make an effort to recognize him. He was simply a skeleton. Eknath shook him; he somehow tried to open his eyes. Eknath said, "I have come to say to you that you are not going to die. Your lifeline is still long enough. I said that you are going to die in seven days as an answer to your question. That was my answer."

The man jumped up. He said, "That was your answer? My God! You had already killed me. I was just looking outside the window for the sun to set and I would have died."

There was rejoicing, but the man asked, "What kind of answer is this? This kind of answer can kill people. You seem to be murderous! We believe in you, and you take advantage of our faith."

Eknath said, "Except that answer, nothing would have helped. I have come to ask you: in seven days have you been fighting with anybody, have you been angry with anybody? Have you been going to the court? – which is your practice; every day you are found in the court." He was a man of that type, that was his business. Even for murders he was ready to be an eyewitness; just pay him enough. In one murder he was an eyewitness in the court, and the court knew that this man could not be an eyewitness to everything – he was a professional witness....

Eknath asked, "What happened to your business? In seven days how many times have you eye witnessed, how much have you earned?"

He said, "What are you talking about? I have not moved from my bed. I have not eaten; there is no appetite, no thirst. I am simply dead. I don't feel any energy, any life in me."

Eknath said, "Now you get up, it is time. Take a good bath, eat well. Tomorrow you have a case in the court. Continue the business. And I have answered your question, because since I have become aware that everybody has to die.... And death can come tomorrow – you had seven days. I don't have even seven days; tomorrow

284

I may not see the sunrise again. I don't have time for stupid things, for stupid ambitions, for greed, for anger, for hate; I simply don't have time – because tomorrow I may not be here. In this small span of life, if I can rejoice in the beauties of existence, the beauties of human beings, if I can share my love, if I can share my songs, perhaps death will not be hard on me."

I have heard from the ancients that those who know how to live, automatically come to know how to die. Their death is a thing of beauty, because they only die outwardly; inwardly the life journey continues.

Your coming to know that you have cancer certainly will be shocking, will bring sadness and despair. But you are my sannyasin; you have to make this opportunity into a great transformation of being. These few days that you will be here should be the days of meditation, love, compassion, friendliness, playfulness, laughter; and if you can do that, you will be rewarded by a conscious death. That is the reward of a conscious life.

An unconscious life comes to die unconsciously. A conscious life is rewarded by existence with a conscious death. And to die consciously is to know the ultimate orgasmic experience of life, and to know simultaneously that nothing dies, only forms change. You are moving into a new house – and of course a better house, on a higher level of consciousness. You use the opportunity to grow. And life is absolutely just, fair. Whatever you earn you never lose it, you are rewarded for it.

Accept that death is just part of your life, and accept the fact that it is good that you have come to know beforehand. Otherwise, death comes and you cannot hear the footsteps, the sounds of death approaching you. That's why I said you are fortunate: death has knocked seven days before. Use these days in deep acceptance. Make these seven days as joyful as possible; make these seven days days of laughter. Die with a joke on your face – the smile, the thankfulness, the gratitude for all that life has given to you.

And this I say to you: death is fiction. There is no death because nothing dies, only things change. And if you are aware, you can make them change for the better. That's how evolution happens. That's how an unconscious man becomes a Gautam Buddha. [104]

?

In December last year they discovered a cancer of my uterus. For me it was like deciding to die and go on suffering, or come out of it. I let you come in totally, and became drowned in your love: the cancer disappeared. The last six months, even when it was not possible to see you, I felt you very close to me. Some friends of mine are sannyasins, and when I tell them this, they say I am running away from reality. Sometimes I think, and have doubts about what I feel. Are they right? What is reality?

Always listen to your own experience, because that is reality. You had cancer. And it often happens that cancer can become a great opportunity, because now death is certain. Now there is no question of holding yourself back – death is going to take you away anyway. And because death was so close, you remembered me more, you loved me more – because there was no more time to postpone. For the first time you allowed me totally to be with you, and the cancer disappeared.

Cancer has many causes. One of the reasons is that your life is meaningless, love-less, that you are not really living – just dragging. You don't have any reason to live, and the trouble is you don't have any reason to commit suicide either. So in a sleepy way – like somnambulists, sleepwalkers – people go on from their cradle to the grave. It is a long journey, yet sleeping, they manage. They reach to the grave – or wherever they reach it turns out to be the grave....

I have been telling you continually to love, to be total. And for these few days there was no other alternative – death was coming already, you loved totally. You allowed me to be within you, and the cancer disappeared. Not that I have done any-thing; *you* have done something. If you had listened to me before, the cancer would not have happened at all. If you had loved with such intensity and totality before, you would not have been available to cancer. Now, after the cancer has disappeared, you are again getting into the mind, thinking that perhaps I have done a miracle. I have not done anything. *You* have done a miracle, and because you have been telling your friends, "My master has done the miracle," they are telling you be more realistic, and then doubts arise in you. Your friends are right. Be realistic – although they them-selves are not realistic. The only real thing is that the cancer disappeared because for the first time you had a totality of being, a togetherness of being which was more powerful than any cancer.

Now doubts are arising, and you will ask friends, and anybody will say, "Don't be foolish. Don't be superstitious" – although they cannot explain how and why the cancer disappeared, and they are asking you to be realistic. You ask them, "Then you be realistic and tell me how the cancer disappeared." Let them have a little experience of cancer! Just let them think it over, let them waste their sleep over it – how did the cancer disappear?...because that is where the reality has to be decided.

And don't expect a miracle from me. That is fiction. You have done a miracle there is no doubt about it. And everybody is capable of doing such miracles. Life is such a mystery that if we really become silent, total, loving, it will change many things in you – in the body, in the mind, in the soul.

But don't get foolish ideas from your friends; otherwise the cancer can appear again – because it is not my doing, it is your doing. If you become doubtful, and if you don't know how it has happened, your doubt can create the cancer. It was your totality which dissolved it; your doubt can make a way for it to come back. And then none of your friends will say, "Be realistic." Then you will have to go back to the same attitude, but it will be more difficult this time.

It is better not to get into the same trouble again. It will be difficult this time because you will be expecting – which was not there before. The first time you had cancer you were not expecting any miracle. Now if it happens, you will be loving, you will be trying to be total – but trying to be total is not total, trying to be loving is not loving. And deep down expecting that the cancer will be dissolved – it is not the same situation. And remember, don't blame me, that the next time I have not helped you. The first time I had not helped you either. It is always you. Whatsoever happens to you, you are responsible.[105]

? *Is there some connection between sex and headache, or migraine?*

No medical researcher has come to the conclusion, but I say it from my own discoveries that I go on and on making – I'm an incurable discoverer, and sooner or later science will have to agree with me. The sex centre exists in the head, not in the genitals – that much science has come to know. And if the sex centre exists in the head and not in the genitals, then sex deprivation can create a headache. It will not create genitalache because there is nothing: it is only an extension of a certain centre in your mind.

Why have people started thinking – and doctors have started even advising their patients – that sex is good for your mental health? And they are right: all the people who have repressed sex in the past in the name of religion, have suffered tremendously with headaches. Even a man like J. Krishnamurti suffered for forty years continuously with such great headaches, migraine, that even he, a man of such understanding, used to think of hitting his head with the wall and be finished – the pain was too much.[106]

It has been discovered that millions of men around the world suffer from migraine after making love. And I was reading a report of a Christian Scientist – because he is Christian, his mind itself is conditioned. He is trying to find all kinds of causes why men suffer from migraines. He has been working on the project continually for one year. Just now he has produced his report, giving many, many causes – physiological, chemical – and the reality is so simple, there is no need of any investigation. The reality is that you have divided men's mind into two parts. One part says, "What you are doing is wrong. Don't do it"; the other part says, "It is impossible to resist the temptation – I'm going to do it." These two parts start struggling, conflicting.

Migraine is nothing but a conflict, a deep conflict, in your mind. No aboriginal suffers from migraine after making love. Catholics suffer more than anybody else, because their conditioning is so deep that it creates a split in their mind. What they have been saying for centuries is without any base, without any evidence, but they go on repeating it. And once...even if a lie is repeated too often, it starts looking as if it is true.

One should be very much aware about words.

A man goes into a bar and begins to tell a Polish joke. The man sitting next to him, a big, hulking, powerhouse of a man, turns and says menacingly, "I'm Polish. Now you just wait a minute till I get my sons."

He then calls out, "Ivan, come out here; and bring your brother." Two men, bigger than the first, appear from the back room. "Joseph," the man calls out, "You and your cousin come in here." Two more men, the biggest of all, come in through the back door. All five men crowd around the man with the joke.

"Now," says the first Polish man, "Do you want to finish that joke?"

"No," says the man.

"No? And why not?" says the Polish man, opening and closing his fist, "Are you scared?"

"No," says the man, "I just don't feel like having to explain it to five men."

People are very clever with words. They can hide any kind of reality. He is afraid – those five men can kill him – but he finds a beautiful excuse: "I don't want to bother myself, explaining to five people the meaning of the joke."

All the religions have been playing with words, and have not allowed man to be intelligent enough to see through the words. They have created a jungle of words and theologies and dogmas and creeds and cults. And poor man is simply carrying the whole load of it in the name of morality.

I want to tell you, never bother about morality. The only concern for a sincere seeker is awareness, more consciousness. And your consciousness will take care of all your acts. Without any effort, your acts will become moral – just like flowers without any act, without any effort they will blossom around you.

Morality is nothing but a conscious man's lifestyle.[107]

?

I understand you have devised a technique to help talk about disease, or a pain such as migraine. I am a doctor and would like to use this method. Can you describe it in detail?

The idea is that people need to be taught how to make friendship with their body. It will be better if the therapist is a woman, who can help people feel where they are tense or are in pain. She should then teach them how to talk to the body, to tell the body, "I have been alienated from you by religions. I want to come closer and be a friend, not an enemy. I feel guilty that I never thought about it – that you have been working for me all these years and I have never thanked you."

First talk to the whole body: "Listen to me, these are the problems – please let them disappear." It is in your power to do it. Then talk to the specific parts where the pain is.

?

Any preparation before doing the talking?

Before the group starts, tell the people that they will be in a trance, but able to talk to the body. They can talk aloud – it is better. The group is to begin with three minutes of people saying the mantra, "Osho." Before starting the mantra, tell the people that as they repeat Osho, "you will be going deeper and slowly falling asleep." Then give them the hypnotic suggestion that they are falling asleep. When all the people are asleep – you can test this by picking up their hands and seeing if they fall – then go to each person individually. The people should be lying far enough apart so that when you are talking to one it won't disturb another. Beforehand, the therapist has found out what each person's problem is; then when they are asleep, the therapist goes up to each person and tells him, "Your mind and your soul are one phenomenon; you have forgotten how to talk to your own mind and body. Your" – whatever is their problem – "will disappear, is disappearing and will not come back."

When everybody has been dealt with in this way, tell them all, "Whatever is said to you under hypnosis you will be able to do it yourself, alone, without hypnosis." Then end the session with the Osho mantra again for three minutes. People should be told to repeat this to themselves every night before falling asleep, for at least one month.

? *I have tried to talk to pain when I experience it, but it has not helped.*

This will be wrong. This disease is not part of the organism, it is something external, in fact something anti. You must talk to the brain/body, not to the disease. You must say to the brain/body, "It is time to leave the pain, the disease." Say this ten to fifteen times and that, "Now you are going to have a good sleep so that you can do your work." And when you wake, tell the body/brain to let go of the pain. And when it is gone, thank the brain and the body for letting the disease go. Tell the brain that now the pain has gone it should not allow it back; otherwise you will be forever telling the pain to go and it will return. Basically, we are talking to the brain, and the brain talks to the body, but we don't know the language.

This is the real trinity – the soul, the mind and the body. The soul can do nothing directly; it is the one asking for the pain to go. The brain has to speak to the body.

This should be part of everybody's education in the schools, but the religions have taught that the body and mind are something separate. Children can quickly learn to send away the pains in the body.

? *Is it always necessary to use hypnosis?*

You can, but it is not necessary.

? *What language should one use?*

Any language will do.

? *How could you use this method for weight control?*

First tell the brain that you are sending a message to the body, and that the brain should pass it on. Then simply tell the body that five pounds or kilos less will be ideal and that, "You digest normally." Do not involve eating at all. Just tell the body that some pounds less are needed. And when you get there, tell the body to stay there, that there is no need to lose any more weight or to gain more weight.

? *Isn't this how Christian Scientists work with health?*

This was the basis of Christian Science, but they went too far. They would tell a blind man that "Now you can see." But neither did the blind man believe it, nor had he any eyes, so how could he see? That was simply stupid. But for simple things like pains here and there, this method can be immensely helpful. [108]

? *As a doctor, in my practice I see many people with the unexotic but very real complaint of constipation. Is constipation another symptom of 'civilization'?*

A man came to me a few years ago – he had been suffering from constipation for a long time. A very rich man, he had tried every medicine, tried every cure, from allopathy to naturopathy – he did everything. He had enough money to waste, enough time, so there was no problem there. He had moved all over the world to get rid of the constipation, but the more he had tried, the worse the constipation had become, deep-rooted. He had come to me and he said, "What to do?"

I told him, "Constipation can only be a symptom, it cannot be the cause. The cause must be somewhere else in your consciousness." So I told him to do a very simple thing. He could not believe it; he said, "How can it be possible? Doing this simple thing you think will help me? Are you fooling me? – because I have done everything, and can such a simple thing help? I cannot believe it." But I said, "You simply try." I told him just to do one thing: to remember continuously, "I am not the body." Nothing else. Of course he could not believe it because how was this going to help?

Man is identified with his body. Too much identification with the body will give you constipation. You cling, you shrink. You don't allow the body to have its way, you don't allow it to flow. That is the meaning of constipation. Constipation is a spiritual disease. Get disidentified with the body. Continuously remember, "I am not

291

the body, I am a witness." For three weeks he tried and said, "It is working. Something is loosening within me."

It is bound to happen. If you are not the body, the body starts functioning. You don't interfere, you don't come in the way, the body goes on working.

Have you seen any animal constipated? No animal in nature is constipated. In zoos you can find animals constipated. Or pet animals, dogs and cats which live with man and are infected with humanity, which are corrupted by human beings, they may get constipation; otherwise in nature there is no constipation. The body has its own way. It flows. It is not frozen, it doesn't have blocks. Blocks come with identification. I told the man, "Just do not be identified with the body. Keep an awareness that you are a witness. And never say 'I am constipated,' just say 'The body is constipated, I am a witness to it.'"

The body became loose. The stomach started functioning – because nothing disturbs the stomach like the mind. If you are worried, the stomach cannot function well. If you are identified with the body, the body cannot flow well. That's why whenever you are very ill deep sleep is needed, because only in deep sleep do you forget the body, and things start flowing.

It changed. But he came and told me that a new thing was happening, "I have always been a miser, and now I don't feel so miserly." It has to be so, because miserliness is deeply connected with constipation. It works both ways: if you are a miser you will be constipated, if you are constipated you will be a miser. Constipation is really a deep miserliness of the body – not to let go of anything, not to allow anything to go out of the body. Keep everything closed!

Change the plane of your consciousness, and problems start changing.[109]

? *Sometimes I'm afraid of going mad. Could you please comment?*

Please don't be afraid of madness – for the simple reason that you are already mad. This world is such a vast madhouse. Every child is born sane, but cannot live sane long; it is impossible. He is brought up by mad people, taught by other mad people, conditioned by other mad people. He is bound to become mad; just to survive he has to become mad.

Only once in a while has there been a sane person – a Buddha, a Zarathustra, Lao Tzu, a Jesus. And the strangest thing is these sane people look mad because the so-called mad are not really mad. The really mad are the so-called sane. The people who are put in the madhouses are simply very sensitive people, vulnerable people, delicate people, not so hard as the others who live in the marketplace. They are not so thick-skinned, that's why they break down. The thick-skinned go on living amongst all kinds of madness, they go on adjusting.

Man has an infinite capacity to adjust himself, and each child learns to adjust to all kinds of things. Just look in your own being at how many superstitions you have become adjusted to, how many stupid beliefs you are carrying. And it is not that there are not moments when you become aware of their stupidity, but those sane moments you put aside because they are dangerous moments. Yes, once in a while the window opens, but you immediately close it. You have to close it. You are afraid the neighbours may see that your window is open. You don't want to show your sanity to anybody....

Don't be afraid of going mad – you cannot. It has already happened!... The whole fear is absolutely unbased. You have already gone mad, otherwise you would not have been able to exist in the society. Whatsoever society you belong to, you have already become distorted. You are no longer innocent, you are already corrupted and poisoned – by the priests, by the politicians, by the pedagogues. They have done the work; my function here is to undo it. And there is no need for me to prove it. You can just look around and you will find a thousand and one proofs.[110]

? *Can you suggest what kind of meditations might be helpful for mentally disturbed people?*

You can help them to do some dynamic types of meditations. That will help very much because mad people need nothing else but catharsis. It is the only treatment, and it is because people have been so suppressed that they are in such a bad space. If everything is allowed, if they are allowed to be mad, then madness will disappear.

The whole world is mad because nobody is allowed to be mad. We must make it a point that everyone has a certain space reserved where he can simply be mad, where there is no need to be worried about anybody else. If a person can be mad each day for half an hour, then for the remaining twenty-three and a half hours he will experience only tremendous sanity.

Madness is also a part of humanity; it is a deep balance. When you become too serious you need a little laughter to bring you down to earth. When you become too tense you need something to help you to relax. In fact, there are many socially accepted ways in which we allow people to be mad.

For example, in a football match or a volleyball match the spectators almost go mad. But it is accepted, and they feel very relaxed. Even watching it on TV they go mad – they jump and become very excited. But it is an accepted thing.

If somebody from Mars was watching for the first time, he would not be able to believe what is happening, because there seems to be no need to be so excited. Just a few people throwing a ball from here to there, and others returning it, and millions of people are so excited! They don't know that this is a socially accepted avenue of release, a device. And each country has its own, creates its own device.

War is also a device that is needed continually so that people can go mad, can hate and destroy. And they can hate and destroy for a great cause, so there is no condemnation! So you destroy and you feel good, you feel happy, and there is no guilt – and you are simply becoming mad. War will continue until and unless we allow everybody to enjoy a certain amount of madness. So you go and do the meditations and let the mad people watch. They will enjoy it tremendously, and they will say that there is not much difference between them and you! Then they will participate and you will be able to help them.

A madman doesn't need a doctor, he needs a friend. A doctor is too impersonal, too far away, too technical. And a doctor always looks at a madman as if he is an object to be treated. In his very look there is condemnation: something is wrong and has to be put right. A madman needs someone who loves, who cares and is friendly, someone who does not make him an objective thing, and accepts his individuality. And not only that, but also accepts his madness, because he accepts deep down that each man has a sane part and an insane part.

Insanity is the night part of man. It is natural, there is nothing wrong in it. When you can say to a madman that not only you are mad but I am too, immediately a bridge is made. And then he is available, and it is possible to help him.[111]

? *I am becoming more and more conscious of the barriers I have built up in myself over the years against being a joyful, self-loving, open being. It feels like the wall in me is getting stronger and stronger the more I am aware of it, and I can't come through. Could you please help me with your understanding?*

The first thing to understand is that the wall is not becoming stronger, it is only that your awareness is becoming clear. There is no reason at all why the wall should become stronger when you are becoming more aware. It is simply like when you bring the light in your dark house you start seeing the cobwebs and the spiders – not that they have suddenly started growing because you have brought light in. The have always been there; it is just that you are becoming aware, alert. But don't think that they are growing. Your light has nothing to do with their growth. Yes, it reveals their presence. Your growing awareness is revealing the presence of your prison walls.

And you say, "I am aware of it and I can't come through." Because these walls are not true walls – they are not made of bricks or stone, they are made of only thoughts – they cannot prevent you. You just have to know the secret of how to come through them. If you start struggling within your thought-processes, which constitute the prison walls, then you will get into a tremendous mess. One can even go insane. That's how people go insane: they are surrounded by so many thoughts and they are trying hard to come out of the crowd and they go on getting deeper and deeper into the crowd, and then naturally a breakdown follows. Their nervous system cannot sustain so much pressure and so much tension. They have opened Pandora's box. It was all hidden there, but they were blissfully unaware of it. Now they have brought a meditative awareness; suddenly they see a great crowd so thick that the more they try, the more they feel their impotence against the walls that are surrounding them.

If you start fighting with them then there is no way; you will become sooner or later tired, tethered, you will find yourself slipping from your sanity. But if you use a right method, instead of a breakdown you will have a breakthrough. The right method to deal with all that you feel you are surrounded with is to be just a witness – not to fight, not to judge, not to condemn. Just remain silent and still, purely witnessing whatever is there.

This is almost a miracle. I have not come across any miracle other than the miracle of meditation, the miracle of witnessing. If you can witness, you will be surprised that the strong wall is becoming thinner, the crowd is dispersing; slowly, slowly you see doors and gaps through which you can get out. But there is no need to get out. Remain where you are. Just go on witnessing. As your witnessing will become stronger, the wall that surrounds you will become weaker. The day your witnessing will be perfect, you will find there has been no wall, nothing is surrounding you, the whole sky is available to you. Rather than fighting with thoughts, fighting against wrong conditionings, just become a pure witness. Fighting, you cannot win. Without fighting, victory is yours. Victory belongs only to those who can witness....

Doctor Klein finished the examination of his patient and then said, "You are in perfect health, Mr. Levinsky. Your heart, lungs, blood pressure, cholesterol level – everything is fine."

"Splendid," said Mr. Levinsky.

"I will see you next year," said Doctor Klein.

They shook hands, but as soon as the patient had left the room, Doctor Klein heard a loud crash. He opened the door and there, flat on his face, lay Mr. Levinsky. The nurse cried, "Doctor, he just collapsed. He fell down like a rock!"

The doctor felt his heart and said, "My God, he is dead." He even put his hands under the corpse's arms.

"Quick," said the doctor, "take his feet!"

"What?" cried the nurse.

"For God's sake," said the doctor, "let us turn him round. We have to make it look like he was coming in!"

Just be a little intelligent. It is said that intelligence is not of much use unless you are intelligent enough to know how to use it.

Just the other day I came across a tremendously great discovery. It says that every idiot you meet in the world is the end-product of millions of years of evolution. Intelligence is certainly rare but the people who have gathered around me – just the fact that they had the courage to be here is enough proof of their intelligence. Now you have to put your intelligence into action.

"My God," sighed Paddy, "I had everything a man could want – the love of a gorgeous woman, a beautiful house, plenty of money, fine clothes."

"What happened?" asked Seamus.

"What happened? Out of the blue without any hint of warning, my wife walked in."

Just be alert – there are dangers on every step. A man who decides to be a meditator has to be very cautious.

Lao Tzu's statement is that a man of meditation walks always as if he is passing through an ice-cold stream in winter, very careful, very alert. Unless you are very careful and very alert, the millions-of-years-old mind and its functioning is going to be difficult to transcend. Although the strategy is simple, sometimes the simple seems to be the most difficult – and particularly when you are absolutely unacquainted with it.

Meditation is only a word to you. It has not become a taste, it has not been a nourishment, it has not been an experience for you; hence I can understand your difficulty. But you have also to understand my difficulty: your diseases may be many, but I have only one medicine, and my difficulty is to go on selling the same medicine for different patients, different diseases. I don't care what your disease is, because I know I have got only one medicine.

Whatever your disease I will discuss it, but finally you have to accept the same medicine. It never changes. As far as I know, in these thirty-five years it has never changed. I have seen millions of people, millions of different questions, and even before I hear their questions, I know the answer. It does not matter what their question is; what matters is how to manage to bring their question to my answer.[112]

CHAPTER 18

AIDS

? *Would you please say something about AIDS?*

Ido not know anything about even the first AIDS, and you are asking me about the last AIDS! But it seems I will have to say something about it. And in a world where people who know nothing about themselves can talk about God, people who know nothing about the geography of the earth can talk about heaven and hell, it is not inconceivable for me to say something about AIDS, although I am not a physician. But neither is the disease now called AIDS just a disease. It is something more, something beyond the limitation of the medical profession.

As I see it, it is not a disease in the same category as other diseases; hence the danger of it. Perhaps it will kill at least two-thirds of humanity. It is, basically, the incapability to resist diseases. One slowly, slowly finds oneself vulnerable to all kinds of infections, and one has no inner resistance to fight those infections.

To me it means humanity is losing the will to live. Whenever a person loses the will to live his resistance falls immediately, because the body follows the mind. The body is a very conservative servant of the mind; it serves the mind in a religious way. If the mind loses the will to live it will be reflected in the body by the dropping of resistance against sickness, against death. Of course the physician will never bother about the will to live – that's why I thought it better that I say something.

It is going to become such an enormous problem all over the world that any insight from any dimension can be of immense help. Just in America, this year, four hundred thousand people are affected by AIDS, and each year the number will double. Next year it will be eight hundred thousand people, and then one million six hundred thousand people; that way it will go on doubling. Just this year America will need five hundred million dollars to help these people, and still there is not much hope of their surviving.

Just in the beginning it was thought to be a homosexual disease. From all around the world researchers supported the idea that it was something homosexual – it was found that it happens more in men than in women. But just yesterday a report from South Africa changes the whole standpoint. South Africa is greatly involved in researching about the disease because South Africa is the most affected area. It seems blacks are almost twice as vulnerable to the disease as white people. South Africa is suffering from a great epidemic of AIDS; hence, they have been researching. It is a question of life and death.

Their report is very strange. It says that AIDS is not a homosexual disease at all, that it is a heterosexual disease, and it happens if people go on changing partners – mixing with many women, with many men, continually changing partners. This continuous changing is the cause of the disease. Homosexuality has nothing to do with it, according to their research. Now all the researchers in Europe and America are on one side, and the South African report is on the opposite side.

To me it is very significant. It has nothing to do with either heterosexuality or with homosexuality. It has certainly something to do with sex. And why has it something to do with sex? – because the will to live is rooted in sex. If the will to live disappears, then sex will be the most vulnerable area of life to invite death.

Remember perfectly well that I am not a medical man, and whatever I am saying is from a totally different point of view. But there is much more possibility of what I am saying being true than what these so-called researchers are saying, because their research is superficial. They think only of cases; they collect data, facts.

That is not my way – I am not a fact-collector. My work is not of research but of insight. I try to see into every problem as deeply as possible. I simply ignore the superficial, which is the area of the researchers. My work you can call insearch, but not research. I try to penetrate deeply, and I see clearly that sex is the phenomenon most related to the will to live. If the will to live declines, sex will be vulnerable; then it is not a question of heterosexuality or homosexuality.

In Europe and in America they started looking into it because it was just a coincidence that the first cases happened in homosexuals; perhaps homosexuals had lost the will to live more than heterosexuals. The whole research was confined to California, and most of the victims were Jews; obviously the researchers found that it is linked to homosexuality. If any heterosexual was also found to have the symptoms then it was naturally assumed that he had got it from some homosexual person.

California is such a stupid part of the world – and as far as sex is concerned, the most perverted part of the world. You can also say avant-garde, progressive, revolutionary, but these beautiful words won't hide the truth: California has become too perverted. Why does it happen, this perversion? And why has it happened in California particularly? – because California is one of the most cultured, civilized, affluent societies. Naturally, they have everything that you can hope for, everything that you can desire – and that's where the problem of the will to live arises.

When you are hungry you think of getting work, food; you don't have time to think about life and death. You don't have time to think about what the meaning of existence is. It is impossible: a hungry man cannot think of beauty, of art, music. Take the hungry man, starving, into a museum filled with beautiful pieces of art: Do you think he will be able to see any beauty there? His hunger will prevent him. These are luxuries. Only when all his basic needs are fulfilled does man come to face the real problems of life. Poor countries don't know the real problems.

Hence, when I say that the richest man is the poorest, you can understand what I mean by saying it. The richest man comes to know the unsolvable problems of life, and he is stuck; there is nowhere to go. The poor man has so much to do, so much to achieve, so much to become. Who cares about philosophy, theology, art? They are too big for him; he is interested in very mundane things, very small things. And it is impossible for him to turn his consciousness upon himself and start thinking and brooding about existence, being – just impossible.

California is, unfortunately, one of the most fortunate parts of the world, in every way: it has the most beautiful people, beautiful land, and it has come to the highest peak of luxury. And there, the question arises. You have done everything; now what else is there to do? That's the point where perversion begins.

You have known many women and you have come to understand that it is all the same. Once you put the light off, every woman is just the same. When the light is off, if the woman goes into the other room and your wife comes in – and you are not aware – you may even make love to your wife, giving her beautiful dialogues, not knowing that she is your wife. What are you doing? If anyone comes to know about it, that you speak these beautiful dialogues – learned from Hollywood movies – to your own wife, they certainly will think that you have gone crazy. These are meant for other people's wives, not for *your* wife. But in darkness there is no difference. Once a man knows many women, a woman knows many men, one thing becomes certain – that it is the same, a repetition. The differences are superficial, and as far as the sexual contact is concerned, they make no difference: a little longer nose, or little blonder hair, a whiter face or a little suntanned – what difference does it make when you come to make love to a woman? Yes, before making love to a woman all these things make a difference. And it continues to make a difference in countries where monogamy is still the rule.

For example, in a country like India, the disease AIDS is not going to happen while India remains monogamous, it is impossible – for the simple reason that people know only their wife, only their husband, their whole life. And they always remain curious about what the neighbour's wife would feel like. It always remains a tremendous curiosity, but there is no possibility for perversion.

Perversion requires the basic condition that you are fed up with changing women, you want something new. Then men start trying men – that seems to be different; women start trying women – that feels a little different. But for how long? Soon that too is the same. Again, the question arises. This is the point where you try all kinds of things, and slowly, slowly one thing becomes settled: that it is all useless. Curiosity disappears. Then, what is the point of living for tomorrow? It was curiosity: tomorrow something new may happen. Now you know that the new never happens. Everything is old under the sky. The new is just a hope, it never happens. You try all kinds of designs in furniture, houses, architecture, clothes – and everything fails finally.

When everything fails and there is no hope for tomorrow, then the will to live cannot go on with the same fervour, force, persistence. It starts dragging. Life seems to lose juice. You are alive because what else to do? You start thinking of committing suicide.

Sigmund Freud is reported to have said, "I have never come across a single man who has not thought, at least once in his life, of committing suicide." But Sigmund Freud is now too old, out of date. He was talking about psychologically sick people; those were the people with whom he was coming in contact.

My own experience is that the poor man never thinks of committing suicide. I have come across thousands of poor people; they never think of committing suicide. They want to live, because they have not lived yet; how can they think of suicide?

Life has so many things to give, and they see that everybody is enjoying all kinds of things and they have not lived yet. There is a great urge, force, to live. Much has to be done, much has to be achieved. There is the whole sky of ambition open, and they have not even begun to scratch the ground. No beggar ever thinks of committing suicide. Logically it should be just the other way: every beggar should think of committing suicide, but no beggar ever thinks of it – even a beggar who has no eyes, is blind, is paralyzed, crippled....

In poor countries nobody thinks of suicide, in poor countries the question of

meaning has not been raised. It is a Western question. What is the meaning of life
In the East nobody asks that. The West has come to a saturation point where every
thing you could live for you have already lived. Now what? If you are courageou
enough, you commit suicide – or murder....

Once this disease, AIDS, spreads – and it is spreading, it is already epidemic, ir
America too. The politicians are keeping quiet, the priests are keeping quiet, because
the problem is too big, and nobody seems to have any suggestion as to how to solve
it, so it is better to keep silent. But how long can you keep silent?

The problem is spreading, and once it spreads and becomes wider, you will be
surprised: the profession that will be the topmost in this business of AIDS will be the
priests, the nuns, the monks. They will be on the topmost, the most affected by
it, because they have been practicing perverted sex longer than anybody else
California is just new. Those monks and nuns have been living in 'California' for cen
turies.

As it appears to me, the disease is spiritual. Man has come to a point where he
finds the way ends. Going back is meaningless because all that he has seen, lived
shows him there was nothing in it; it has all proved meaningless. Going back has nc
meaning; going ahead there is no road: facing him is the abyss. In this situation if he
loses the desire, the will to live, it is not unexpected.

It has been experimentally proved that if a child is not brought up by loving
people – the mother, the father, the other small children in the family – if the child
is not brought up by loving people, you can give him every nourishment but some
how his body goes on shrinking. You are giving everything necessary – medical need
are fulfilled, much care is being taken – but the child goes on shrinking. Is it
disease? Yes, to the medical mind everything is a disease; something must be wrong
They will go on researching the facts, why it is happening. But it is not a disease.

The child's will to live has not even arisen. It needs loving warmth, joyful faces
dancing children, the warmth of the mother's body – a certain milieu which make
him feel that life has tremendous treasures to be explored, that there is so much joy
dance, play; that life is not just a desert, that there are immense possibilities. He
should be able to see those possibilities in the eyes around him, in the bodies around
him. Only then will the will to live spring up – it is almost like a spring. Otherwise
he will shrink and die – not with any physical disease, he will simply shrink and die

I have been to orphanages; one of my friends, Rekhchand Parekh, in Chanda
Maharashtra, used to run an orphanage – nearabout one hundred to one hundred and
ten orphans were there. And orphans would come, two days old, three days old
people would just leave them in front of the orphanage. He wanted me to come to
see the orphanage. I said, "Sometime later on I will see it, because I know whatever

is there will make me unnecessarily sad." But he insisted, so one time I went, and what I saw.... They were taking every care, he was pouring his money on those children, but they were all ready to die just any moment. Doctors were there, nurses were there, medical facilities were there, food was there, everything was there. He had given his own beautiful bungalow – he had moved to a smaller bungalow – a beautiful garden and everything was there; but the will to live was not there.

I told him, "These children will go on dying slowly."

He said, "You are telling *me?* I have been running this orphanage for twelve years; hundreds have died. We have tried every possible way to keep them alive, but nothing seems to work. They go on shrinking and one day simply they are no longer there." If there was a disease the doctor could help, but there was no disease; simply, the child had no desire to live. When I said this to him it became clear to him. He immediately, that very day, gave the orphanage to the government, and he said, "I have been trying to help these children for twelve years; now I know it is not possible. What they need I cannot give, so it is better that the government takes it over." He said to me, "I had come to this point many times, but I am not an articulate man so I could not figure out what it was. But in a vague way I was feeling that something was missing and that goes on killing them."

AIDS is the same phenomenon at the other end. The orphan child shrinks and dies because his will to live never sprouts, never springs up, never becomes a flowing current. AIDS is at the other end: You suddenly feel you are an existential orphan. This existential feeling of being an orphan causes your will to live to disappear. And when the will to live disappears, sex will be the first thing to be affected because your life starts with sex; it is a by-product of sex.

So while you are living, throbbing, hoping, ambitious, and the tomorrow remains the utopia – so that you can forget all the yesterdays which were meaningless, you can forget today which is also meaningless...but tomorrow when the sun rises and everything will be different.... All the religions have been giving you that hope.

Those religions have failed. Although you go on keeping the label – Christian, Jew, Hindu – it is only a label. Inside, you have lost hope, the hope has disappeared. Religions could not help; they were pseudo. Politicians could not help. They were never intending to help; it was just a strategy to exploit you. But how long can this false utopia – political or religious – help you? Sooner or later, one day man will become mature; and that's what is happening. Man is becoming mature, aware that he has been cheated by the priests, by the parents, by the politicians, by the pedagogues. He has been simply cheated by everybody, and they have been feeding him on false hopes. The day he matures and realizes this, the desire to live falls apart. And the first thing wounded by it will be your sexuality. To me that is AIDS.

When your sexuality starts shrinking you are really hoping that something will happen and you will go into eternal silence, into eternal disappearance. Your resistance is not there. AIDS has no other symptoms except that your resistance goes on dropping. At the most you can live two years if you are fortunate and don't get accidentally infected. Each infection will be incurable, and each infection will be weakening you more and more. Two years is the longest the AIDS patient can live; and he may disappear sometime before that. And no treatment is going to help, because no treatment can bring back your will to live.

What I am doing here is multidimensional. You are not fully aware of what I am trying to do; perhaps you may become aware only when I am gone. I am trying to give you not a hope in the future – because that has failed – I am trying to give you a hope herenow. Why bother about tomorrow?...because tomorrow has not helped. For centuries the tomorrow has been keeping you somehow dragging, and it has failed you so many times that now you cannot go on clinging to it. That would be sheer stupidity. Those who are clinging to it still are only proving that they are retarded in their minds.

I am trying to make this very moment fulfillment, a contentment so deep that there is no need for the will to live. The will to live is needed because you are not alive. The will keeps picking you up: you go on slipping down, the will keeps picking you up. I am not trying to give you a new will to live, I am simply trying to teach you to live without any will, to live joyously. It is the tomorrow that goes on poisoning you. Forget yesterdays, forget tomorrows. This is our day – let us celebrate it and live it. And just by living it you will be strong enough so that without the will to live you will be able to resist all kinds of diseases, all suicidal attitudes.

Just being fully alive is such a power that not only can you live, you can make others aflame, afire.

This has been a well-known fact. When there are great epidemics have you not wondered why the doctors and nurses and others don't get infected? They are human beings just like you, and they are overworked, more vulnerable to infection because they are continually tired. When there is an epidemic you cannot insist on a five-hour day or six-hour day, and a five-day week. An epidemic is an epidemic; it does not bother about your holidays and your overtime. You have to work – people work sixteen hours, eighteen hours, every day, for months. Still, the doctors, the nurses, the Red Cross people, they don't get infected.

What is the problem? Why are others getting infected? These are similar kinds of people. If just having a Red Cross on your shirt...then put the Red Cross on everybody's shirt; on every house the Red Cross. If the Red Cross is preventing infection it would be so easy – but that is not the thing.

No, these people are so much involved in helping others, they don't have any tomorrow. This moment is so involving, they don't have any yesterday. They don't have any time to think or even worry, "I may get infected." Their involvement... When millions of people are dying, can you think of yourself, and your life, and your death? Your whole energy is moving to help people, to do whatever you can do. You have forgotten yourself, and because you have forgotten yourself you cannot be infected. The person who could have been infected is absent: he is so involved in doing something, he is so lost in some work.

It does not matter whether you are painting or sculpting, or you are serving a dying human being – it does not matter what you are doing, what matters is: Are you totally involved in the herenow? If you are involved in the herenow you are completely out of the area where infection is possible. When you are so much involved, your life becomes such a torrential force. And you will see: even a lazy doctor, in a time of epidemic, when hundreds of people are dying, suddenly forgets his laziness. An old doctor suddenly forgets his age....

Only meditation can release your energy herenow. And then there is no need for any hope, for any utopia, for any paradise anywhere. Each moment is a paradise unto itself. But as far as my qualifications are concerned, I am not qualified to say anything about AIDS. I have never even taken the course on first-aid. So please forgive my entering into something which is not my business. But I go on doing that, and I am going to continue to do that.[113]

CHAPTER 19

HEALTH AND ENLIGHTENMENT

? *What is the difference between madness and enlightenment?*

There is a great difference and also a great similarity. The similarity has to be understood first, because without understanding it, it will be difficult to understand the difference.

Both are beyond the mind – madness *and* enlightenment. Enlightenment is above the mind. But both are out of the mind. Hence, you have the expression for a madman 'out of his mind'. The same expression can be used for the enlightened person; he is also out of his mind.

Mind functions logically, rationally, intellectually. Neither madness nor enlightenment function intellectually. They are similar: madness has fallen below reason, and enlightenment has gone above reason, but both are irrational; hence, sometimes in the East a madman is misunderstood as being an enlightened man. These similarities are there.

And in the West, once in a while – it is not an everyday phenomenon, but once in a while – an enlightened person has been understood as being mad, because the West understands only one thing: if you are out of your mind, you are mad. It has no category for above the mind; it has only one category – below the mind.

In the East the misunderstanding happens because for centuries the East ha known people who are out of their mind and at the same time above the mind; hence, they are similar to madmen. For the Eastern masses it creates a confusion, it creates a problem. They have decided it is better to misunderstand a madman as being an enlightened man, than to misunderstand an enlightened man as being a madman – because what are you losing by misunderstanding a madman as being an enlightened man? You are not losing anything. But by misunderstanding an enlightened man as being a madman you are certainly losing a tremendous opportunity. But the misunderstanding is possible because of the similarities....

A madman sometimes can have glimpses which the rational man cannot have because the madman has stepped out of the mechanism of mind; of course on the wrong side, from the back door, but still he is out of the mind. Even from the back door he can have some glimpses which are not available to the people who never come out of the house. Certainly he is not as fortunate as to have come from the front door: that needs tremendous effort.

Madness is disease. It happens to you – you don't have to make an effort to be mad. It is a sickness and it is curable. Enlightenment happens through tremendous awareness and arduous effort.

Enlightenment is the supreme health.

You should understand the word 'health' carefully. It is not only physiologically meaningful. Of course physiologically it is meaningful, but not only physiologically; it has a far higher meaning too. Health means healing the wounds. It comes from the root which means healing. If your physiology needs some healing then medicine is offered. If your spirituality needs some healing, then meditation is offered. Strangely, 'health' comes from the same root from which comes the word 'wholeness'.

Health means the body is whole, nothing is missing. And from wholeness comes the word holy: the spirit is whole, nothing is missing. Similarly, the word medicine and the word meditation come from the same root – that which cures. Medicine cures wounds in your physiology, and meditation cures wounds in your spiritual existence, in your ultimate being....

Sufis call the madman *masta;* masta means intoxicated. The madman and the enlightened man both have to pass through a certain state, that is, getting out of reason, out of their mind. They have to cross the same boundary: by the wrong door or right door, they both cross the same boundary, and while they are crossing the boundary they both become mastas – intoxicated. But the enlightened person soon regains his balance because he has made the effort to get out of the mind; he is prepared to get out of the mind, he is ready to get out of the mind. The madman has got out of his mind unprepared. He was not ready. He has simply fallen out of his mind – it is an accident. Enlightenment is never an accident....

The enlightened man is also always blissful. I am using a different word just so you don't get confused. The madman is always happy. But there is a possibility he can be cured; then he will become unhappy, then he will start worrying. He will worry more than you because he will see that he had gone mad: now he will worry about madness. When he was mad he had no worry at all, he could not care less. Now he will worry that he had gone mad and he will worry that tomorrow it can happen again because it *has* happened....

Just see the point: even if you fall below the mind you are happy. It is the mind that is causing you all kinds of misery, suffering, jealousies, hatred, anger, violence, greed; and they all go on making you more and more a pain to yourself. You start hurting all over, everybody is hurting all over. Even to fall below the mind – which is falling below humanity, because that is the only difference between you and the animals... A madman is really back in the world of animals. He has dropped out of evolution. He has gone back; he has turned his back on Charles Darwin. He has said, "Good-bye. Good-bye to your evolution!" He has simply fallen back to a subhuman level.

Animals are not happy, but they are not unhappy. Have you seen any animal unhappy? Yes, you will not see them happy – they cannot be happy because they don't know what unhappiness is. But when a man falls from the human level to the sub-human level, he becomes happy because he knows what unhappiness is. So he is not exactly the same animal that he was before he became man. He is a totally different kind of animal; a happy animal. There are no happy buffalos, no happy donkeys, no happy monkeys, no happy Yankees! Animals are not happy because they don't know unhappiness. But a madman is just happy for no reason at all. That gives tremendous proof of what I have been teaching you, that if you can get out of the mind – but not by an accident, not by a shock – you will be blissful....

The enlightened man is out of his mind but he has full control of his mind. And he does not need a switchboard – just his awareness is enough. If you observe any-thing minutely, you will have a little experience of the enlightened man – not the full experience but a little taste, just a tongue-tip taste. If you observe your anger minutely, anger disappears. You are feeling a sexual urge: watch it closely, and soon it disappears. If just by your watching, things evaporate, what to say about the man who is continually above the mind, simply aware of the whole mind? Then all those ugly things that you would like to drop simply evaporate. And remember, they all have energy. Anger is energy. When anger evaporates, the energy which is left behind turns into compassion. It is the same energy. Through observation the anger has left – that was the mode, the form surrounding the energy – but the energy remains. Now, the energy of anger, without anger, is compassion. When sex disappears the tremendous energy of love is left behind. Each ugly thing in your mind, disappearing, leaves a great treasure behind.

The enlightened man has no need to drop anything and has no need to practice anything. All that is wrong drops of its own accord because it cannot stand up to his awareness, and all that is good evolves of its own accord because awareness is nourishment for it.

The madman can be helped very easily because he has tasted something out of the mind, but he needs to be shown the right door. In a better world our madhouses will not only be trying to make those people sane – that is meaningless – our madhouses will be trying to help those people to use that opportunity to move through the right door. A madman going into a madhouse will come out enlightened – not just the same old self again, miserable, suffering.

So, to me, madness has immense significance. It can become a way towards enlightenment.[114]

? *If faith can move mountains, why can you not heal your own body?*

I don't have any body.

This feeling that you have a body is absolutely wrong. The body belongs to the universe; you don't have it, it is not yours. So if the body is ill or if the body is healthy the universe will take care of it. And a person who is in meditation should remain a witness, whether the body is healthy or ill.

The desire to be healthy is part of ignorance. The desire not to be ill is also part of ignorance. And this is not a new question – this is one of the oldest questions. It has been asked of Buddha, it has been asked of Mahavira; ever since there have been enlightened persons, the unenlightened have always asked this question.

Look... Jesus said faith can move mountains, but he died on the cross. He couldn't move the cross. You or someone like you must have been present there waiting. The disciples were waiting because they knew Jesus, and he had been saying again and again that faith could move mountains. So they were waiting for some miracle to happen – and Jesus simply died on the cross. But this was the miracle: he could be a witness to his own death. And the moment of witnessing one's own death is the greatest moment of being alive.

Buddha died of food poisoning. He suffered for six months continuously, and there were many disciples who were waiting for him to do a miracle. But he suffered silently and died silently. He accepted death.

There were disciples there who were trying to cure him, many medicines were given to him. A great physician of those days, Jivaka, was Buddha's personal physician. He used to move with him wherever he went. Many times people must have asked, "Why does this Jivaka go with you?" But it was Jivaka's own attachment. Jivaka was moving with Buddha because of his own attachment, and the disciples who were trying to help Buddha's body remain alive longer in this world, even if only for a few days more, were also attached. For Buddha himself, illness and health were the same.

That doesn't mean that illness will not give pain. It will! Pain is a physical phenomenon, it will happen. But it will not disturb the inner consciousness. The inner consciousness will remain undisturbed, it will remain as balanced as ever. The body will suffer, but the inner being will remain just a witness of the whole suffering. There will be no identification – and this I call the miracle. This is possible through faith. And no mountain is bigger than identification – remember. The Himalayas are nothing; your identification with your body is a greater mountain. The Himalayas may be moved or not moved through faith, that is irrelevant, but your identification can be destroyed. But we cannot conceive of anything which we do not know, we can think only according to our minds. We think according to where we are; the pattern remains the same.

Sometimes my body is ill, and people come to me and they say, "Why are you ill? You should not be ill; an enlightened person should not be ill." But who told you that it is so? I have never heard about any enlightened person who was not ill. Illness belongs to the body. It has no concern with your consciousness or whether you are enlightened or not.

And sometimes it happens that enlightened persons are more ill than unenlightened ones. There are reasons. Now that they don't belong to the body, they don't cooperate with the body; deep down they have broken themselves from the body. So the body remains but the attachment and the bridge is broken. Many illnesses happen because of the separation that has happened. They are in the body but their cooperation is no longer there. That is why we say an enlightened person will never be born again – because now he cannot make any bridge with any body again. The bridge is broken. While he is in the body, then too, really, he is dead.

Buddha attained enlightenment when he was nearabout forty. He died when he was eighty, so he lived forty years more. On the day he was dying, Ananda started crying and said, "What will happen to us? Without you we will fall into darkness. You are dying and we have not yet become enlightened. Our own light is not yet lit and you are dying. Do not leave us!"

Buddha is reported to have said, "What? What are you saying, Ananda? I died forty years ago. This existence was just a phantom existence, a shadow existence. It was running along somehow, but the force was not there. It was just a momentum from the past."

If you are pedaling a bicycle, and then you stop and there is no pedaling, you are not giving any cooperation to the cycle, it will go on moving for a little while just because of the momentum, the energy that you gave it in the past.

The moment someone becomes enlightened, the cooperation is broken. Now the body will take its own course. It has a momentum. From many lives in the past, momentum has been given to it. It has a life span of its own which will be completed, but now, because the inner force is no longer with it, the body is prone to be more ill than ordinarily. Ramakrishna died of cancer; Ramana died of cancer. To the disciples it was a great shock, but because of their ignorance they could not understand.

One thing more has to be understood. When a person becomes enlightened, this is going to be his last life. So all the past karmas and the whole continuum has to be fulfilled in this life. The suffering – if he has anything to suffer – will become intense. For you there is no hurry, your suffering will be spread out over many lives. But for Ramana this is the last. All that is there from the past has to be completed. There will be an intensity of everything, of all karmas. This life will become a condensed life. Sometimes it is possible – this is difficult to understand – to suffer in a single moment the sufferings of many lives. In a single moment the intensity becomes such...because time can be condensed or spread out.

You know already that sometimes when you sleep you see a dream, and when you are awake again you know that you have been asleep for only a few seconds. But you have seen such a long dream. It is possible that even a whole life can be seen in a single dream. What has happened? In such a small period of time how could you see such a long dream? There is not a single layer of time as we ordinarily understand, there are many layers of time. Dream time has its own existence. Even while awake time goes on changing. It may not change according to the clock because a clock is a mechanical thing, but psychological time goes on changing.

When you are happy, the time flows fast. When you are unhappy, the time slows down. A single night can be eternity if you are in suffering, and a whole life can become a single moment if you are happy and blissful.

When a person becomes enlightened, everything has to be closed; this is a closing time. Many millions of lives have to be closed and all the accounts have to be cleared, because there will be no chance anymore. After his enlightenment an enlightened person lives in a different time altogether and whatsoever happens to him is qualitatively different. But he remains a witness.

Mahavira died of stomach pain, something like an ulcer – for many years he suffered. His disciples must have been in difficulty because they have created a story around it. They could not understand why Mahavira should suffer, so they have created a story which shows something about the disciples, not about Mahavira. They say that a person who had a very evil spirit, Goshalak, was the cause of Mahavira's suffering. He threw his evil force on Mahavira and Mahavira absorbed it only because of his compassion – and that is why he suffered. This shows nothing about Mahavira but something about the difficulty of the disciples. They cannot conceive of Mahavira suffering so they had to find a cause somewhere else.

One day I was suffering from a cold – it is my constant companion. So somebody came and he said, "You must have taken somebody else's cold." That doesn't show anything about me, it shows something about him. It is difficult for him to conceive of me suffering. So he said, "You must have somebody else's cold." I tried to convince him, but it is impossible to convince disciples. The more you try to convince them, the more they believe that they are right. In the end he said to me, "Whatsoever you say I am not going to listen. I know! You have taken somebody else's illness."

What to do? The body's health and illness is its own affair. If you want to do something about it, you are still attached to it. It will take its own course; you need not be much worried about it.

I am only a witness. The body is born, the body will die; only the witnessing will be there. It will remain forever. Only witnessing is something absolutely eternal – everything else goes on changing, everything else is a flux.[115]

CHAPTER 20
A LOOK INTO THE FUTURE

? *Recently you spoke of science and how we could produce a new man — more intelligent, creative, healthier and freer. It sounds fascinating and at the same time it is scary because of the feeling of some sort of mass product. Can you say something about the fear I am feeling?*

It is absolutely fascinating, and there is no need to feel any fear about it. In fact, what we have been doing for millions of years is mass production — accidental mass production.

Do you know what kind of a child you are going to give birth to? Do you know if he will be blind, crippled, retarded, sick, weak, vulnerable to all kinds of diseases for his whole life? Does your lover know what he is doing? While you are making love you have no conception, not even a possibility of guessing. You are giving birth to children just like animals, and you don't feel scared about it, you don't feel any fear about it. And you see the whole world full of retarded people, crippled, blind, deaf, dumb. All this rubbish! Who is responsible for it? And is it not mass production?

My conception of giving scientific birth to a child is that, conscious, alert, knowingly, we are bringing a visitor to the earth. We know who he is, what he is and what he is to become finally; how long he will live, how much intelligence he will have. We are discarding all possibilities of blind children, deaf children, dumb children, retarded in any way – physically, psychologically – and you are feeling fear? Don't be stupid.

The scientific birth of a child is not animalistic. You are transcending the animal

313

by giving birth to a child scientifically. It is fascinating, the greatest, most fascinating thing around. We can manage it, it is already a scientific reality. We can manage healthier people, who will live as long as we want, and we can give them as much intelligence as is needed for their work.

A couple comes to a scientific lab and tells them that they want a child like Albert Einstein, but better than him, living two hundred years; and he should never suffer any disease, he should be strong. The scientific lab finds the right egg from the bank, the right semen from the bank, and the child is produced in a test-tube with all precautions.

You will have to adopt the child, you cannot produce the child. Production of children is animalistic. Adoption of children of your own imagination.... Everybody wants a Shakespeare to be born, wants their child to be a great poet, a great musician, a great dancer. Every mother thinks that her child is going to be in some way a superhuman being, and every mother is frustrated – the child turns out to be just rotten. He just gets lost in this whole crowd on an overpopulated planet. This is mass production. But adopting a child, you can contemplate on all the qualities that you need. You can ask the advice of the experts as to what other qualities will be helpful in his life, how much he will be capable of love.... You want a Romeo? – you can get a Romeo. It is only a question of chemistry. Romeo has more male hormones than anybody else, he is richer; that's why one woman is not enough for him.

You want a poet who will transcend all the poets of the past? A scientist in comparison to whom all the scientists of the past will look like pygmies? A musician who brings the unknown, the invisible, through sounds to you? A poet who sings songs of joy and celebration as nobody else has ever done? You can ask anything, and they have just to work out, calculate which female egg, which male semen will produce such a human being. That semen is not yours, that egg is not your wife's, you adopt the child. In this way you can get what humanity has always dreamed about, the birth of the superman, a man who is made almost of steel. Your Muhammad Ali the Great will not be able to face him – just one punch on his nose and he will be finished.

What makes you afraid? Don't you want to get above animals? The desire that it will be your semen, that it will be your wife's egg, is simply ugly. Children belong to the universe. What speciality has it got that it is your semen? What is the point of creating a crippled person, just because it is your semen? Science can manage to raise you above animality – and it is not mass production, it will be just the opposite. There is not going to be an assembly line the way cars are produced. It is going to be very individual because every couple has the choice and the freedom to decide what kind of child they want.

How has the idea of mass production come into your mind? Do you think everybody would like the same kind of child? You are wrong. Do you think science labs will go on producing children according to their own desire, and you have to adopt them? Then it will be mass production. I am not for it. You are absolutely free to choose. Right now you are absolutely blind and doing whatsoever you are doing in utter darkness. You are simply a slave of blind biology.

Don't you want freedom from blind biology? Don't you want to go above this stupid attachment to the idea that the child is born out of your semen and your wife's egg? Those eggs don't know to whom they belong. And what is special about your semen? You don't know anything about it. You are completely unaware of what kind of people are struggling within you to be born. You have no choice, you are simply a slave.

What I am saying about scientific birth makes you go beyond slavery, blindness, darkness. It makes you in a certain way more spiritual, because you are no longer concerned that your semen, your wife's egg, are absolutely needed for your child. You give your requirements; you adopt the child. And you can ask experts what will be the best for the child. Would you not like your child to be a unique genius? For futile attachments you are satisfied with a crippled child. And giving birth to a crippled child, a blind child, are you doing any favour to the child? He will never forgive you! You are responsible. And he will have to live a life which is not life at all.

My vision gives total freedom to you and, of course, great responsibility. Right now you are producing children without any responsibility. You have means available to determine what colour the child should be, what kind of face – Greek, Roman?... You can create children who will look like sculptures, utterly beautiful, with genius in some dimension of life, living a life of love, intelligent enough to discard all the priests and all the politicians. They will not become followers of a leader, they will be enough unto themselves.

Right now, what are you doing? First you create in blindness, darkness, a child, not knowing what he is going to turn out like. Then you force him to become a slave by making him a Christian, Hindu, Mohammedan, or politically giving him a certain ideology – socialism, fascism, communism. And he is not intelligent enough to rebel against all these slaveries.

The child of my vision will be absolute freedom. He will not belong to any political party, he will not belong to any organized religion. He will have his own religion, he will have his own political ideology. What is the need for him to hang around Karl Marx and be a communist? He can think better than Karl Marx – and Karl Marx is not a great thinker. He can live so long that he is not in a hurry about anything; patient, ready to wait – he has time enough. Just think of Albert Einstein

living three hundred years. He would have given miracles to the world. But becaus
he was living in an accidental body, he had to die.

We can discard disease, old age. We can program life in every way. We can eve
program the life of the child, so that when *he* wants to die only then will he die
otherwise he can go on living. If he feels that there are still juices that he has not taste
if he feels there are still dimensions that he has not explored, if he feels that mor
time is needed, then he is the master to decide how long to live.

Up to now, you have lived seventy years on average – that includes people wh
live one hundred and fifty years in some places of the world. In Russia there ar
people who have passed one hundred and fifty years, and they are still young. Ther
are people in a certain part of Kashmir, which Pakistan has invaded, who live ver
easily to one hundred and fifty, sixty, seventy. And it is a surprising fact – I have bee
to those people – a one-hundred-and-fifty-year-old person is just working in the fiel
the same way he was working when he was fifty, with the same strength, with th
same gusto.

All that is needed is better planning, better crossbreeding. It is a known an
applied fact about animals. Do you see the many kinds of beautiful dogs around th
earth? – small, big, powerful, or just beautiful. Just to see them jump around you
such a joy. Do you think they came out of blind nature? No, for centuries we hav
been crossbreeding dogs.

You know it as a fact – the whole world accepts it – that a man should not g
married to his own sister. Why? That should be the most simple thing, to g
married to your own sister. You love her already, you have been together since birt
you know each other. But why have all cultures prohibited it? All cultures have sa
that marriage should be with distant people, people who don't come from the sam
family tree, because the bigger the distance, the better the product. If a whit
American marries a Negro, the child will be far better than a white America
marrying another white American, or a Negro marrying another Negro, because th
distance between those two is immense – different centuries. They have grown
different atmospheres, their programming is totally different from each other. S
when these two totally different cultures, traditions, conventions, lifestyles mee
they give birth to a better man, who has a double heritage: the heritage of the Negro
and the heritage of the white Americans.... In a scientific lab it will be possible
find eggs and semen cells as distant as possible. And we can create through th
crossbreeding a totally new man.

There is nothing scary about it. It is not mass production. The couple has to s
what kind of person they would like to have as their child. It avoids all accidents. An
we will be creating the universal man – not the Chinese, not the Indian, not th

English, but the universal man. So please, just feel fascinated, don't feel scared and afraid. There is nothing to be afraid of.

You have seen the way children have been produced in the past. For millions of years you have been doing the same thing – what is the outcome? The outcome decides the value of what you have been doing. Once in a while there is an Albert Einstein or a Bertrand Russell – once in a while! This is not right. It should be the ordinary phenomenon, usual. Once in a while perhaps there will be a person who is born out of some unawareness, unalertness on the part of the scientist; otherwise everybody should be a genius. Just think: the whole world full of people like Rabindranath, Jean-Paul Sartre, Jaspers, Heidegger! And we can prevent people like Adolph Hitler, Mussolini, Joseph Stalin from being born, because they have been calamities here. We can close the door completely on all Genghis Khans, Tamerlanes, Nadir Shahs – all those ugly monsters whose whole life consisted of killing people, destroying people, burning people.

The way we have lived has not proved right. We have only a crowd of pygmies all around – *this* is what you should be scared of! But having a garden of geniuses, creative people, a garden from where we have removed all fanatics, idiots, politicians – in short, we have taken out all that was poisonous, all pollution…. There is so much in the idea. Now, how many people are suffering because they have a snubbed nose? Their whole life they feel inferior. How many people are suffering because they have *only* a nose? If you look at them, everything else is so small and the nose is so big….

I have heard: one millionaire had a very big nose and very small eyes, but he was the richest man in the community. People used to laugh behind him, but nobody ever dared…. He was invited by a family for dinner. The family was concerned about only one thing: their child, who was a born philosopher, asked about everything.

From the morning they were teaching him, "You can ask anything, but when the rich man comes, you are not to ask about his nose." They told him so many times that he became immensely interested: "What is so great about his nose?" They had never prevented him from asking any question. Why was this nose so important? He was really excited, eagerly waiting for the millionaire to come. When he came in, the child laughed. He said to his parents, "He has only a nose, nothing else! And why were you preventing me…? He is a rare specimen!" He destroyed the whole effort.

But people…almost everyone is suffering from something or other. Somebody is suffering from his colour, somebody is suffering from his tallness; somebody is too tall, somebody is too small. What have you produced? *This* is mass production –

accidental, produced in darkness. At least human beings – who are the crown in existence – should not suffer any more from an inferiority complex. The only way is scientific production of children. And there are immense possibilities in it.

For example, if the child is produced in a scientific lab they can produce similar child simultaneously. The other child will be kept in the lab growing simultaneously; exactly as the one who has gone out to be adopted by a family, the other will be growing in the scientific lab. Just the existence of the other gives great opportunities. For example, you get a fractured leg. Now no need to bother to fix the fracture – the leg from the other fellow can be taken and given to you. Something goes wrong, berserk, in your head – now there is no need for all the psychologists, psychoanalysts, psychiatrists. Your head is just removed, you get fresh head. The other person will remain in anaesthesia his whole life, in a deep freeze. He will not know anything of what is happening. He is just there in case something goes wrong with you – and many things go wrong in life, even with every precaution. Something can always go wrong; life is a long affair. You may have a car accident...now, that cannot be prevented by scientific reproduction of children.

But all depends on whether we have courage enough to rise over our fearful selves. We have to rise above the scary feeling. Be fascinated with the new man! The new man must have a new kind of birth. The new man must have a new kind of life, a new kind of love, a new kind of death. He will be new in every possible way. He will replace the old models who are overcrowding the earth – junkyards. They are not needed.

It is a simple process of programming the first cell. And only the first cell can be programmed, because then it goes on reproducing itself – that is an autonomous process. You can program it for everything. Right now it is difficult; it is programmed for all kinds of diseases, it is programmed for death, old age. You can't have any control over it. There is no way to change the program now, because all the cells have the same program. If they are programmed for a particular disease that you get by inheritance, you will suffer from that disease. It could have been changed, but only in the first meeting of the male and the female cells. Everything can be programmed and an exact copy of you can be kept in the lab. If your heart is not functioning well the new heart is available – which will fit you exactly, because it comes from your copy, your twin.

Any new thing scares, but it scares only cowards. Any new thing fascinates, but it fascinates only the brave ones. Be brave, because we need a new, brave world.[116]

318

?

I am a research scientist. For eleven years I have been involved in a medical research programme to develop artificial organs, including hearts, skin, and blood. I enjoy my work, but I do not have a right sense about what I am doing, as natural organs are always better. I have a deep love and respect for nature, and there is much to do to keep the natural balance of which you speak; but I cannot find any institution or organization where research is done with respect or love. Please help me to find a way out or a better way in.

I can understand your difficulty.

There is no organization or institute on the whole planet earth where research is being done with respect and love towards nature. Just the contrary is the case. The research is being done to *conquer* nature. A man has even written a book, *Conquest of Nature*. It is simply unbelievable that you are part of nature, a small part, a tiny part, trying to conquer the whole – as if one of my fingers is trying to take possession of my whole body. Man is nature too. So wherever you are, do not bother about the organization or the institution or their attitude; but you work with deep love, respect. You are not working against nature.

And remember one thing: why have you been given intelligence? It is the natural growth. Nature is trying to improve upon itself through your intelligence. Right now it may be that natural organs are superior to artificial organs. But remember, the artificial organs can be superior to the natural organs, for the simple reason that nature works blindly. Through man nature is trying to have eyes.

The natural heart can certainly be replaced by an artificial heart. The artificial heart will not have heart attacks. And the artificial heart will be easily removable, replaceable. Human blood is going to be a great need soon. You have to improve upon nature, because as the religious disease, AIDS, is spreading throughout the world, blood transfusion is becoming more and more dangerous. Through a blood transfusion you can become a victim of AIDS. Artificial blood will be purer because artificial blood is not going to be religious and homosexual, it is not going to be the source of your death. And what a death! – ugly; in your own eyes you fall down.

So don't feel that you are working against nature. Nobody can succeed against nature. All the successes of science are not conquests, the way they have been described. All that we have discovered is through the compassion of nature allowing us its secrets. We are part of nature, the best part of it. And nature wants through human consciousness to reach newer heights.

Science is not against nature, cannot be. It has to follow natural laws, it cannot go against the natural laws. So all discovery, all research is to find out how nature functions, what its laws are. And you have intelligence that is given by nature; nature is ready to reveal its secrets to that intelligence. Follow the laws of nature, and you will be able to improve upon nature itself. Intelligence is nature trying to improve upon itself; up to now it has worked blindly. In man's intelligence there is a hope. So don't be worried that you are doing something against nature. Do it with great love, respect, with great gratitude, meditativeness; and be certain that it is nature trying to improve upon itself through you. In the beginning, of course, your artificial organs will not be so good. But it is only the beginning: there is immense possibility of going on improving.

Blood will be needed soon, and artificial blood will be better. Perhaps if things like AIDS become a wildfire, then the only alternative we have is to reproduce children in the test-tubes, where they can be protected; otherwise they will bring AIDS from their very birth. Three children in Europe have been found with AIDS. What an ugly world we are creating for our children! – that AIDS has come through natural birth. 'Natural birth' does not mean that we cannot improve upon it....

Every woman and every man should be standing in a queue before hospitals to be tested. If he is declared a positive case of AIDS, then something has to be done for the poor man; something so that he does not need sex anymore, some biological change. Otherwise, he is going to live two years – what is he going to do with his biology, with his physiology, with his male sperm? Something has to be done, and that can be done only by scientific investigation into how to divert the old blind biological process of creating sperm in man. If for two years we can stop the production of sperm in the man, he can live without repression – he can enjoy these two years more than anybody else. Everybody is going to die. He is a rare person because death is giving him notice.

You may die tomorrow. Everything remains incomplete. Everybody has been dying on the earth leaving things incomplete because nobody knows when death will come and knock on your door. But the man with AIDS – if science can help him not to produce sexual energy, or can channel it into different directions of creativity because it *is* creative energy – perhaps for these two years he will be grateful. He will not feel bad about AIDS; he may even feel proud of it, because for these two years he will be able to paint, play music, write the novel he always wanted to but there were so many things to do...and now there is a clean two years of time. He can meditate. It is difficult in the ordinary world to find such a long stretch of time – two years – to sit silently, do nothing, and just be a witness. He can do that. Then AIDS becomes a blessing in disguise.

The men whose sperm is found not to be carrying any AIDS or other diseases can donate their sperm to the hospital. Just like blood banks, there should be sperm banks. If we want humanity to continue, and certainly we want to continue, then artificial insemination will be the only way to produce children – either in the test-tubes or, if the woman is happy and ready, then in her womb....

So you are in the great service of humanity and nature. Go deeper into the research. Don't just do it as a job, let it be your worship. These things are going to be needed. Nowadays if you have a fracture, then for six weeks you are carrying the cast – unnecessarily! If we can create artificial organs, limbs...if a leg has a fracture, it is better to replace it. Why bother with rotten old things? Just replace it with a new, brand-new leg, and that can be done very easily. And the artificial leg can be made as strong as we want; it can be absolute steel, with no fear of any fracture.

It is perfectly in tune with nature. Just remember one criterion: whatever you do should not be in the service of destruction, it should be in the service of creativity.[117]

? *Do you see experiments on human life, such as artificial birth and the exchange of hearts and brains, as an advance, or as an action against nature?*

It all depends who is going to do it. If the politicians are going to do it, or the so-called religions are going to do it, then it is against nature. They cannot do anything natural, they are against nature. But if it is being done by an international academy of scientists – I say *international* academy of scientists – it can be a tremendous, progressive step, and it will not be against nature. It will be nature's growth. But it all depends on who is doing it. The experiments themselves are neutral. No experiment has any vested interest, it is neutral. You can use poison to kill you; the same poison can be used by medical people to save you. It all depends who is doing it.

For example, the discovery of atomic energy was a step of tremendously great progress, a quantum leap. We had found a key to transform the earth into paradise – so much energy in such a small atom. And they are in everything... just in a dew-drop there are millions of atoms. Any atom, if it is exploded, releases so much energy that you can make the whole earth live in luxury. Or you can create Hiroshima and Nagasaki – thousands of people dead within seconds. But because atomic energy, after its invention, went into the hands of the politicians, it became a servant of death. Now there are even more advanced nuclear weapons which can destroy the whole earth. The already existing weapons are enough to destroy this earth seven times. One simply wonders why nations are going to develop more and more nuclear power. Seven times destroying the earth is not enough? In fact, you can destroy the earth only once.

But scientific progress falls into the hands of the politicians because only they can provide enough finance to make these discoveries possible. The scientists of the whole world should think it over: their genius is being used by idiots! The scientists should disconnect themselves from any nation – whether it is the Soviet Union or America. They should create an international academy of sciences. And it is not difficult. If all the scientists of the world are together, finances can be made available, and these discoveries can help man tremendously....

Science should not be the monopoly of any nation, any country. The whole idea is stupid. How can science be monopolized? And every country is trying to monopolize the scientists, keep their inventions secret. This is against humanity, against nature, against existence. Whatever a genius discovers should be in the service of the whole.

You are asking whether discoveries like changing human hearts or human brains are progressive steps. They are of great importance to bring a new humanity on the earth. If Einstein's body is no longer capable of living, do you think it would not be good if his whole brain is transplanted into a young, healthy man? The new man will become an Einstein, because all the genius of Einstein is transplanted to a younger body.

This way bodies may go on changing, but we can keep the genius of Albert Einstein growing for centuries. And if a man in a seventy-year life can give so much, you can imagine if his brain continues for centuries how much benefit it will be for humanity, for the whole universe. This is really a wastage: the container gets rotten and you throw the contents also. The body is only a container. If the container has become dirty, old, unusable, change the container, but don't throw away the contents. The genius mind can live for eternity in different bodies; that is nothing against nature. You heart, if it starts failing, and if you are of immense value to humanity...what is the fear of exchanging the heart? Somebody may be dying from cancer, but his heart is perfectly healthy; that heart can be planted in a man who is talented, a genius, and is healthy, but whose heart is not strong. This is simple; there is nothing in it against nature.

But with politicians and the power in their hands, of course every advance has gone against nature. Everything that human genius has discovered, invented, finally is in the service of death. So are the priests. Now science is no longer a child, that it has to depend on others. Science is now grown-up enough, it is adult. Just a little courage....

I give the invitation to all the scientists of the world; we have the place, we have intelligent people here to help you in every possible way. It will be a great revolution in the history of man. The whole power will be in the hands of the scientists, who

ve never done any harm to anybody. And once all the power is in the hands of the
ientists, politicians will fade away of their own accord. They have been exploiting
ientists for their own purposes, and to be exploited by anybody is not an act of
gnity.

The scientists should recognize their dignity, they should recognize their
dividuality. They should recognize that they have been exploited down the ages by
e priests and the politicians. Now it is time to declare that science is going to stand
its own feet. This will be a great freedom. Then all these experiments, such as
boratory babies, will be of a different caliber, because you can arrange what kind
genius you want. Up to now it has been just accidental, and because it has been
cidental, ninety-nine percent of the people have nothing to contribute. They
ntribute only problems to the world. Now, what has Ethiopia contributed to the
orld? What have the poor countries contributed to the world – or even the rich
untries? Except problems, wars, there is no contribution on their part.

But if you can give birth to a child in a scientific lab.... It is possible, there is no
oblem in it.... Sex, for the first time, will be simply fun! Children will be produced
the lab. They will belong to all. And because you are not going to produce
ildren in the old way – it should be illegal and criminal to do so, you will be behind
rs if you do it – then many problems of your life will be simply dissolved.

Why is the man so insistent? Throughout the ages the insistence has remained
ere: he wants to be certain that the child born out of his wife's womb is his. Why?
ho are you anyway? It is a question of property, because your child will become
e inheritor of all that you have accumulated. You want to be certain that it is your
ild, not your neighbour's child. Women have been kept almost imprisoned for the
mple fear that if they start mixing with people it will be difficult to decide whose
ild it is. Only the mother will know, or even she may not know.

Once production of life goes into the hands of science sex will be transformed. Then
u are not jealous, then you are not a monopolist, then monogamy is absurd. Then
x is just fun, the way you enjoy tennis. And you don't bother that the partners
ould remain monogamous – two bodies enjoying each other.... And there will be
fear that the wife may get pregnant and there will be problems, financial and other.
x will no longer be a problem for the world population; it will no longer be a prob-
m for the priest. In fact, if children are produced in the scientific lab many of the
oubles of the world will dissolve. And we can create the best people: beautiful,
althy, capable of living as long as we want. Old age is not necessary – a man can
main young, healthy, without sickness. All these hospitals and so many people, so
uch money involved. Do you know – America spends more money on laxatives
an on education. Great idea! Who cares about education? The question is laxatives!

But the basic thing should be remembered: scientists have to be courageous enough and declare that they don't belong to any nation, to any religion, that whatsoever they will be doing will be for the whole of humanity. And I don't see that there is anything impossible in it. I am absolutely for those progressive inventions which can make man happier, live longer, be younger, healthier, and which make his life more of a play, fun, and less of a tortuous journey from the cradle to the grave.[11]

CHAPTER 21

LAUGHTER AND HEALTH

? *Could you speak to us on laughter, its meditative powers, its chemistry on the brain, its power of transformation and healing?*

aughter has meditative powers and medicinal powers. It certainly changes your very chemistry; it changes your brain waves, it changes your intelligence – you become more intelligent. The parts of your mind that have been asleep suddenly wake up. The laughter reaches to the innermost part of your brain, to your heart. A man of laughter cannot have a heart attack. A man of laughter cannot commit suicide. A man of laughter automatically comes to know the world of silence, because when laughter ceases suddenly there is silence. And each time laughter becomes deeper it is followed by deeper silence.

It certainly clarifies you – from the traditions, from the garbage of the past. It gives you a new vision of life. It makes you more alive and radiant, more creative.[119]

Now, even medical science says that laughter is one of the most deep-going medicines nature has provided man with. If you can laugh when you are ill you will get your health back sooner. If you cannot laugh, even if you are healthy, sooner or later you will lose your health and you will become ill. Laughter brings some energy from your inner source to your surface. Energy starts flowing, follows laughter like a shadow. Have you watched it? – when you really laugh, for those few moments you are in a deep meditative state. Thinking stops. It is impossible to laugh and think together. They are diametrically opposite: either you can laugh or you can

think. If you really laugh, thinking stops. If you are still thinking, laughter will be ju
so-so, it will be *just* so-so, lagging behind. It will be a crippled laughter. When yo
really laugh, suddenly mind disappears. And the whole Zen methodology is how t
get into no-mind – laughter is one of the beautiful doors to get to it.

As far as I know, dancing and laughter are the best, natural, easily approachab
doors. If you really dance, thinking stops. You go on and on, you whirl and whir
and you become a whirlpool – all boundaries, all divisions are lost. You don't eve
know where your body ends and where the existence begins. You melt into existenc
and the existence melts into you; there is an overlapping of boundaries. And if yo
are really dancing – not managing it but allowing it to manage you, allowing it t
possess you – if you are possessed by dance, thinking stops. The same happens wi
laughter. If you are possessed by laughter, thinking stops. And if you know a fe
moments of no-mind, those glimpses will promise you many more rewards th
are going to come. You just have to become more and more of the sort, of th
quality, of no-mind. More and more, thinking has to be dropped. Laughter can be
beautiful introduction to a non-thinking state....

In a few Zen monasteries every monk has to start his morning with laughter ar
has to end his night with laughter – the first thing and the last thing! You try it. It
very beautiful. It will look a little crazy – because so many serious people are a
around. They will not understand. If you are happy, they always ask why. Th
question is foolish! If you are sad, they never ask why. They take it for granted –
you are sad, it's okay. Everybody is sad. What is new in it? Even if you want to te
them they are not interested because they know all about it, they themselves are sa
So what is the point of telling a long story? – cut it short! But if you are laughing f
no reason then they become alert – something has gone wrong. This man seems
be a little crazy because only crazy people enjoy laughter; only in madhouses will yo
find crazy people laughing. This is unfortunate, but this is so.

It will be difficult, if you are a husband or a wife it will be difficult for you
suddenly laugh early in the morning. But try it – it pays tremendously. It is one of th
most beautiful moods to get up with, to get out of the bed with. For *no* reason!
because there is no reason. Simply you are again there, still alive – it is a miracle.
seems ridiculous – why are you alive? And again the world is there. Your wife is st
snoring, and the same room, and the same house. In this constantly changing wor
– what Hindus call the *maya* – at least for one night nothing has changed? Everythi
is there: you can hear the milkman and the traffic has started, and the same noises
it is worth laughing for!

One day you will not get up in the morning. One day the milkman will knock
the door, the wife will be snoring, but you will not be there. One day death w

come. Before it knocks you down have a good laugh – while there is time have a good laugh. And look at the whole ridiculousness: again the same day starts; you have done the same things again and again for your whole life. Again you will get into your slippers, rush to the bathroom – for what? Brushing your teeth, taking a shower – for what? Where are you going? Getting ready and nowhere to go! Dressing, rushing to the office – for what? Just to do the same thing again tomorrow?

Look at the whole ridiculousness of it – and have a good laugh. Don't open your eyes. The moment you feel that sleep is gone, first start laughing, then open the eyes – and that will set a trend for the whole day. If you can laugh early in the morning you will laugh the whole day. You have created a chain effect; one thing leads to another. Laughter leads to more laughter. And almost always I have seen people doing just the wrong thing. From the very early morning they get out of bed complaining, gloomy, sad, depressed, miserable. Then one thing leads to another – and for *nothing* – and they get angry. It is very bad because it will change your climate for the whole day, it will set a pattern for the whole day.

Zen people are more sane. In their insanity they are saner than you. They start with laughter…and then the whole day you will feel laughter bubbling, welling up. There are so many ridiculous things happening all over! God must be dying of his laughter – down the centuries, for eternity, seeing this ridiculousness of the world. The people that he has created, and all the absurdities – it is really a comedy. He must be laughing. If you become silent after your laughter, one day you will hear God also laughing, you will hear the whole existence laughing – trees and stones and stars with you.

The Zen monk goes to sleep in the night again with laughter. The day is over, the drama is closed again – with laughter he says, "Good-bye, and if I survive again tomorrow morning I will greet you again with laughter."

Try it! Start and finish your day with laughter, and you will see, by and by, in between these two more and more laughter starts happening. And the more laughing you become, the more religious. [120]

Millions of people have forgotten how to laugh. In the Soviet Union psychologists are preparing manuals for people to be taught in schools, colleges, hospitals, in how to laugh, because they have discovered what I have been saying to you continually: love and laughter go together, and laughter is one of the greatest medicines. At the same time it is also a great meditation. Only in the Soviet Union are they working very deeply to find out what happens when people laugh. Their blood flow changes, their brain cells become more active, their heartbeat becomes more rhythmic. Something like laughter has been found by the scientists to be of tremendous importance – but they are being immensely stupid about it. They think it has to be a training; every schoolchild has to be trained how to laugh.

And if in the Soviet Union everybody is trained how to laugh, no laughter will exist at all. Now they are saying that in every hospital there should be a special ward, a humour ward where all the patients should tell jokes and laugh. It is very calculated: what their medicines cannot do, laughter can do. But to me, if laughter comes as a training it may do something, but it cannot be a total transformation where in a single moment your whole being is thrilled, vast, rejuvenated, and there are no side-effects.

Just today I came to know that one-third of the diseases in the world are created by the doctors. Not knowingly – just because of their medicines, which are going to have after-effects. For the moment they may be useful, but they may create something in your chemistry, in your hormones, in your biology. And you may never connect them. You had taken the aspirin only for your headache – to be exactly true, only for your wife! – but that aspirin is going to have its own effects, and you are a complex phenomenon.

It is a poor humanity who needs training to laugh. The day would be very ugly when birds ask, "First train us, then we will sing the song." And the peacocks will say, "We don't care about the clouds. First train us; then we will open our wings." But the peacocks dance as the first clouds of rain start coming; there is no training for it, no training school for peacocks. No training for the birds, no training for the flowers – why should man be trained for everything? Why should he not be allowed to be spontaneous?

There is some fear in spontaneousness, because the spontaneous behaviour is unpredictable. You may laugh at somebody and he may simply look at you as if you are an idiot. There is no need for him to laugh in response – he is being spontaneous, he is feeling like looking at you as an idiot. Nothing is wrong in it; it is his problem. You were laughing – that was your problem. Why get mixed up? To avoid such situations, people have been trained for everything: how to walk, how to talk, what to say, when to say it. Naturally, by and by they become very phony – just actors in a drama, repeating dialogues.

I was visiting a theological college which is the biggest in Asia, which trains missionaries to go all over the poor East to convert people to Christianity. The principal was a friend, and he took me around their campus. In one class, I could not believe my eyes. What I saw being done was such an absurdity that I was almost stunned. The professor was teaching nearabout sixty students who were ready, almost ready to go for their missionary work. He was telling them, when they repeat a certain statement of Jesus, what kind of gesture, what kind of facial expression to use...when is the time to hit hard on the table, and when is the time to whisper silently that God is love. "And when you describe paradise, don't just describe it in prose. Let your face be radiant; let each of your words be pure honey, just poetry."

And at that time one student asked, "And when we are describing hell, what are we supposed to do?"

The professor said, "As far as hell is concerned...as you are, it is perfectly okay." There is no training for hell because you already look like you are in hell!

I asked the principal, "Can't you see this nonsense? These people don't have any feeling, and you are imposing on them that when they say something a certain expression on the face, in the eyes, in the hands, is needed."

I have never been in any training, but when it is needed the hands know what to do. The words know when to stop and when to let silence take over. The eyes flash by themselves when you are describing your own experience. Then there is no effort....

All that is needed is to tell people: Be spontaneous! When laughter comes, don't stop it. In this world, everything has become fake, because you believe in the fake. Be simple, be just yourself. There is no need to act. Whatever action comes spontaneously, let it come; enjoy its spontaneity. Then you will see a beauty, a centredness, a simplicity. Something authentic – not fake, not pseudo. All this is so simple.

A farmer once had on his farm a rooster that was one of the laziest creatures that ever lived. Instead of crowing as it was supposed to do, when the sun came up in the morning, it merely waited until some other rooster crowed – and then it nodded its head in agreement.

But if it is spontaneous, it has its own beauty. Why bother? – somebody else is going to do it. I am in absolute agreement with that rooster; I have never done anything in my life. If somebody happens to do it....

To celebrate their golden wedding anniversary, Saul and Sylvia Shulman decide to repeat the same things they did on their honeymoon. They go to the same hotel and book into the same room. Sylvia puts on the same perfume and the same nightgown. Just as he did on the honeymoon night, Saul goes into the bathroom and Sylvia hears him laughing – just as he had done fifty years before. So when he comes back Sylvia says, "Honey, it is really beautiful – everything is the same. I can remember it as if it were yesterday. Fifty years ago you went to the bathroom and laughed in the same way. At the time I did not have enough courage to ask you, but now, tell me. Why did you laugh?"

"Well, it is like this, darling," says Paul. "That night fifty years ago, when I went to piss, I wet the ceiling. And tonight I wet my feet!"

Just be innocently simple. This man must have been a very spontaneous man. He told the truth – there is nothing to hide about it. But most of you would not have dared to tell the truth. Truth is very simple; it needs no training, no preparation, no homework. You simply are what you are. Just accept it and expose it to the world.[121]

REFERENCES

1   Beyond Enlightenment, Ch. 28
2   From Bondage to Freedom, Ch. 28
3   Sermons in Stones, Ch. 10
4   Meditation: The First and Last Freedom
5   A Bird on the Wing, Ch. 1
6   Zen: The Path of Paradox, Vol. 3, Ch. 6
7   Yoga: The Alpha and the Omega, Vol. 3, Ch. 2
8   Don't Let Yourself Be Upset By The Sutra, Ch. 6
9   Hidden Mysteries, Ch. 5 (unpublished)
10 From Misery to Enlightenment, Ch. 25
11 Socrates Poisoned Again After 25 Centuries, Ch. 20
12 Sermons in Stones, Ch. 2
13 Take it Easy, Vol. 1 Ch. 7
14 Sat Chit Anand, Ch. 2
15 Yoga: The Alpha and the Omega, Vol. 10, Ch. 7
16 Far Beyond the Stars, Ch. 15
17 The Shadow of the Whip. Ch. 20
18 Only Losers Can Win, Ch. 11
19 The No Book, Ch. 29
20 Get Out of Your Own Way, Ch. 2
21 Satyam-Shivam-Sundram, Ch. 29
22 The Transmission of the Lamp, Ch. 22
23 Beyond Psychology, Ch. 40
24 Just Like That, Ch. 5
25 God's Got a Thing About You, Ch. 8

67 The Shadow of the Whip, Ch. 9

68 Nothing to Lose But Your Head, Ch. 17

69 A Rose is a Rose is a Rose, Ch. 22

70 Answer to Personal Question

71 The Passion for the Impossible, Ch. 25

72 Far Beyond the Stars, Ch. 25

73 That Art Thou, Ch. 16

74 The Revolution, Ch. 6

75 Philosophia Perrennis, Vol. 1, Ch. 2

76 Above All Don't Wobble, Ch. 12

77 The Secret of Secrets, Vol. 1, Ch.13

78 And Now and Here, Vol 1, Ch. 4

79 Vigyan Bhairav Tantra, Vol. 1, Ch. 15

80 Ancient Music in the Pines, Ch. 1

81 Sufis: The People of the Path, Vol. 2, Ch. 5

82 Don't Just Do Something, Sit There, Ch. 14

83 Hammer on the Rock, Ch. 4

84 The Rebellious Spirit, Ch. 25

85 For Madmen Only (Price of Admission: Your Mind), Ch. 19

86 From Unconsciousness to Consciousness, Ch. 17

87 The Great Pilgrimage: From Here to Here, Ch. 25

88 The Razor's Edge, Ch. 26

89 The Rebel, Ch. 23

90 From Unconsciousness to Consciousness, Ch. 25

91 The Golden Future, Ch. 16

92 Beyond Psychology, Ch. 11

93 Sufis: The People of the Path, Vol. 2, Ch. 6

94 The Razor's Edge, Ch. 3

95 Socrates Poisoned Again After 25 Centuries, Ch. 1

96 Believing the Impossible Before Breakfast, Ch. 3

97 From the False to the Truth, Ch. 19

98 Zen, Zest, Zip, Zap, Zing, Ch. 15

99 The Zen Manifesto: Freedom From Oneself, Ch. 7

100 The Golden Future, Ch. 6

101 The Golden Future, Ch. 3

102 The Open Secret, Ch. 24

103 Sufis: The People of the Path, Vol. 2, Ch. 14

104 The Osho Upanishad, Ch. 8

105 The Osho Upanishad, Ch. 19

106 The Great Pilgrimage: From Here to Here, Ch. 8

107 The Razor's Edge, Ch.19

INDEX

FOR FURTHER INFORMATION

M any of Osho's books have been translated and published in a variety of languages worldwide. For information about Osho, his meditations, books, tapes and the address of an Osho meditation/information centre near you, contact:

Osho International
24 St James's St.
St James's
London SW1A 1HA
Tel: 0171 9251900
Fax: 0171 9251901

Osho Commune International
17 Koregaon Park
Poona 411001, India

Chidvilas Inc.
P.O. Box 17550, Boulder
CO 80308, U.S.A.

OSHO COMMUNE INTERNATIONAL

The Osho Commune International in Poona, India, guided by the vision of the enlightened master Osho, might be described as a laboratory, an experiment in creating the "New Man" — a human being who lives in harmony with himself and his environment, and who is free from all ideologies and belief systems which now divide humanity.

The Commune's Osho Multiversity offers hundreds of workshops, groups and trainings, presented by its nine different faculties:

Osho School for Centering and Zen Martial Arts
Osho School of Creative Arts
Osho International Academy of Healing Arts
Osho Meditation Academy
Osho Institute for Love and Consciousness
Osho School of Mysticism
Osho Institute of Tibetan Pulsing Healing
Osho Center for Transformation
Osho Club Meditation: Creative Leisure

All these programs are designed to help people to find the knack of meditation: the passive witnessing of thoughts, emotions, and actions, without judgement or identification. Unlike many traditional Eastern disciplines, meditation at Osho Commune is an inseparable part of everyday life — working, relating or just being. The result is that people do not renounce the world but bring to it a spirit of awareness and celebration, in a deep reverence for life.

The highlight of the day at the Commune is the meeting of the Osho White Robe Brotherhood. This two-hour celebration of music, dance and silence, with a discourse from Osho, is unique — a complete meditation in itself where thousands of seekers, in Osho's words, "dissolve into a sea of consciousness."